Case Files™:
Microbiology

NOTICE

Medicine is an ever-changing science. As new research and clinical experience broaden our knowledge, changes in treatment and drug therapy are required. The authors and the publisher of this work have checked with sources believed to be reliable in their efforts to provide information that is complete and generally in accord with the standard accepted at the time of publication. However, in view of the possibility of human error or changes in medical sciences, neither the editors nor the publisher nor any other party who has been involved in the preparation or publication of this work warrants that the information contained herein is in every respect accurate or complete, and they disclaim all responsibility for any errors or omissions or for the results obtained from use of the information contained in this work. Readers are encouraged to confirm the information contained herein with other sources. For example and in particular, readers are advised to check the product information sheet included in the package of each drug they plan to administer to be certain that the information contained in this work is accurate and that changes have not been made in the recommended dose or in the contraindications for administration. This recommendation is of particular importance in connection with new or infrequently used drugs.

Case Files™:
Microbiology

EUGENE C. TOY, MD
THE JOHN S. DUNN, SR. ACADEMIC CHAIR AND
PROGRAM DIRECTOR
CHRISTUS ST. JOSEPH HOSPITAL, OBSTETRICS
AND GYNECOLOGY RESIDENCY PROGRAM
HOUSTON, TEXAS
CLERKSHIP DIRECTOR, ASSISTANT CLINICAL
PROFESSOR
DEPARTMENT OF OBSTETRICS/GYNECOLOGY
UNIVERSITY OF TEXAS AT HOUSTON MEDICAL SCHOOL
HOUSTON, TEXAS

CYNTHIA DEBORD, PHD
INSTRUCTOR AND COURSE DIRECTOR
OF MEDICAL MICROBIOLOGY
DEPARTMENT OF MICROBIOLOGY
AND MOLECULAR GENETICS
UNIVERSITY OF TEXAS AT HOUSTON MEDICAL SCHOOL
HOUSTON, TEXAS

AUDREY WANGER, PHD
ASSOCIATE PROFESSOR
DEPARTMENT OF PATHOLOGY
UNIVERSITY OF TEXAS AT HOUSTON MEDICAL SCHOOL
HOUSTON, TEXAS

GILBERT CASTRO, PHD
PROFESSOR
DEPARTMENT OF INTEGRATIVE BIOLOGY
AND PHARMACOLOGY
UNIVERSITY OF TEXAS AT HOUSTON MEDICAL SCHOOL
AND VICE PRESIDENT FOR INTER-INSTITUTIONAL RELATIONS
THE UNIVERSITY OF TEXAS HEALTH SCIENCE CENTER AT
HOUSTON
HOUSTON, TEXAS

JAMES D. KETTERING, PHD
PROFESSOR AND ASSOCIATE CHAIR
DEPARTMENT OF BIOCHEMISTRY
AND MICROBIOLOGY
LOMA LINDA UNIVERSITY SCHOOL OF MEDICINE
LOMA LINDA, CALIFORNIA

DONALD BRISCOE, MD
ASSOCIATE PROGRAM DIRECTOR
FAMILY PRACTICE RESIDENCY
CHRISTUS ST. JOSEPH HOSPITAL
HOUSTON, TEXAS

Lange Medical Books/McGraw-Hill

MEDICAL PUBLISHING DIVISION

New York   Chicago San Francisco
Lisbon   London Madrid Mexico City
Milan New Delhi San Juan Seoul
Singapore Sydney Toronto

The **McGraw·Hill** Companies

Case Files™: Microbiology

Copyright © 2005 by the McGraw-Hill Companies, Inc. All rights reserved. Printed in the United States of America. Except as permitted under the United States Copyright Act of 1976, no part of this publication may be reproduced or distributed in any form or by any means, or stored in a data base or retrieval system, without the prior written permission of the publisher.

Case Files™ is a trademark of The McGraw-Hill Companies, Inc.

34567890 DOC/DOC 09876

ISBN: 0-07-144574-9

This book was set in Times New Roman by Fine Composition.
The editors were Catherine A. Johnson and Penny Linskey.
The production supervisor was Catherine H. Saggese.
The cover designer was Aimee Nordin.
The index was prepared by Pamela J. Edwards.
RR Donnelley was printer and binder.

This book is printed on acid-free paper.

Library of Congress Cataloging-in-Publication Data

Case files™ : Microbiology / Eugene C. Toy... [et al.].
    p. ; cm.
  Includes index.
  ISBN 0-07-144574-9
  1. Medical Microbiology—Case studies. I. Title: Microbiology. II.Toy, Eugene C.
  [DNLM: 1. Microbiology—Case Reports. 2. Microbiology—Problems and Exercises.
3. Anti-Infective Agents—Case Reports. 4. Anti-Infective Agents—Problems and Exercises.
5. Clinical Medicine—Case Reports. 6. Clinical Medicine—Problems and Exercises.
QW 18.2 C337 2005]
QR46.C356 2005
616.9′041—dc22

2004065583

❖ DEDICATION

To the wonderful students of the University of Texas Medical School at Houston who taught me so much and enrich my life daily.

— ECT

To my parents, Darrell and Ruth, for their ongoing support; to my loving husband, Wes, who encouraged and enabled me to complete this project; and to our newborn babies, Emily and Elliot.

— CD

To my wife, Georgia, and daughters, Theresa and Mitzi, who have always been the ultimate movitation for me to do my work, and enjoy it.

— GC

To my patient wife, Betty, and children, Brian, Pamela, and David.

— JK

To Cal, Casey, Peter, Ben, Kristen, Leonard, Eric, and all of their parents.

— DB

❖ CONTENTS

SECTION IV

❖ CONTRIBUTORS

Carrie Danner, MS III
Medical Student
University of Texas at Houston Medical School
Houston, TX
Mycoplasma pneumoniae
Hepatitis
Chlamydia trachomatis
Treponema pallidum
Adenovirus
Molluscum contagiosum
Smallpox

Kristian Delgado, MS III
Medical Student
University of Texas at Houston Medical School
Houston, TX
Chlamydia trachomatis
Treponema pallidum
Adenovirus
Molluscum contagiosum
Smallpox
Cryptococcus neoformans

Sarah Kott, MS III
Medical Student
University of Texas at Houston Medical School
Houston, TX
Helicobacter pylori

Anita Red, MS III
Medical Student
University of Texas at Houston Medical School
Houston, TX
Human Papillomavirus
Herpes Simplex Virus
Cytomegalovirus
Varicella-Zoster Virus
Epstein-Barr virus

Gary C. Rosenfeld, PhD
Professor
Department of Integrative Biology and Pharmacology
Assistant Dean for Educational Programs
The University of Texas Medical School at Houston
Houston, TX
Antimicrobial Therapy

Craig A. Seheult, M.S. (Microbiology)
MD/PhD Student
Loma Linda University School of Medicine
Loma Linda, California
Bacteriology

❖ INTRODUCTION

Often, the medical student will cringe at the "drudgery" of the basic science courses and see little connection between a field such as microbiology and clinical problems. Clinicians, however, often wish they knew more about the basic sciences, because it is through the science that we can begin to understand the complexities of the human body and thus have rational methods of diagnosis and treatment.

Mastering the knowledge in a discipline such as microbiology is a formidable task. It is even more difficult to retain this information and to recall it when the clinical setting is encountered. To accomplish this synthesis, microbiology is optimally taught in the context of medical situations, and this is reinforced later during the clinical rotations. The gulf between the basic sciences and the patient arena is wide. Perhaps one way to bridge this gulf is with carefully constructed clinical cases that ask basic science-oriented questions. In an attempt to achieve this goal, we have designed a collection of patient cases to teach microbiological related points. More important, the explanations for these cases emphasize the underlying mechanisms and relate the clinical setting to the basic science data. We explore the principles rather than emphasize rote memorization.

This book is organized for versatility: to allow the student "in a rush" to go quickly through the scenarios and check the corresponding answers, and to provide more detailed information for the student who wants thought-provoking explanations. The answers are arranged from simple to complex: a summary of the pertinent points, the bare answers, a clinical correlation, an approach to the microbiology topic, a comprehension test at the end for reinforcement or emphasis, and a list of references for further reading. The clinical cases are arranged by system to better reflect the organization within the basic science. Finally, to encourage thinking about mechanisms and relationships, we intentionally used open-ended questions with the clinical cases. Nevertheless, several multiple-choice questions are included at the end of each scenario to reinforce concepts or introduce related topics.

HOW TO GET THE MOST OUT OF THIS BOOK

Each case is designed to introduce a clinically related issue and includes open-ended questions usually asking a basic science question, but at times, to break up the monotony, there will be a clinical question. The answers are organized into four different parts:

PART I

1. **Summary**

2. A **straightforward answer** is given for each open-ended question

3. **Clinical Correlation**—A discussion of the relevant points relating the basic science to the clinical manifestations, and perhaps introducing the student to issues such as diagnosis and treatment.

PART II

An **approach to the basic science concept** consisting of three parts

1. **Objectives**—A listing of the two to four main principles that are critical for understanding the underlying microbiology to answer the question and relate to the clinical situation

2. **Definitions of basic terminology**

3. **Discussion of topic**

PART III

Comprehension Questions—Each case includes several multiple-choice questions that reinforce the material or introduces new and related concepts. Questions about the material not found in the text are explained in the answers.

PART IV

Microbiology Pearls—A listing of several important points, many clinically relevant reiterated as a summation of the text and to allow for easy review, such as before an examination

❖ ACKNOWLEDGMENTS

The inspiration for this basic science series occurred at an educational retreat led by Dr. Maximilian Buja, who at the time was the Dean of the University of Texas at Houston Medical School. It has been such a joy to work together with Drs. DeBord, Wanger, and Castro, who are accomplished scientists and teachers, as well as the other excellent authors and contributors. It has been rewarding to collaborate with Dr. Donald Briscoe, a brilliant faculty member. Dr. James Kettering is an inspiring author, phenomenal scientist, and virologist. I would like to thank McGraw-Hill for believing in the concept of teaching by clinical cases. I owe a great debt to Catherine Johnson, who has been a fantastically encouraging and enthusiastic editor. I appreciate Penelope Linskey for her copyediting expertise. At the University of Texas–Houston Medical School, I would like to recognize Dr. Samuel Kaplan, Professor and Chair of the Department of Microbiology and Molecular Genetics, for his support. At CHRISTUS St. Joseph Hospital, I would like to recognize the finest administrators I have encountered: Jeff Webster, Michael Brown, and Benton Baker, III, MD. I appreciate Dottie Mersinger's excellent advice and assistance. Without the help from my colleagues, this book could not have been written. Most important, I am humbled by the love, affection, and encouragement from my lovely wife Terri and our four children, Andy, Michael, Allison, and Christina.

Eugene C. Toy

Applying the Basic Sciences to Clinical Medicine

PART 1. APPROACH TO LEARNING MICROBIOLOGY

The student of microbiology should be aware of the scientific characteristics of each microbe, with a particular interest in the relevance to clinical manifestations. The following is a systematic three-pronged approach:

1. **What can be done if a person is infected?** This translates to knowing the best treatment and method of prevention of infection. In other words, once a patient is known to be infected with a certain microbe, what is the best treatment? The student is best served by learning more than one antimicrobial therapy and some of the advantages and disadvantages of each therapeutic choice. For example, a urinary tract infection caused by *Escherichia coli* may be treated empirically with a variety of antibiotics; however, a quinolone antibiotic such as ciprofloxacin is contraindicated in pediatric patients, and gentamicin is relatively contraindicated in those with renal insufficiency.

2. **Where and how is a person infected?** This question translates to understanding about the mechanisms of disease transmission. For example, if a patient is found to be infected with the hepatitis B virus, the student should be aware that the most common methods of disease acquisition are intravenous drug use, sexual transmission, and vertical transmission. Blood transfusion at one time was a common modality, but now with screening of banked blood, the incidence is very low.

3. **How does one know that a person is infected?** The clinician may have a suspicion of a certain etiologic agent based on clinical clues, but this educated guess must be corroborated by laboratory confirmation. This necessitates an understanding of the basis for presumptive and definitive diagnosis. Possible laboratory tests include culture, PCR of DNA or RNA, antigen tests, or antibody tests.

Likewise, the student should have a systematic approach to classifying microorganisms: viruses, bacteria, protozoa, and fungi.

Virus: A noncellular organism having genetic nucleic acid that requires a host to replicate. They are usually 15 to 450 nanometers (nm) in diameter. Viruses do not have a cell membrane or cell wall, but they have a rigid protein coat called the "capsid." The inner cavity contains DNA or RNA. Viruses come in various shapes including spherical, tetrahedral, polygonal, rod shaped, and polyhedral. One end is usually broader (head), and one end narrower (tail). The tail often has antigenic proteins for attachment to the host. Because viruses do not reproduce without a host, they are considered obligate parasites and not living. See Figure I-1 for a schematic of viruses.

			Genome size (kb)	Envelope	Capsid symmetry
Positive-strand RNA Viruses	🦠	Picornaviridae	7.2-8.4	No	Icosahedral
	🦠	Caliciviridae	8	No	Icosahedral
	◎	Togaviridae	12	Yes	Icosahedral
	◎	Flaviviridae	10	Yes	Icosahedral
	🦠	Coronaviridae	16-21	Yes	Helical
Negative-strand RNA Viruses	🦠	Rhabdoviridae	13-16	Yes	Helical
	〰️	Filoviridae	13	Yes	Helical
	🦠	Paramyxoviridae	16-20	Yes	Helical
Segmented Negative-strand RNA Viruses	🦠	Orthomyxoviridae	14	Yes	Helical
	🦠	Bunyaviridae	13-21	Yes	Helical
	🦠	Arenaviridae	10-14	Yes	Helical
Segmented Double-strand RNA Viruses	⬡	Reoviridae	16-27	No	Icosahedral
Retroviruses	◯	Retroviridae	3-9	Yes	Icosahedral
DNA Viruses	🦠	Parvoviridae	5	No	Icosahedral
	⬡	Papovaviridae	5-9	No	Icosahedral
	🦠	Adenoviridae	36-38	No	Icosahedral
	🦠	Herpesviridae	100-250	Yes	Icosahedral
	🦠	Poxviridae	240	Yes	Complex

Figure I-1. Schematic diagram of selected virus families that are pathogenic to humans, approximately to size.

Bacteria: These single-celled organisms belong in the kingdom Prokaryotae, and they usually have a cell wall as an outer covering consisting of a complex of sugar and amino acids, and often a cell mem-

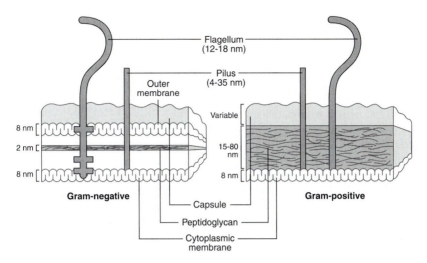

Figure I-2. Schematic diagram of cell walls of gram-negative versus gram-positive bacteria.

brane surrounding the cytoplasm. Being prokaryotes, bacteria do not have a membrane around their nuclei. Some bacteria have flagella, which are cytoplasmic fibrous structures for locomotion. Bacteria may be classified according to shape (cocci, bacilli, or vibrio [comma-shaped], or spirilla [corkscrew]). Bacteria may also be classified by Gram stain characteristics, metabolism requirements (anaerobic versus aerobic), and presence or absence of cell wall [*Mycoplasma* do not have a cell wall]. See Figure I-2 for cell wall characteristics of gram-negative versus gram-positive bacteria.

Parasites: Usually consisting of the protozoa and helminths. Helminths are parasitic worms usually subdivided into flat worms, or platyhelminths, and round worms, or nemathelminths.

Protozoa: Parasites in humans belonging to the Kingdom Protozoa are classified into three phyla: Sarcomastigophora (flagellates and amebas), Ciliophora (the ciliates), and Apicomplexa (containing the sporozoans).

Fungi: Eukaryotic organisms growing in two basic forms: yeasts and molds. The mold form usually consists of multicellular filamentous colonies. Branching cylinder-like tubules form, called hyphae. The yeast form are single cells, usually spherical or ellipsoid in shape. Most yeast reproduce by budding. When the yeast cells bud but fail to break off, they can form elongated yeast cells, called pseudohyphae. Fungi can be classified according to their ability to produce superficial versus deep invasive infection, or by their appearance or sexual reproduction characteristics.

PART 2. APPROACH TO DISEASE

Physicians usually approach clinical situations by taking a history (asking questions), performing a physical examination, obtaining selective laboratory and imaging tests, and then formulating a diagnosis. The conglomeration of the history, physician examination, and laboratory tests is called the **clinical database.** After reaching a diagnosis, a treatment plan is usually initiated, and the patient is followed for a clinical response. Rational understanding of disease and plans for treatment are best acquired by learning about the normal human processes on a basic science level, and likewise, being aware of how disease alters the normal physiological processes is understood on a basic science level.

Clinicians should be aware of the laboratory methods of diagnosis, including the advantages and disadvantages, cost, time requirements, and potential morbidity to the patient. Various laboratory techniques include detecting DNA or RNA sequences, identifying certain protein components of the microorganism (antigen), or unique enzyme or toxin; microscopic examination such as Gram stain (most bacteria), acid-fast stain (*Mycobacterium*), and immunofluorescence techniques (used to detect difficult-to-culture organisms such as *Legionella*). Cultures are the traditional method of diagnosis, and they must be taken in such a way as to minimize contamination and placed on the appropriate media (or mammalian cell for viruses), with temperature and atmospheric conditions for optimal amplification. Thereafter, the correct identification process should be used to assess characteristics such as colony morphology both grossly and under the microscope hemolytic pattern on agar, fermentation profile, Gram stain appearance, and the like.

Once the organism is identified, then susceptibility testing is generally performed to assess the likelihood that certain antimicrobial agents will be effective against the particular strain of pathogen. For example, isolates of *Staphylococcus aureus* should be tested against beta-lactam antibiotics such as methicillin to aid the clinician in treating with methicillin versus vancomycin. Susceptibility is generally performed in a qualitative manner (susceptible, intermediate, resistant), or quantitative with minimum inhibitory concentrations (MIC) or minimum bactericidal concentrations (MBC) as determined by successive dilutions of the isolate bathed in antimicrobial mixtures.

PART 3. APPROACH TO READING

There are seven key questions that help to stimulate the application of basic science information to the clinical setting.

1. **Given a particular microorganism, what is the most likely clinical manifestation?**
2. **Given a particular microorganism, what is the mechanism whereby clinical or subclinical findings arise?**

3. **Given clinical symptoms of infection, what is the most likely causative microorganism?**
4. **Given clinical findings, what are the most likely associated features of the microorganism (such as cell wall characteristics or viral genome)?**
5. **Given the clinical findings, what is the most likely vector of transmission?**
6. **Given the clinical findings, what is the most likely laboratory culture findings?**
7. **Given a particular microorganism, what is the most likely mechanism of resistance acquisition?**

1. **Given a particular microorganism, what is the most likely clinical manifestation?**

    This is the fundamental knowledge that the student must learn in the broad scope of microbiology, that is, the most likely presentation of clinical disease. Each organism has certain typical patterns of clinical manifestations, based on its characteristics. The interaction between microbe and host, including replication cycle, enzymes released, and host immune response all play roles in the overt symptoms and signs. The student should have an understanding of the common presentations of disease. Likewise, the student should be aware of the mechanisms of the clinical manifestations.

2. **Given a particular microorganism, what is the mechanism whereby clinical or subclinical findings arise?**

    The student of microbiology is often tempted to memorize the extensive list of microorganisms and clinical disease. Unfortunately, this haphazard approach leads to quick forgetfulness and lack of understanding of the basic science underlying this discipline. Instead, the student should approach the field of microbiology by linking the microorganism, and its particular characteristics, to the mechanisms of disease. It is the ability of the student to understand the mechanisms that allows for rational approaches to diagnosis and treatment.

3. **Given clinical symptoms of infection, what is the most likely causative microorganism?**

    The student of microbiology first learns antegrade from microbe toward disease, but patients present instead with disease symptoms and signs. Thus, the student must be able to work backward from clinical presentation to a differential diagnosis (a list of the most likely etiologies) to the probable causative organism. Again, rather than memorization, the student should incorporate mechanisms in the learning process. Thus, the student would best be served to give a reason why the suspected microorganism causes a certain clinical presentation.

    Microorganism → Host defenses → Clinical signs
    Clinical signs → Most likely microbe

4. **Given clinical findings, what are the most likely associated features of the microorganism (such as cell wall characteristics or viral genome)?**

    This is similar to question 3, but it goes back to the underlying basic science peculiarities of the microbe. First, the student must use the clinical information to discern the likely microorganism, and then the student must be able to relate the characteristics of the microbe. Because a common and effective method of classifying viruses includes the viral genome, this is an important differentiating point. Likewise, bacteria are often subdivided by their cell wall characteristics, which lead to their Gram stain findings. For example, the clinical information may be: "A 66-year-old male complains of blisters erupting on the right chest wall region associated with pain and tingling." The student should be able to remember that a vesicular rash that is unilateral associated with pain and tingling is characteristic for herpes zoster. The etiologic agent is varicella zoster, which causes chickenpox. The virus is can lay dormant in the dorsal root ganglia and, then during times of stress or immunocompromised states, travel down the nerve and cause local eruption on the dermatome distribution. The pain and tingling are caused by the stimulation of the nerve. The student may recall that varicella is a herpes virus, and thus is a double-stranded DNA virus.

5. **Given the clinical findings, what is the most likely vector of transmission?**

    Again, the student must first discern the most likely etiologic agent based on the clinical findings. Then, an understanding of how the microbe causes disease, such as vector of transmission, is important. A related topic is preventive or treatment related, such as how to sterilize equipment exposed to the patient, or the best antibiotic therapy for the described patient.

6. **Given the clinical findings, what are the most likely laboratory findings?**

    Based on the clinical presentation, the student should discern the most likely microbe and then its laboratory characteristics. These laboratory findings should be correlated to its mechanisms of disease. For example, the clinical findings are: "A 10-year-old boy presents with sore throat and fever. On examination, there is exudate in the oropharynx. A Gram stain reveals gram-positive cocci in chains." The student should be aware that a culture would reveal beta-hemolytic pattern on blood agar media. Furthermore, the mechanism should be learned, that is, that the group A *Streptococcus* gives off *hemolysin,* which leads to *hemolysin* of the red blood cells.

7. **Given a particular microorganism, what is the most likely mechanism of resistance acquisition?**

Patterns of antimicrobial resistance are enormous concerns for all involved in medical sciences. Bacteria and viruses are increasingly acquiring mechanisms of resistance, which spurs scientists to design new antibiotics or chemicals that disable the microbial method of resistance. For example, if the mechanism of resistance is a beta-lactamase enzyme, then the addition of a beta-lactamase inhibitor such as sulbactam may lead to increased efficacy of a beta-lactam such as ampicillin.

MICROBIAL PEARLS

- There are seven key questions to stimulate the application of basic science information to the clinical arena.
- The student of microbiology should approach the discipline in a systematic manner, by organizing first by bacteria, viruses, fungi, and protozoa, and then subdividing by major characteristics.
- Learning microbiology can be summarized as a threefold approach: (1) Treatment and prevention of infection (i.e., what can be done if a person is infected), (2) disease transmission (i.e., where and how a person is infected), (3) basis for presumptive and definitive diagnosis (i.e., understanding how one knows that a person is infected).
- The skilled clinician must be able to translate back and forth between the basic sciences and the clinical sciences.

REFERENCES

Brooks GF, Butel JS, Morse SA. The science of microbiology. In: Medical microbiology. New York: McGraw-Hill, 2004:1–7.

Madoff LC, Kasper DL. Introduction to infectious disease. In: Kasper DL, Fauci AS, Longo DL, eds. Harrison's principles of internal medicine, 16th ed. New York: McGraw-Hill, 2005:695–99.

SECTION II

Antimicrobial Therapy

Antimicrobial agents consist of **antibacterial, antiviral, antifungal, and antiparasitic medications.** These drugs take advantage of the different structures or metabolism of the microbes versus human cells. The student should group classes of drugs together rather than memorize each individual agent. A systematic approach includes learning the agent, the mechanism of action, and the spectrum of activity.

PART 1. ANTIBACTERIAL AGENTS

Antibacterial agents, which target specific components of microorganisms that are unique or more essential to their function than they are to humans, are classified according to their mechanisms of action. The component targets include **enzymes necessary for bacterial cell wall synthesis, the bacterial ribosome, and enzymes necessary for nucleotide synthesis and DNA replication.**

Resistance of pathogens to antibacterial and other chemotherapeutic agents may be the result of a natural resistance or may be acquired. In either case, it occurs through **mutation, adaptation, or gene transfer.** The mechanisms of resistance for any antibacterial agent vary, but are consequences of either changes in uptake of drug into, or its removal from, the bacterial cell, or to changes in the bacterial cell target site of the drug from a gene mutation. **Multiple drug resistance** is also a major impediment to antibacterial therapy and may be **chromosomal or plasmid mediated** where genetic elements from resistant bacteria that code for enzymes that inactivate antibacterial agents are transferred to nonresistant bacteria. The emergence of drug resistance is to a large degree the result of the widespread and often unnecessary or inappropriate use of antibiotics in humans.

The **penicillins** include natural penicillins, penicillins that are resistant to staphylococcal beta lactamase, and extended-spectrum penicillins (see Table II-1). The **cephalosporins** are classified as first to fourth generation according to their antibacterial spectrum (see Table II-2). **Aztreonam,** which is relatively β-lactamase resistant, is the only available **monobactam.** It is nonallergenic and is active only against aerobic gram-negative bacilli (e.g., *Pseudomonas, Serratia*). See Table II-3 for a listing of selected antibacterial agents. The **carbapenems** (imipenem, meropenem, and ertapenem), which are resistant to most β-lactamases, have a wide spectrum of activity against gram-positive and gram-negative rods and anaerobes. To **prevent its metabolism to a nephrotoxic metabolite, imipenem** is administered with an **inhibitor of renal tubule dehydropeptidase, cilastatin. Vancomycin,** which is unaffected by β-lactamases, **inhibits bacterial cell wall synthesis** by covalent binding to the terminal two D-alanine residues of nascent peptidoglycan pentapeptide to prevent their elongation and cross-linking, thus increasing the susceptibility of the cell to lysis. It is **active against gram-positive bacteria.**

Table II-1
PARTIAL LISTING OF PENCILLINS

Natural penicillins: Penicillins G (prototype); Penicillin V

β-lactamase resistant: Nafcillin; Oxacillin; Cloxacillin; Dicloxacillin

Extended-spectrum
Aminopenicillin: Ampicillin; Amoxicillin
Ureidopenicillins: Mezlocillin; Piperacillin
Carboxypenicillin: Ticarcillin

Table II-2
SELECTED LISTING OF CEPHALOSPORINS

REPRESENTATIVE CEPHALOSPORINS (ROUTE)	NOTES
1st generation – Cefazolin (iv) – Cephalexin (po) – Cepadroxil (po)	Active against gram-positive cocci, including staphylococci, pneumococci, and streptococci. They are particularly good for soft tissue and skin infections.
2nd generation – Cefuroxime (po) – Cefotoxitin (iv) – Cefotetan (iv)	Marked differences in spectrum of activity; generally, active against certain aerobic gram-negative bacteria and somewhat less active against many gram-positive organisms sensitive to 1st generation cephalosporins. Cefuroxime more active against *haemophilus influenza, and cefoxitin more* active against bacteroides fragilis.
3rd generation – Cefotaxime (iv) – Ceftazidime (iv) – Ceftriaxone (iv)	Expanded aerobic gram-negative spectrum and cross and blood-brain barrier. Useful to treat bacterial strains resistant to other drugs.
4th generation – Cefepime (iv)	Generally similar activity to 3rd generation cephalosporins but more resistant to β-lactamases.

iv = intravenous; po = oral.

Table II-3
PARTIAL LISTING OF ANTIBACTERIAL AGENTS

ANTIBACTERIAL AGENTS	MECHANISM OF ACTION
BETA-LACTAM ANTIBIOTICS Penicillins Cephalosporins Monobactams – aztreonam (p) Carbapenems – imipenem (p) – meropenem (p) – ertapenem (p)	Inhibit synthesis of the bacterial cell wall
Vancomycin (o,p)	
Chloramphenicol *Tetracyclines* – tetracycline (o,p) – oxytetracycline (o,p) – doxycycline (o,p) – methacycline (o) – minocycline (o,p) *Macrolides* – erythromycin (o,p) – clarithromycin (o) – azithromycin (o) *Ketolides* – telithromycin (o) *Oxazolidones* – linezolid (o,p) *Aminoglycosides* *Spectinomycin* (p) *Lincomycins* – clindamycin (o,p)	Bind to bacterial ribosomes to inhibit protein synthesis
SULFONAMIDES – sulfadiazine (o) – sulfamethizole (o) – sulfamethoxazole (o) – sulfanilamide (t) – sulfisoxazole (t,o) *Trimethoprim*	*Sulfonamides:* Structural analogs of p-aminobenzoic acid that inhibit bacterial dihydropteroate synthase to block folic acid synthesis and cell growth. *Trimethoprim:* Selectively inhibits dihydrofolic acid eductase to block folic acid synthesis and cell growth. Acts synergistically with sulfmethoxazole.
Fluoroquinolones (selected) – ciprofloxacin (t,o,p) – levofloxacin (t,o,p) – ofloxacin (t,o,p) – gatifloxacin (o,p) – moxifloxacin (o,p)	Inhibit activity of bacterial topoisomerase (DNA gyrase) that is necessary for replication

t = topical, o = oral, p = parenteral

PART 2. ANTIVIRAL AGENTS

The **three major classes of antiviral agents** are **DNA polymerase inhibitors, reverse transcriptase inhibitors, and protease inhibitors.** It should be noted that HIV treatment usually includes the use of at least two reverse transcriptase inhibitors and one protease inhibitors. DNA polymerase inhibitors are subdivided into nucleoside and non-nucleoside. Drugs may target viral nucleic acid replication such as DNA polymerase either via nucleoside (purine or pyrimidine analogs) such as acyclovir or ribavirin, or by attacking a unique viral process needed in nucleic acid synthesis such as viral pyrophosphate (nonnucleoside type). Antiviral drugs used to treat herpes simplex virus (HSV), varicella-zoster virus (VZV), and *Cytomegalovirus* (CMV), can be classified as either nucleosides or nonnucleosides, or according to their site of action in the viral replicative cycle or according to their clinical use.

Common Antiviral Agents

Influenza. **Amantadine and rimantadine** are primarily used against infections caused by the **influenza A virus.** Their mechanism of action is interfering with **viral uncoating.** Both agents are fairly well absorbed orally and cause some minor central nervous system (CNS) effects (rimantadine less so) and minor gastrointestinal (GI) effects (see Table II-4 for partial listing).

Table II-4
PARTIAL LISTING OF ANTIVIRAL MEDICATIONS

Hepatitis B and C	Lamivudine, adefovir, interferon alfa and ribavirin.
Influenza	Amantadine and rimantadine (non-nucleosides that inhibit uncoating), zanamivir and oseltamivir (non-nucleosides that inhibit release and budding).
HIV-1	Nucleoside reverse transcriptase inhibitors (NRTIs; abacavir, didanosine, lamivudine, stavudine, zalcitabine, zidovudine) Nucleotide inhibitors (tenofovir), Non-nucleotide reverse transcriptase inhibitors (NNRTIs; delavirdine, efavirenz, nevirapine) Protease inhibitors (ampreavir, idinavir, nelfinavir, ritonavir saquinavir) Fusion inhibitors (enfuvirtide)

Herpes Virus

Acyclovir is used against **herpes simplex virus 1 and 2.** Acyclovir, a **nucleoside DNA polymerase inhibitor,** is a **deoxyguanosine triphosphate (dGTP) analog,** which is incorporated into the viral DNA and causes DNA chain termination. Its specificity is a result of the presence of **herpes specific thymidine kinase** in infected cells, which phosphorylates acyclovir 100 times more efficiently than by uninfected cells. Acyclovir can be used topically, orally for recurrent genital herpes, and intravenously for immunocompromised patients or herpes encephalitis. Its adverse effects include headache, nausea, and rarely nephrotoxicity with IV use. **Valacyclovir** is an analog of acyclovir and is converted to acyclovir in the body. Its advantage is **better bioavailability.** See Table II-5 for listing of agents against herpes viruses.

Table II-5
AGENTS USED TO TREAT HERPES VIRUSES
(Route of Administration)

AGENTS	VIRAL INFECTIONS
Acyclovir (t,o,p)	HSV, VZV
Cidofovir (p)	VZV, CMV
Famciclovir (o)	HSV, VZV
Ganciclovir (o,p)	CMV
Penciclovir (t)	HSV, VZV
Idoxuridine (o)	HSV
Valacyclovir (o)	HSV, VZV
Trifluridine (t)	HSV
Foscarnet (p)	HSV, CMV
Fomivirsen (p)	CMV

HSV = Herpes simplex virus; CMV = Cytomegalovirus; VZV = Varicella-zoster virus;
t = topical, o = oral, p = parenteral

Penciclovir is converted to the triphosphate form and inhibits viral DNA polymerase. **Famciclovir** is converted to the active agent penciclovir in the body. Their main use is to treat **localized herpes zoster in immunocompromised patients.** Headache and GI effects are common. **Ganciclovir** is structurally similar to acyclovir and must be converted to the triphosphate form to be active; it competes with dGTP for incorporation into viral DNA, thereby inhibiting DNA polymerase. Its primary role is against **Cytomegalovirus** and is **far more effective than acyclovir against CMV.** Ganciclovir can induce serious **myelosuppression.**

Forcarnet is a **synthetic non-nucleoside analog of pyrophosphate** and inhibits DNA polymerase or HIV reverse transcriptase by directly binding to the pyrophosphate binding site. Its use is usually for **acyclovir resistant herpes or CMV retinitis.** Significant **nephrotoxicity** may occur with its use.

Sorivudine is a **pyrimidine nucleoside analog** and, on being converted to the triphosphate form, is active against herpes DNA synthesis. It is effective against **varicella zoster** and is usually well tolerated. **Idoxuridine** is an **iodinated thymidine analog,** which **inhibits herpes DNA synthesis** in its triphosphate form. It is used primarily topically for **herpes keratitis.** Adverse effects include pain and inflammation. **Vidarabine** is an **adenosine analog,** which also needs to be in its triphosphate form and blocks **herpes specific DNA polymerase.** It has been used for **herpes encephalitis or zoster in immunocompromised individuals,** but because of its **nephrotoxicity,** it has largely been supplanted by acyclovir. **Trifluridine** is a **fluorinated pyrimidine nucleoside analog.** Its monophosphate form inhibits thymidylate synthetase and triphosphate form inhibits DNA polymerase. It is active against herpes 1 and 2 and CMV, and it is used primarily against keratoconjunctivitis and recurrent keratitis.

Anti-HIV Agents

Retrovir (azidothymidine [AZT] or zidovudine [ZDV]) inhibits viral reverse transcriptase when its triphosphate form is incorporated into the nucleic acid and **blocks further DNA chain elongation,** leading to **termination of the DNA.** Also, the monophosphate form of Retrovir may block deoxythymidine kinase and inhibit the production of normal dTTp. Its principal role is treating HIV infection, and adverse effects include headache, **bone marrow suppression,** fever, and abdominal pain.

Didanosine is also a **nucleoside reverse transcriptase inhibitor,** primarily used as an **adjunct to Retrovir,** or for those patients with HIV infection intolerant or unresponsive to zidovudine. **Peripheral neuropathy** and **pancreatic damage** are its side effects. **Stavudine** is a thymidine nucleoside analog that inhibits HIV-1 replication and that is used in HIV patients unresponsive to other therapies.

Protease Inhibitors

Invirase or saquinavir blocks **HIV protease activity,** rendering the virus unable to generate essential proteins and enzymes including reverse transcriptase. It is used in combination with a conventional reverse transcriptase inhibitor.

PART 3. ANTIFUNGAL AGENTS

In addition to the pyrimidine analog, **flucytosine,** and the penicillium-derived antifungal agent, **griseofulvin,** the three major classes of antifungal agents are the **polyene macrolides, azoles, and allylamines** (Table II-6).

Of all the available antifungal agents, **amphotericin B** has the **broadest spectrum of activity,** including **activity against yeast, mycoses, and molds.** It is the **drug of choice for disseminated or invasive fungal infections** in **immunocompromised** patients. The **major adverse effect** resulting from amphotericin B administration is the almost invariable **renal toxicity** that

Table II-6
SELECTED ANTIFUNGAL DRUGS

POLYENE MACROLIDES
Nystatin (o)
Natamycin (t)
Amphoterecin B (t, o for GI tract, p)

AZOLES
Miconazole (t)
Ketaconazole (t,o)
Clotrimazole (t)
Itraconazole (o,p)
Fluconazole (o,p)
Voriconazole (o,p)

ALLYLAMINES
Naftifine (t)
Terbinafine (o,t)

OTHER ANTIFUNGAL AGENTS
Flucytosine (o)
Griseofulvin (o)

t = topical; o = oral; p = parenteral

results from decreased renal blood flow and from tubular and basement membrane destruction that may be irreversible and may require dialysis. Other adverse effects of amphotericin B relate to its intravenous infusion and include fever, chills, vomiting, hypotension, and headache that can be ameliorated somewhat by careful monitoring and slow infusion.

The **azole antifungal agents** have a **broad spectrum of activity,** including activity against **candidiasis, mycoses, and dermatophytes,** among many others. As topical agents they are relatively safe. Administered orally, their **most common adverse effect is gastrointestinal (GI) dysfunction.** Hepatic dysfunction may rarely occur. Oral azoles are **contraindicated for use with midazolam and triazolam** because of potentiation of their **hypnotic and sedative effects,** and with beta-hydroxy-beta-methylglutaryl-coenzyme A **(HMG CoA) reductase inhibitors** because of an **increased risk of rhabdomyolysis. Itraconazole** has been associated with **heart failure when used to treat onychomycosis** and, therefore, **should not be used in patients with ventricular abnormalities.** Monitoring patients who receive itraconazole for potential **hepatic toxicity** is also highly recommended. **Voriconazole** frequently causes an **acute blurring of vision** with changes in color perception that resolves quickly.

The **allylamine antifungal agents, naftifine and terbinafine,** are used **topically** to treat dermatophytes. Contact with mucous membranes may lead to local irritation and erythema and should be avoided. **Terbinafine** administered orally is effective against the **onychomycosis. Monitoring for potential hepatic toxicity is highly recommended.**

Flucytosine is active against only a **relatively restricted range of fungal infections.** Because of rapid development of resistance, it is used concomitantly for its synergistic effects with other antifungal agents. The most commonly reported adverse effect is **bone marrow suppression,** probably because of the **toxicity of the metabolite fluorouracil,** that should be continuously monitored. Other reported less common adverse effects include reversible hepatotoxicity, enterocolitis, and hair loss.

Griseofulvin, the use of which is declining relative to terbinafine and itraconazole, is an effective antifungal agent that is used only **systemically** to treat a very **limited range of dermatophyte infections.** The most common adverse effects include **hypersensitivity** (fever, skin rash, serum-sickness–like syndrome) and **headache.** It is **teratogenic.**

Mechanism of Action

Nystatin and amphotericin B bind to ergosterol, a major component of fungal cell membranes. This disrupts the stability of the cell by forming pores in the cell membrane that result in leakage of intracellular constituents. Bacteria are not susceptible to these agents because they lack ergosterol.

Azoles (imidazoles less so) have a greater affinity for fungal than human **cytochrome P$_{450}$ enzymes** and, therefore, more effectively reduce the synthesis of fungal cell ergosterol than human cell cholesterol.

The allylamine antifungal agents, naftifine and terbinafine, decrease ergosterol synthesis and increase fungal membrane disruption by inhibiting the enzyme squalene epoxidase.

Flucytosine must first be transported into fungal cells via a cytosine permease and converted to 5-fluorouracil and then sequentially converted to 5-fluorodeoxyuridylic acid, which disrupts DNA synthesis by inhibiting thymidylate synthetase. Human cells are unable to synthesize the active flucytosine metabolites.

The mechanism of antifungal action of griseofulvin is not definitely known. It acts only on growing skin cells and has been reported to inhibit cell wall synthesis, interfere with nucleic acid synthesis, and disrupt microtubule function, among other activities.

Administration

Amphotericin B is insoluble in water and, therefore, is generally administered as a colloidal suspension with sodium deoxycholate. Because of its poor absorption from the GI tract, amphotericin B must be given intravenously to treat systemic disease, although it is effective orally for fungal infections within the GI lumen. Likewise, nystatin is poorly absorbed but may also be used for fungal infection of the GI tract. It is too toxic for systemic use and, therefore, is mostly used topically to treat fungal infections of the skin and mucous membranes (e.g., oropharyngeal thrush, vaginal candidiasis). Costly lipid formulations of amphotericin B are available for intravenous use which reduce its nonspecific binding to cholesterol of human cell membranes and, therefore, its potential to cause renal damage. Griseofulvin is administered in a microparticulate form to improve absorption.

PART 4. ANTIPARASITIC AGENTS

Parasitic infections affect half the world's population and are particularly prevalent in developing countries. Immunocompromised individuals such as those with HIV infection are also prone to parasitic disease. These medications can be categorized as active against malaria, toxoplasmosis, cyclospora, cryptosporidia, pneumocystis, amebiasis, leishmaniasis, helminths, trematodes, and cestodes (see Table II-7).

Table II-7
DRUGS FOR PARASITES

	PROPHYLAXIS	TREATMENT
Malaria (erythrocytic)	• Chloroquine • Mefloquine • Doxycycline	• Chloroquine 2nd drug for falciparum: • Quinine • Fansidar • Quinidine • Doxycycline • Clindamycin
Malaria (hepatic)	• Primaquine • Etaquine	• Primaquine
Toxoplasmosis	• Trimethoprim/ Sulfamethoxazole	• Pyrimethamine/Sulfadiazine • Pyrimethamine/Clindamycin
Cyclospora	• Trimethoprim/ Sulfamethoxazole	• Trimethoprim/Sulfamethoxazole • Pyrimethamine/Sulfadiazine
Cryptosporidiosis		• Antiretrovirals • Paramomycin/Azithromycin
Pneumocystis	• Trimethoprim/ Sulfamethoxazole • Dapsone • Pentamidine (inhaled) • Atovaquone	• Trimethoprim/Sulfamethoxazole • Trimethoprim/Dapsone • Clindamycin/Primaquine • Atozaquine • Pentamidine (IV)
Amebiasis		Metronidazole Iodoquinol Paraomomycin
Giardiasis		Metronidazole Paramycin
Leishmaniasis		Pentamidine Amphotericin B Azole antifungal drugs
Antihelminthics (intestinal worms)		Mebendazole Albendazole Thiabendazole Pyrantel pamoate
Antitrematodes & Anticestodes (Flukes, Shistosomiases)		Praziquantel Albenazole

Source: Harrison's Internal Medicine, 2004; 1202–8.

ANTIMICROBIAL PEARLS

❖ β-lactam antibiotics inactivate bacterial transpeptidases and prevent the cross-linking of peptidoglycan polymers essential for cell-wall integrity.

❖ Both penicillin and amoxicillin are susceptible to β-lactamases.

❖ To prevent its metabolism to a nephrotoxic metabolite, imipenem is administered with an inhibitor of renal tubule dehydropeptidase, cilastatin.

❖ Vancomycin, which is unaffected by β-lactamases, is active against gram-positive bacteria.

❖ Chloramphenicol can cause GI disturbances, reversible suppression of bone marrow, and rarely plastic anemia.

❖ Aminoglycosides may cause ototoxicity or nephrotoxicity and should be used with caution in those patients who have renal insufficiency or who are elderly.

❖ The primary strategy of antiviral agents is to attack a unique but vital viral enzyme or process.

❖ The three major types of antiviral agents include DNA polymerase inhibitors, reverse transcriptase inhibitors, and protease inhibitors.

❖ HIV therapy usually uses at least two reverse transcriptase inhibitors and one protease inhibitor.

❖ Didanosine is also a nucleoside reverse transcriptase inhibitor for HIV infections and is associated with peripheral neuropathy and pancreatic damage.

❖ Foscarnet is a synthetic nonnucleoside analog of pyrophosphate and is associated with reversible nephrotoxicity; hypo- or hypercalcemia and phosphatemia that may lead to neural and cardiac dysfunction. Also, hallucinations, genital ulceration, and anemia may occur.

❖ Itraconazole has been associated with heart failure when used to treat onychomycosis and, therefore, should not be used in patients with ventricular abnormalities.

❖ A common side effect of griseofulvin is hypersensitivity.

❖ Because of renal toxicity, amphotericin B is often used to initiate a clinical response before substituting a continuing maintenance dose of an azole.

REFERENCES

Gale EF, Cundliffe E, Reynolds PE, et al. The molecular basis of antibiotic action, 2nd ed. London: Wiley, 1981.

Groll A, Piscitelli SC, Walsh TJ. Clinical pharmacology of systemic antifungal agents: a comprehensive review of agents in clinical use, current investigational compounds, and putative targets for antifungal drug development. Adv Pharmacol 1998;44:343.

Levy SB. The challenge of antimicrobial resistance. Sci Am 1998;278:46.

Sarosi GA, Davies SF. Therapy for fungal infections. Mayo Clin Proc 1994;69:1111.

Stevens DA, Bennett JE. Antifungal agents. In: Mandell GL, Bennett JE, Dolin R, eds. Principles and practices of infectious diseases, 5th ed. Philadelphia: Churchill Livingstone, 2000:448.

Wright AJ. The penicillins. Mayo Clin Proc 1999;74:290.

Clinical Cases

A 53-year-old male farmer presents for evaluation of a growth on his arm. About a week previously, he noticed some mildly itchy red bumps on his arm. They started to blister a day or two later and then ruptured. During this time he had a low-grade fever, but otherwise felt well. Further questioning reveals that he has had no ill contacts and never had anything like this before. He has cows, horses, goats, sheep, and chickens on his farm. On examination of his right upper arm, you find a 4.5-cm circular black eschar surrounded by several vesicles (blisters) and edema. He has tender axillary lymph node enlargement (adenopathy). A Gram stain of fluid drained from a vesicle and a biopsy from the eschar both show chains of gram-positive bacilli on microscopy.

◆ **What organism is the likely cause of this disease?**

◆ **What are the primary virulence factors of this organism?**

ANSWERS TO CASE 1: *Bacillus anthracis*

Summary: A 53-year-old male farmer has a 4.5 cm circular skin lesion of black eschar surrounded by vesicles and edema. The Gram stain on microscopy shows gram positive bacilli in chains.

◆   **Organism most likely causing disease:** *Bacillus anthracis.*

◆   **Primarily virulence factors:** Capsular polypeptide and anthrax toxin.

CLINICAL CORRELATION

Bacillus anthracis is the etiologic agent of cutaneous, gastrointestinal, and inhalational anthrax. Approximately 95% of anthrax disease is cutaneous. *B. anthracis* is distributed worldwide, and all animals are susceptible, but it is more prevalent in herbivores. Infected animals often develop a fatal infection and contaminate the soil and water with *B. anthracis* that can sporulate and continue to survive in the environment for many years. Oxygen is required for sporulation, and the spores will grow on culture plates, in soil, or in the tissue of dead animals. Human infections are caused by either penetration of these spores through the skin barrier (cutaneous), ingestion of the spores (rare), or inhalation of the spores (so-called wool-sorters' disease), which usually occurs while processing animal products. Person-to-person transmission of anthrax has not been described. Cutaneous anthrax, the most common clinical manifestation, occurs within 2–3 days of exposure to an infected animal or animal product. A papule develops at the site of inoculation, which progresses to form a vesicle. A characteristic black eschar is formed after rupture of the vesicle and development of necrosis in the area. In rare cases the disease progresses and becomes systemic with local edema and bacteremia, which can be fatal if untreated.

The only other *Bacillus* species frequently associated with human disease is ***Bacillus cereus,*** which is a cause of gastroenteritis following ingestion of a contaminated food product, most commonly **fried rice.** The spores of *B. cereus* can also survive in the soil and be responsible for traumatic wound infections, particularly to the eye, when soil contamination is involved.

Approach to Suspected Anthrax Infection

Definitions

Eschar: Skin lesion associated with cutaneous anthrax and resembling a black, necrotic sore.

Wool-sorters' disease: Disease associated with inhalation of anthrax spores from infected animal products, most often associated with sheep wool.

Differential diagnosis: Listing of the possible diseases or conditions that may be responsible for the patient's clinical presentation.

Objectives

1. Know the structure and characteristics of *Bacillus anthracis*.
2. Know the clinical diseases caused by and virulence of *B. anthracis*.
3. Know the structure and characteristics of *B. cereus*.
4. Know the clinical diseases caused by and virulence of *B. cereus*.

Discussion

Characteristics of *Bacillus* Species

Bacillus species are **large, motile, facultative anaerobic, gram-positive rods with a central spore.** The spore is quite resistant to extreme conditions and can survive in nature for prolonged periods of time. *B. anthracis* is nonmotile and on Gram stain is often seen in chains. **The virulent forms of *B. anthracis* is more likely to be surrounded by a capsule.** The organism can be cultured as large colonies on blood agar plates within 24 hours, often resembling a "Medusa head" (irregular appearance to the colony with swirling projections). The **principal virulence factors** of *B. anthracis* are the **capsular polypeptide and anthrax toxin.** The capsule consists of **poly-D-glutamic acid,** which is thought to **allow the organism to resist phagocytosis. Anthrax toxin** consists of three proteins: **protective antigen, edema factor, and lethal factor.** Protective antigen is named for its ability to confer immunity in experimental situations. Edema factor and lethal factor bind to protective antigen to form edema toxin and lethal toxin. The bound proteins are transported across cell membranes and are released in the cytoplasm where they exert their effects. Once the spores enter the body they are taken up by macrophages. Because of both lethal and edema factors, the spores survive killing, and subsequently germinate.

Diagnosis

The differential diagnosis of a patient (farmer) with fever, adenopathy, and black eschar include other cutaneous lesions such as **furuncles** (staphylococci), **ecthyma gangrenosum** (*Pseudomonas aeruginosa*), and **spider bites.** However, none of these etiologies are known to cause **eschar formation with surrounding edema.** The specific diagnosis of anthrax is made by growth of the organism from blood (inhalation anthrax), or wound (cutaneous anthrax).

Bacillus anthracis grows easily on most bacteriological culture media within 18–24 hours at 35°C (95°F). The organism is a **nonmotile, spore-forming gram-positive bacillus** that is **nonhemolytic** when grown on blood containing agar medium and produces **lecithinase** on egg yolk agar. Lecithinase is an enzyme produced by both *B. anthracis* and *B. cereus* that **degrades the lecithin in the egg yolk agar leaving a white precipitate.**

Careful review of a Gram stain from a primary specimen of a patient with suspected anthrax is necessary, because the organisms have the propensity to easily decolorize and appear gram-negative. However, the presence of **spores** is a key to the identification of the organism as a gram-positive bacillus. Based on these few tests (large gram-positive bacilli, nonhemolytic, lecithinase positive) a presumptive identification of *Bacillus anthracis* can be made. As a result of the recent events in the world leading to concerns over bioterrorism, definitive diagnosis of anthrax must be performed in a public health laboratory. **Confirmatory testing involves the use of fluorescently labeled monoclonal antibodies as well as DNA amplification assays.** The use of **India ink** can also help to determine the presence of a capsule, a relatively unique aspect. The **capsule of *B. anthracis* is not stained by the India ink,** which can be easily visualized against the dark background.

Treatment and Prevention

Ciprofloxacin is the drug of choice for anthrax, following the identification of weaponized strains that were resistant to penicillin as a result of the production of a β-lactamase. **Prevention** of anthrax involves **vaccination** of animals as well as humans at high risk of exposure (military personnel). Prophylaxis is not recommended for asymptomatic persons. When deemed necessary, prophylaxis with ciprofloxacin must be maintained for up to 30 days because of the potential delay in germination of inhaled spores.

Comprehension Questions

[1.1]   A wound specimen obtained from a person working with wool from a Caribbean island demonstrated a large gram-positive rod from a non-hemolytic colony with swirling projections on blood agar. The most likely method to demonstrate **spores** would be which of the following?

A. Acid-fast stain
B. Gram stain
C. India ink stain
D. Malachite green stain

[1.2]   Which of the following is the current preferred antimicrobial treatment of cutaneous anthrax?

A. Aminoglycosides
B. Ciprofloxacin
C. Penicillin
D. Tetracyclines

[1.3]   *Bacillus anthracis* is unique to other bacteria. It is the only bacteria to possess which of the following?

A. An endotoxin
B. An exotoxin
C. A polypeptide capsule
D. A polysaccharide capsule
E. Lipopolysaccharide in its outer cell wall
F. Teichoic Acid in its outer cell wall

Answers

[1.1]   **D.** Spores can be observed as intracellular refractile bodies in unstained cell suspensions. Also, they are commonly observed by staining with malachite green or carbolfuchsin. The spore wall is relatively impermeable, but heating of the preparation allows dyes to penetrate. Alcohol treatment then serves to prevent spore decolorization. Finally, the spores are counterstained.

[1.2]   **B.** Penicillin G was considered to be the first choice treatment for patients with cutaneous anthrax and when used should be continued for 7–10 days. However, because some naturally occurring isolates have been reported to be penicillin resistant (but still ciprofloxacin sensitive) and some patients are allergic to penicillin, ciprofloxacin is now considered to be the drug of choice for cutaneous anthrax. Ciprofloxacin belongs to the family of quinolones. As a fluorinated quinolone, it has greater antibacterial activity, lower toxicity, and is able to achieve clinically useful levels in blood and tissues compared to nonfluorinated quinolones. They act against many gram-positive and gram-negative bacteria by inhibiting bacterial DNA synthesis via the blockage of DNA gyrase. Despite the use of antibiotics in the treatment of anthrax, clinically manifested inhalational anthrax is usually fatal. If anthrax is suspected, public health authorities should be notified immediately. Aminoglycosides and tetracyclines have different mechanisms of action and have preferred uses in other disease states and infections. Aminoglycosides inhibit bacterial protein synthesis by attaching to and inhibiting the function of the 30S subunit of the bacterial ribosome. Their clinical usefulness has declined with the advent of cephalosporins and quinolones. Tetracyclines also inhibit bacterial protein synthesis; however they do so by inhibiting the binding of aminoacyl-tRNA to the 30S subunit of bacterial ribosomes.

[1.3]   **C.** Virulent forms of *B. anthracis,* the causative agent of anthrax, are more likely to be surrounded by a capsule. This capsule is a polypeptide, composed of a polymer of glutamic acid, and is a unique feature of *B. anthracis.* Lipopolysaccharides (LPS/endotoxin) are unique to gram-negative bacteria (*B. anthracis* is a gram-positive rod). In addition, whereas *B. anthracis* is associated with both teichoic acid (cell wall) and a potent exotoxin, these are not unique features of this bacterium. Other gram positives (i.e., staphylococci) release exotoxins and have teichoic acid in their cell walls.

MICROBIOLOGY PEARLS

❖ The most common form of anthrax is cutaneous anthrax in which penetration of the skin by *B. anthracis* spores causes eschar formation with regional lymphadenopathy.

❖ The organism is a **nonmotile, spore-forming gram-positive bacilli** that is **nonhemolytic** and produces **lecithinase.**

❖ Inhalation anthrax is a matter of public health concern.

❖ The drug of choice for treating anthrax is ciprofloxacin.

❖ The two main methods of anthrax virulence are its capsule and toxin.

❖ An eschar surrounded by edema is suspicious for anthrax.

REFERENCES

Logan NA, Turnbull PCB. Bacillus and other aerobic endospore-forming bacteria: manual of clinical microbiology. ASM, 2003.

Murray PR, Rosenthal KS, Kobayashi GS, Pfaller MA. Bacillus. In: Murray PR, Rosenthal KS, Kobayashi GS, Pfaller MA. Medical microbiology, 4th ed. St. Louis: Mosby, 2002:240–44.

Ryan KJ. Sherris medical microbiology: an introduction to infectious diseases, 3rd ed. New York: McGraw-Hill, 2003.

Swartz MN. Recognition and management of anthrax—an update NEJM 2001.

A 60-year-old man presents to the emergency room with severe abdominal pain. He has had mild, left lower abdominal cramping pain for about 3 days, which has worsened in the past 8 hours. He has also had nausea, fever, and chills. On examination he is in obvious pain, has a fever of 38.6°C (101.5°F) and has an elevated heart rate (tachycardia). His abdominal examination is notable for absent bowel sounds, diffuse tenderness, and rigidity when palpated. An x-ray reveals the presence of free air in the abdominal cavity. He is taken for emergency surgery and found to have severe diverticulitis with a perforated colon. Cloudy peritoneal fluid is collected. An anaerobic culture grows *Bacteroides fragilis*.

◆ **What characteristics are noted on Gram staining of *B. fragilis*?**

◆ **What are its primary mechanisms for resisting phagocytosis?**

ANSWERS TO CASE 2: *Bacteroides fragilis*

Summary: A 60-year-old man has a ruptured diverticulitis leading to peritonitis. The cultures of the purulent drainage reveal *Bacteroides fragilis.*

◆ **Characteristics on gram staining:** *B. fragilis* appears encapsulated, with irregular staining, pleomorphism, and vacuolization.

◆ **Primary mechanisms of resisting phagocytosis:** The capsular polysaccharide and succinic acid production.

CLINICAL CORRELATION

B. fragilis is one of the most clinically significant **anaerobic** organisms. It is part of the **normal flora of the gastrointestinal (GI) tract** and causes clinical infections when it escapes from this environment following surgery, traumatic bowel perforation, or other diseases, such as **diverticulitis.** Although many anaerobes are part of the normal gastrointestinal flora, *B. fragilis* is the most common cause of intraabdominal infections. *B. fragilis* is also associated with respiratory tract infections (sinusitis, otitis), genital tract infections, brain, skin, and soft tissue infections.

Diverticulitis is an inflammation of a small food and particle collecting sac in the large intestine, it may lead to colonic rupture and therefore allow the organisms normally present in the GI tract to penetrate the peritoneal cavity and possibly the bloodstream. These infections usually involve a mixture of both aerobes and anaerobes.

Approach to Suspected Anthrax Infection

Definitions

Anaerobes: Organisms that do not require oxygen for growth and may die in its presence.

Bacteroides bile esculin (BBE) agar: Media selective for *B. fragilis* on which the colonies appear black.

Diverticulitis: Inflammation of a diverticulum, which is a small bulging sac in the colon wall which can trap food particles and become inflamed and painful.

Objectives

1. Know the microbiologic characteristics of *Bacteroides fragilis* and other *Bacteroides* species.
2. Know the virulence factors associated with *B. fragilis.*

Discussion

Characteristics of *Bacteroides* Species

Bacteroides species include the *B. fragilis* group as well as many other species. Two new genera were recently created, *Prevotella* and *Porphyromas,* to remove the pigmented, bile-sensitive anaerobes previously in the genus *Bacteroides.* All are **small, anaerobic, gram-negative bacilli** and many strains are encapsulated. **Vacuolization, irregular staining, and pleomorphism** are common.

B. fragilis has a distinct **capsule** composed of two **polysaccharides,** which appears to **inhibit phagocytosis and allow adherence to peritoneal surfaces.** Other virulence factors for this bacterium include the presence of **pili,** which promote adherence to epithelial cells and the production of **succinic acid, which inhibits phagocytosis.** *B. fragilis* produces an endotoxin that has little biologic activity. It also produces **superoxide dismutase,** an enzyme, **which allows the organism to survive in the presence of small amounts of oxygen.**

Diagnosis

Anaerobes are not usually the primary cause of an infection, but are involved in a mixed aerobic, anaerobic infection. Often diagnosis of **anaerobic infections** is based on clinical features including a **foul smelling wound** with the **presence of gas** in the involved tissue usually located in close proximity to a mucosal surface. Infections that involve spillage of GI material into the peritoneum are likely to involve aerobes and anaerobes. The **most commonly associated anaerobe is *B. fragilis.*** Patients with severe diverticulitis, appendicitis, or colonic injury often develop *B. fragilis* peritonitis.

To increase the chances of recovery of anaerobes from a specimen, the sample must be appropriately collected to allow survival of anaerobes. Anaerobes are organisms that do not require oxygen for growth. Sensitivity of the anaerobic organism can vary from those that **cannot tolerate any oxygen (strict anaerobes)** to those that can grow in the presence of **small amounts of oxygen (oxygen tolerant).** Anaerobes are therefore grown under atmospheric conditions that limit the presence of oxygen and include predominantly nitrogen, as well as hydrogen and carbon dioxide. Tissues or fluids collected and transported under anaerobic conditions are the most optimal; however, if necessary an anaerobic transport swab can also be used.

Bacteroides species produce **small colonies on anaerobic blood agar** medium within 24 hours. Selective media such as kanamycin/gentamicin laked blood agar will support growth of gram-negative anaerobes only. Presumptive identification of *B. fragilis* can be made by growth of **black pigmented colonies on *Bacteroides* bile esculin agar,** and resistance to kanamycin, colistin, and vancomycin special potency antimicrobial disks. Definitive identification of anaerobes or *B. fragilis* is made with commercial identification systems that are based on the presence of preformed enzymes or in reference laboratories using gas liquid chromatography to determine the specific gases produced by the organism.

Treatment and Prevention

Surgical debridement is usually necessary at least in part for the treatment of anaerobic infections. **β-lactamase activity is common in *Bacteroides* species,** especially *B. fragilis,* which results in **resistance to penicillin and cephalosporin antibiotics.** Drugs of choice for *Bacteroides* species include β-lactam–β-lactamase inhibitor combinations, such as piperacillin/tazobactam, metronidazole, and imipenem.

Comprehension Questions

[2.1] During an emergency surgery, a 60-year-old male is found to have severe peritonitis and a perforated colon. Foul-smelling cloudy peritoneal fluid is collected. Subsequent analysis reveals the growth of black pigmented colonies on *Bacteroides* bile esculin agar. No growth is detected in the presence of kanamycin, colistin, or vancomycin. Which of the following microorganisms is most likely involved in this case?

A. *Actinomyces israelii*
B. *Bacteroides fragilis*
C. *Clostridium difficile*
D. *Enterococcus faecalis*
E. *Porphyromonas gingivalis*
F. *Prevotella melaninogenica*

[2.2] Which of the following is the treatment of choice to control this infection in this patient (described in question [2.1])?

A. Cephalothin
B. Erythromycin
C. Metronidazole
D. Penicillin

[2.3] Among the many virulence factors produced, *B. fragilis* produces an enzyme that allows the organism to survive in the presence of small amounts of oxygen. Which of the enzymes listed below catalyzes the following reaction?

$$2O_2^- + 2H^+ \rightarrow H_2O_2 + O_2$$

A. Beta lactamase
B. Myeloperoxidase
C. Nicotinamide adenine dinucleotide phosphate (NADPH) oxidase
D. NO synthase
E. Oxidase
F. Superoxide dismutase

[2.4]   A foul-smelling specimen was obtained from a 26-year-old woman with a pelvic abscess. Culture grew both aerobic and anaerobic gram-negative bacteria. The most likely organisms are which of the following?

    A. *Actinomyces israelii* and *Escherichia coli*
    B. *Bacteroides fragilis* and *Listeria monocytogenes*
    C. *Bacteroides fragilis* and *Neisseria gonorrhoeae*
    D. *Clostridium perfringens* and *Bacteroides fragilis*
    E. *Escherichia coli* and *Peptostreptococcus*

Answers

[2.1]   **B.** *Bacteroides* species are normal inhabitants of the bowel and other sites. Normal stools contain large numbers of *B. fragilis* (10^{11} organisms per gram). As a result, they are very important anaerobes that can cause human infection. Members of the *B. fragilis* group are most commonly isolated from infections associated with contamination by the contents of the colon, where they may cause suppuration, for example, peritonitis after bowel injury. Classification is based on colonial and biochemical features and on characteristic short-chain fatty acid patterns in gas chromatography. These short-chain fatty acids also contribute to the foul-smelling odor emanating from the wound in the above case.

[2.2]   **C.** Metronidazole, mainly used as an antiprotozoal agent, is also highly effective against anaerobic bacterial infections, such as those infections caused by *Bacteroides* species. It is the drug of first choice for gastrointestinal strains of *Bacteroides*. Two other effective antibiotics are imipenem and piperacillin/tazobactam. *Bacteroides* species, such as *B. fragilis,* commonly possess β-lactamase activity resulting in resistance to penicillin and cephalosporin (e.g., cephalothin) antibiotics. Erythromycin is not indicated in the treatment of *Bacteroides* species.

[2.3]   **F.** A key feature of obligate anaerobes such as *Clostridium, Bacteroides,* and *Actinomyces* is that they lack catalase and/or superoxide dismutase (SOD) and are therefore susceptible to oxidative damage. *B. fragilis,* however, is able to survive (not grow) in environments with low oxygen content because of its ability to produce small amounts of both SOD and catalase. Anaerobes that possess SOD and/or catalase are able to negate the toxic effects of oxygen radicals and hydrogen peroxide and thus tolerate oxygen. Other common enzymes listed above catalyze the following reactions:

Catalase/superoxide dismutase catalyzes: $2H_2O_2 \rightarrow 2H_2O + O_2$
Myeloperoxidase catalyzes: $Cl^- + H_2O_2 \rightarrow ClO^- + H_2O$
NADPH oxidase catalyzes: $NADPH + 2O_2 \rightarrow 2O_2^- + H^+ \ NADP^+$
NO synthase catalyzes: $\frac{1}{2}O_2 + arginine \rightarrow NO + citrulline$
Oxidase catalyzes: $2H^+ + 2e^- + \frac{1}{2}O_2 \rightarrow H_2O$

[2.4]   **C.** In infections, such as intraabdominal abscesses, *Bacteroides* species are often associated with other organisms. The only other organism in the list above that is solely aerobic and gram-negative is *N. gonorrhoeae*. *Clostridium* and *Listeria* are both gram-positive. *E. coli* is gram-negative and a facultative anaerobe.

MICROBIOLOGY PEARLS

❖ The treatment of choice of *B. fragilis* is surgical debridement in addition to metronidazole, imipenem, or piperacillin/tazobactam.

❖ Most anaerobes are part of mixed infections at mucosal surfaces.

❖ *B. fragilis* is the most common anaerobe in the human GI tract.

❖ *Bacteroides fragilis* usually express superoxide dismutase, an enzyme, which allows the organism to survive in the presence of small amounts of oxygen.

REFERENCES

Brook I, Frazier EH. Aerobic and anaerobic microbiology in intraabdominal infections associated with diverticulitis. J Med Microbiol 2000;49:827–30.

Engelkirk PG, Duben-Engelkirk JD, Dowell VR. Principles and practice of clinical anaerobic bacteriology. Star Publishing, 1992.

Murray PR, Rosenthal KS, Kobayashi GS, Pfaller MA. Anaerobic gram negative bacilli. In: Murray PR, Rosenthal KS, Kobayashi GS, Pfaller MA. Medical microbiology, 4th ed. St. Louis: Mosby, 2002:354–58.

A 28-year-old woman presents to the office for the evaluation of a rash. She had just returned from a weeklong camping trip in the New England area, when she noted the presence of a circular, red rash on her lower abdomen. Also, she has had a low-grade fever, and some achiness and fatigue. Examination of her abdomen reveals a 10-cm flat, red, circular patch with some central clearing. No other skin rashes are noted, and the remainder of the examination is normal. The blood cultures are negative. You make the presumptive diagnosis of erythema migrans and send blood for confirmatory serologic studies.

◆ **What organism is the etiologic agent of erythema migrans?**

◆ **What are the primary reservoir and vector of transmission of this agent?**

ANSWERS TO CASE 3: *Borrelia burgdorferi*

Summary: A 28-year-old woman who has been recently camping in the New England area complains of fever and a skin rash consistent with erythema migrans. Confirmatory serologies are sent.

◆ **Etiologic agent of erythema migrans:** *Borrelia burgdorferi.*

◆ **Primary reservoir of infection:** Small rodents, primarily the white-footed mouse.

◆ **Primary vector of transmission:** *Ixodes* tick.

CLINICAL CORRELATION

Borrelia burgdorferi is the causative agent of Lyme disease and is transmitted to humans by *Ixodes* ticks. This disease was first recognized in Old Lyme, Connecticut, with the identification of cluster cases of arthritis in children. The infection is characterized by a **"bull's eye" skin lesion,** which develops from the site of the tick bite, 1–4 weeks postinfection. Additional initial symptoms include fever, fatigue, headache, joint pain, or mild stiffness of the neck. **Lyme disease is the most common vector-born disease in the United States,** and if left undiagnosed and untreated, the infection usually progresses to involve the nervous or vascular systems and cause fluctuating or chronic arthritis.

Approach to *Borrelia* Species

Definitions

Erythema migrans: Skin lesion composed of redness (erythema) with central clearing (target lesion).

Spirochetes: Thin spiral bacteria of which three genera cause significant disease in humans: *Leptospira, Borrelia,* and *Treponema,* which lead to leptospirosis, lyme disease, and syphilis, respectively (see Table 3–1 for an abbreviated listing).

Objectives

1. Know the characteristics and virulence factors of *B. burgdorferi.*
2. Know the reservoir, vector, and host involved in the transmission of *B. burgdorferi.*

Discussion

B. burgdorferi belongs to the **spirochete** family of **prokaryotes.** It stains **gram-negative,** although spirochetes are considered neither gram positive nor gram-negative. Spirochetes consist of a **flexible, multilayer outer cell mem-**

Table 3-1
ABBREVIATED LISTING OF SPIROCHETES

SPIROCHETE	DISEASE	TREATMENT	COMMENT
Treponema	Venereal syphilis, Yaws, pinta, endemic syphilis	Penicillin	Veneral syphilis usually is sexually or vertically (to fetus/neonate) transmitted, whereas yaws, pinta, endemic syphillis is by skin or shared utensils, usually affecting children
Leptospires	Weil syndrome (severe hepatic renal failure) Anicteric leptospirosis (without jaundice)	Doxycycline or ampicillin	Coiled, highly motile with hooked ends and flagella allowing burrowing into tissue
Borrelia	Relapsing fever Lyme disease	Erythromycin, tetracycline	Usually human or rodent reservoir transmitted by tick bite

Source: Harrison's Internal Medicine, 2004.

brane and a **more rigid, peptidoglycan-containing cytoplasmic membrane.** Between these two layers are **endoflagella** that insert at the ends of the spirochete. **Rotation of these flagella** creates the **characteristic cork-screw shape** of these organisms. This provides for motility of the organism and hides the normally antigenic flagella from host defenses. These organisms are **microaerophilic** and have a doubling time of 8–24 hours. The disease is endemic in several regions of the United States including **Northeastern, Midwest, and Pacific coast** states. However, most reported cases occur in **New York, Connecticut, Pennsylvania, and New Jersey.**

The spirochetes that cause Lyme disease have been divided into genospecies. Three genospecies, *B. burgdorferi* sensu stricto, *B. garinii* and *B. afzelii,* are known to cause Lyme disease and are known collectively as *B. burgdorferi* sensu lato. The outer membrane of *B. burgdorferi* contains unique outer surface proteins (Osps), which are thought to play a role in their virulence. **Small rodents,** particularly the white-footed mouse, are the **primary reservoirs** of *B. burgdorferi,* and the vector of transmission is the *Ixodes* tick. The larva of the tick is born uninfected. The **ticks become infected with**

the spirochete on feeding on an infected animal. This usually occurs during the nymph stage of the tick's life cycle. The spirochetes **multiply in the gastrointestinal (GI) tract** of the **tick,** and then are transmitted to the animal host by regurgitation or salivation during a subsequent feeding. *B. burgdorferi* are next **transmitted to humans via tick bite** followed by dissemination through the bloodstream to the joints, heart, and central nervous system (CNS). The nymphal stage of the tick is more infective than the adult and larval stages. Most exposures to *Borrelia* occur between the months of May and July, when the nymphs are most active.

Clinically there are three stages of *B. burgdorferi* infection: **stage 1,** which occurs in the first 1–4 weeks postinfection, involves the initial characteristic skin lesion referred to as **"erythema migrans"; stage 2** follows months postinfection with **neurologic and cardiac** involvement; and **stage 3** results in **chronic arthritis** of the joints.

Diagnosis

The diagnosis of Lyme disease is made primarily by **clinical presentation** and patient history of exposure. Confirmation of a clinical **diagnosis is made serologically** via the detection of **antibody** by enzyme-linked immunoabsorbance or indirect immunofluorescence. However, serologic tests are most reliable 2–4 weeks post infection, because of cross-reactivity with normal flora, and Western blot analysis should be used to confirm a positive serologic test. Alternately, **new PCR-based tests** are available to detect *B. burgdorferi* DNA. *B. burgdorferi* is difficult to grow in culture, requiring complex culture media and a microaerophilic environment. It is also difficult to visualize under light microscopy, but can be seen under darkfield microscopy or when stained with Giemsa or silver stains.

Treatment and Prevention

Initial stages of infection with *B. burgdorferi* can be effectively treated with **doxycycline** or **amoxicillin,** while **later stages of disease** are better treated with **penicillin G or ceftriaxone. Prevention** of infection involves limiting exposure to ticks by **wearing protective clothing in endemic areas,** including long sleeves and long pants tucked into socks. Careful search for and removal of ticks is also an important preventative measure. Use of **repellants** is also helpful and administration of insecticides may reduce the number of active nymphal ticks for a given season. A **vaccine** containing recombinant OspA protein was developed for persons with the highest risk of exposure. The vaccine is approved for adults and shows approximately 75 percent efficacy.

Comprehension Questions

[3.1]   A 9-year-old boy presents with a migratory rash with central clearing on the back of his neck. The child had recently been on vacation with his family in Oregon and had gone hiking. The child's pediatrician observes the rash and suspects an infection with *Borrelia burgdorferi.* Which of the following is thought to be a virulence factor of this organism?

A. Intracellular growth in leukocytes
B. Endotoxin release
C. Localization in reticuloendothelial cells
D. Antiphagocytic capsular antigen
E. Expression of outer surface proteins

[3.2]   If the child's infection is left untreated, which of the following symptoms would most likely appear?

A. Urethritis
B. Centripetal spread of rash
C. Biphasic illness with fever and chills
D. Stiffness in the knees
E. Swelling of lymph nodes

[3.3]   A small tick, of the genus *Ixodes,* most commonly transmits *Borrelia burgdorferi.* Which of the following diseases is also transmitted by a tick?

A. Q fever
B. Leptospirosis
C. Ehrlichiosis
D. Yellow fever
E. Eastern equine encephalitis

Answers

[3.1]   **E.** Differential expression of outer surface proteins is thought to be involved with virulence; answers A, B, C, and D are incorrect: (A) intracellular growth in leukocytes is a virulence factor of *Ehrlichia;* (B) endotoxins are characteristic of gram-negative organisms, not *Borrelia;* (C) localization in reticuloendothelial cells occurs in infections with *Francisella tularensis;* (D) an antiphagocytic capsular antigen is not a virulence factor of *Borrelia.*

[3.2]   **D.** Later stages of infection with *Borrelia burgdorferi* include arthritis, meningitis, nerve palsies, and cardiovascular abnormalities; answers A, B, C, E, are incorrect: (A) arthritis, not urethritis, is a later manifestation of infection with *Borrelia burgdorferi;* (B) the skin rash or erythema migrans expands centrifugally, not centripetally; (C) biphasic illness with fever and chills occurs more commonly with *Leptospira* infections; (E) swelling of lymph nodes is more commonly associated with *Yersinia* infections.

[3.3]   **C.** Similar to Lyme disease, Ehrlichiosis is also transmitted via a tick vector; answers A, B, D, and E are incorrect: (A) Q fever is most commonly transmitted via inhalation of dried feces or urine contaminated with rickettsiae; (B) Leptospirosis is typically transmitted via ingestion of contaminated food or water; (D and E) both yellow fever and eastern equine encephalitis are transmitted by mosquitoes.

MICROBIOLOGY PEARLS

❖ *B. burgdorferi* is a microaerophilic spirochete.
❖ Primary reservoirs of *B. burgdorferi* are small rodents (e.g., white-footed mouse), and the vector of transmission is the *Ixodes* tick.
❖ States with highest incidence include: New York, Connecticut, Pennsylvania, and New Jersey.
❖ Primary treatment is doxycycline or amoxicillin.
❖ Prevention consists of wearing protective clothing, use of insect repellants or insecticides, and a recombinant OspA protein vaccine.

REFERENCES

Brooks GF, Butel JS, Morse SA. Jawetz, Melnick, & Adelberg's medical microbiology, 23rd ed. New York: McGraw-Hill, 2004:336–338.
Murray PR, Rosenthal KS, Kobayashi GS, Pfaller MA. Medical microbiology, 4th ed. St. Louis: Mosby, 2002:384–390.
Ryan JR, Ray CG. Sherris medical microbiology, 4th ed. New York: McGraw-Hill, 2004:431–434.
Wilske B, Schriefer ME. Borrelia. In: Murray PR et al., eds. Manual of clinical microbiology, 8th ed. ASM Press, 2003.

A 19-year-old male college student presents to the student health department with abdominal pain, diarrhea, and fever. He says that his symptoms started one day ago. He has had 10 stools in the past day and has noted blood mixed in with the stool on several occasions. He usually eats at home but reports having eaten chicken in the college cafeteria three days ago. He has no history of gastrointestinal (GI) disease. On examination he has a temperature of 37.8°C (100°F) and appears to be in pain. His abdomen has hyperactive bowel sounds and is diffusely tender but without rigidity, rebound tenderness, or guarding. A general surgeon is consulted and is considering the diagnosis of acute appendicitis versus bacterial gastroenteritis possibly related to the chicken eaten. A stool sample tests positive for blood and fecal leukocytes. Stool cultures are sent and are subsequently positive for a pathologic organism.

◆ **What is the most likely pathologic organism?**

◆ **In what atmospheric environment does this organism grow?**

ANSWERS TO CASE 4: *Campylobacter jejuni*

Summary: A 19-year-old man presents with a bacterial gastroenteritis that mimics appendicitis.

◆ **Most likely etiology of this infection:** *Campylobacter jejuni.*

◆ **Preferred atmospheric environment:** Microaerophilic (presence of increased levels of carbon dioxide).

CLINICAL CORRELATION

More than 50 serotypes of *C. jejuni* have been identified based on heat labile (capsular and flagellar) antigens. *C. jejuni* is endemic worldwide, and most cases of infection are associated with eating chicken, although milk, water and other meats have also been implicated. Human-to-human transmission is rare. **C. jejuni is one of the most frequent causes of bacterial diarrhea occurring most often in the summer or early fall.** The incubation period is 1–3 days followed initially by symptoms of fever, malaise, and abdominal pain. *C. jejuni* can cause bloody diarrhea, mucosal inflammation, and bacteremia, suggesting that it is invasive to the lining of the intestine. Most cases of *Campylobacter* gastroenteritis is self-limited, with symptoms resolving within 7 days; however, relapses can occur in 5–10 percent of cases which are untreated.

Complications of *Campylobacter* gastroenteritis include pancreatitis, peritonitis, or more uncommonly arthritis, osteomyelitis, and sepsis. A serious postinfection sequelae of *Campylobacter* gastroenteritis is Guillain-Barré syndrome, an acute demyelinating disease. Antigenic similarities between the lipopolysaccharides on the surface of some serotypes of *C. jejuni* and myelin proteins are thought to be responsible for Guillain-Barré disease.

Other *Campylobacter* species such as *C. coli* also cause gastroenteritis, which is clinically indistinguishable from *C. jejuni* infection. *C. fetus* is primarily a cause of bacteremia, septic arthritis, peritonitis, abscesses, meningitis, and endocarditis in immunocompromised patients.

Approach to Suspected *Campylobacter* Infection

Definitions

Guillain-Barré syndrome: A demyelinating disease resulting from similarities between the host and the surface of the *Campylobacter* organism.
Fecal leukocytes: White blood cells present in the stool, which correlate loosely with the presence of an invasive pathogen.

Objectives

1. Know the characteristics, virulence factors, and preferred growth environments of *C. jejuni.*

2. Know the sources of infection with and mechanism of transmission of *C. jejuni.*

Discussion

Characteristics of *Campylobacter*

Campylobacter species are **small motile, nonspore-forming, comma-shaped, gram-negative bacilli.** Its motility is the result of a single **flagellum** located at one or both poles of the organism. Campylobacter does not grow in aerobic or anaerobic environments. It is **microaerophilic,** requiring 5–10 percent oxygen and high concentrations of carbon dioxide for growth. *C. jejuni* grows better at 42°C (107.6°F) than 37°C (98.6°F). *C. jejuni* multiplies more slowly than other enteric bacteria, making isolation difficult from stool samples unless selective media are used. When **selective media** are used, the colonies that grow tend to be **gray, mucoid, and wet appearing.** Its outer membrane contains lipopolysaccharides with endotoxic activity. Extracellular toxins with cytopathic activity have also been found; however, little is known regarding the pathogenesis of this organism and the role of these putative virulence factors in disease. The organisms are sensitive to decreased pH, so it is hypothesized that factors that neutralize gastric acid enhance the organisms chances for survival.

Diagnosis

The differential diagnosis of acute gastroenteritis would include *Salmonella, Shigella, Yersinia,* as well as *Campylobacter.* Because of the feature of abdominal pain and cramps, sometimes in the absence of diarrhea, *Campylobacter* gastroenteritis can be misdiagnosed as appendicitis or irritable bowel syndrome. The presence of bloody diarrhea may also suggest enterohemorrhagic *E. coli.*

   Definitive diagnosis would be made by **culture of the stool and growth of** *Campylobacter. Campylobacter* are more fastidious than most other causes of bacterial gastroenteritis and specimens should be transported to the laboratory in media such as **Cary-Blair.** Selective media such as camp blood agar or Skirrow's medium, which includes antibiotics to inhibit the normal stool flora, allows for growth of *Campylobacter* within 48–72 hours. Presumptive identification can be made by growth of **oxidase positive colonies on selective media at 42°C** (107.6°F) **after 48–72 hours** with the characteristic **comma-shaped, small, gram-negative bacilli.** Confirmation of identification of either *C. jejuni* or *C. coli* can be made by resistance to cephalothin and susceptibility to nalidixic acid antimicrobial disks. As a result of the fastidious nature of these pathogens, a commercial assay for detection of *Campylobacter* antigen in the stool is frequently used for diagnosis.

Treatment and Prevention

Most often *Campylobacter jejuni* infection is self-limited and does not require specific antimicrobial therapy. Supportive care, that is, hydration, is often the only treatment needed. If specific therapy is needed for severe disease, or infection in immunocompromised patients, **erythromycin** is the drug of choice, because of the recent increase in resistance to fluoroquinolones.

Prevention involves care in food preparation. Foods, especially chicken, should be completely cooked, and exposure to raw or undercooked chicken or unpasteurized milk should be limited, especially in pregnant or immunocompromised persons.

Comprehension Questions

[4.1]   Which of the following are the special laboratory conditions needed to recover *Campylobacter jejuni?*

A. 37°C (98.6°F) aerobic on blood agar plates
B. 37°C (98.6°F) anaerobic on blood agar plates
C. 42°C (107.6°F) microaerophilic on Skirrow's medium
D. 42°C (107.6°F) aerobic on Skirrow's medium

[4.2]   A 21 year-old woman presents to the emergency room with shortness of breath 2 weeks after recovering from a "stomach flu." Physical exam reveals ascending muscle weakness that began in her toes. Cardiac irregularities are also notable. A review of the patient's chart revealed that a bacterial stool culture 2 weeks earlier, during the patient's "flu" episode, found comma-shaped organisms growing at 42°C (107.6°F). Which of the following pairs represents the causative agent of this patient's flu and the postflu condition, respectively?

A. *Campylobacter jejuni,* Guillain-Barré syndrome
B. *Clostridium botulinum,* botulism
C. JC virus, progressive multifocal leukoencephalopathy (PML)
D. Poliovirus, poliomyelitis

[4.3]   In a nonimmunocompromised patient with *Campylobacter jejuni* as the causative agent of their food poisoning, which of the following is the treatment most often required?

A. Metronidazole
B. Vancomycin
C. Cephalosporin
D. TMP-SMZ
E. Supportive care and hydration

[4.4] A 20-year-old college student develops diarrhea that lasts for approximately 1 week. Stool cultures reveal a motile, microaerophilic gram-negative rod that is isolated by incubation at 41°C (105.8°F) on medium containing antibiotics. This organism is most likely to be which of the following?

   A. *Escherichia coli*
   B. *Vibrio parahaemolyticus*
   C. *Yersinia enterocolitica*
   D. *Campylobacter jejuni*
   E. *Proteus vulgaris*

Answers

[4.1] **C.** The isolation and identification of *Campylobacter jejuni* can be achieved using special culture characteristics. Three requirements must be met. First, a selective medium is needed. There are several selective media in widespread use: Skirrow's medium uses vancomycin, polymyxin B, and trimethoprim; other selective media contain cefoperazone, other antimicrobials, and inhibitory compounds. The selective media are suitable for isolation of *C. jejuni* at 42°C (107.6°F); when incubated at 36–37°C (96.8–98.6°F), other *Campylobacters* and bacteria may be isolated. Finally, incubation must be in an atmosphere with reduced oxygen and added carbon dioxide. The colonies appear to be colorless or gray and may be watery and spreading or round and convex.

[4.2] **A.** Guillain-Barré syndrome (acute idiopathic polyneuritis) is associated with infections such as herpesvirus and *Campylobacter jejuni* (comma-shaped bacteria that grows at 42°C [107.6°F]). It is believed that some *C. jejuni* serotypes have surface lipopolysaccharides that are antigenically similar to myelin protein leading to the inflammation and demyelination of peripheral nerves and ventral root motor fibers. Suspected Guillain-Barré in a patient is always a medical emergency because respiratory distress or failure can ensue, and the patient should always be admitted to the hospital for careful treatment and observation. The other answers contain correct matching of the causative agent with the resulting condition, but do not reflect the clinical scenario described.

[4.3] **E.** Most infections with *C. jejuni* are self-limiting and thus do not require specific antimicrobial therapy, except in cases of severe disease and infection in immunocompromised individuals. Therefore, most often the only required therapy is hydration and supportive care. When specific antimicrobial therapy is indicated, the drug of first choice is erythromycin, with alternate drugs being tetracycline, ciprofloxacin, and ofloxacin.

[4.4]   **D.** Based on the culture characteristics indicated above, the only possible answer is *Campylobacter jejuni*. Please also refer to the discussion for Question 4.1.

MICROBIOLOGY PEARLS

❖ *Campylobacter* species are small motile, non–spore-forming, comma-shaped, gram-negative bacilli, best grown in a microaerophilic environment at 42°C (107.6°F).

❖ Guillain-Barré is a rare neurological complication of *C. jejuni* gastroenteritis.

❖ *C. jejuni* gastroenteritis is usually self-limited; however, if necessary, erythromycin is the drug of choice.

❖ *Campylobacter* infection most often occurs several days after consumption of undercooked chicken.

❖ Symptom of fever and abdominal pain may initially mimic appendicitis.

REFERENCES

Allos BM. *Campylobacter jejuni* infections: update on emerging issues and trends. CID 2001;32:1201–206.

Murray PR, Rosenthal KS, Kobayashi GS, Pfaller MA. *Campylobacter* and *Helicobacter.* In: Murray PR, Rosenthal KS, Kobayashi GS, Pfaller MA. Medical microbiology, 4th ed. St. Louis: Mosby, 2002:288–96.

A 19-year-old woman presents for the evaluation of pelvic pain. The pain has progressively worsened over the past week. She has also been having some burning with urination and a vaginal discharge. She is sexually active, has had 4 lifetime partners, takes oral contraceptive pills, and occasionally uses condoms. On examination, she appears in no acute distress and does not have a fever. Her abdomen is soft with moderate lower abdominal tenderness. On pelvic examination, she is noted to have a yellow cervical discharge and significant cervical motion tenderness. No uterine or adnexal masses are palpated, but mild tenderness is also noted. A Gram stain of the cervical discharge reveals only multiple polymorphonuclear leukocytes. A direct DNA probe test subsequently comes back positive for *Chlamydia trachomatis*.

◆ **How does *C. trachomatis* enter a target cell?**

◆ **What are the two stages of the *C. trachomatis* life cycle?**

ANSWERS TO CASE 5: *Chlamydia trachomatis*

Summary: A 19-year-old woman with probable pelvic inflammatory disease has a positive assay for *Chlamydia trachomatis.*

◆ **How *C. trachomatis* enters a target cell:** the elementary body of *C. trachomatis* binds to receptors on the host and induces endocytosis.

◆ **Two stages of the *C. trachomatis* life cycle:** the elementary body and the reticulate body.

CLINICAL CORRELATION

Chlamydia trachomatis is the causative agent of the most common sexually transmitted disease in the United States, and it is also the greatest cause of preventable blindness around the world. Chlamydial disease affects women five times more often than men, and approximately two-thirds of those affected lack symptoms and thus, do not know that they are infected. Many of those infected with gonorrheal disease are also infected with chlamydia, as both organisms infect the columnar epithelial cells of the mucous membranes. Chlamydial disease usually affects the poor and is prevalent in underdeveloped countries. Children are also a main reservoir, transmitting the disease by hand-to-hand transfer of infected eye fluids or by sharing contaminated towels or clothing.

Approach to Suspected Chlamydial Infection

Definitions

Elementary body: Nondividing 300-nm infectious particle. This particle has an outer membrane with disulfide linkages which allows it to survive extracellularly.

Chandelier sign: Cervical motion tenderness during the bimanual exam, characteristic of pelvic inflammatory disease (PID).

Exudate: Material, such as fluids, cells or debris, which has extravasated from vessels and has been deposited on tissue surfaces or in tissue.

Papule: Small palpable elevated lesion that is less than 1 cm.

Discussion

Characteristics of *Chlamydia trachomatis*

Chlamydia trachomatis is a **gram-negative obligate intracellular parasite** with a unique life cycle. It is coccoid in morphology and is very small, usually about 350 nm in diameter. Although *C. trachomatis* is classified as a gram-negative bacteria, it **lacks a peptidoglycan layer and muramic acid,** which are present in other gram-negative organisms. There are many disulfide linkages present in the outer membrane which stabilize the organism. Its **extracellular form is called the elementary body,** which has a small, spore-like structure. It attaches to columnar, cuboidal or transitional epithelial cells in structures lined by mucous membranes. The elementary body binds to receptors on susceptible cells and induces endocytosis into the host. These membrane-protected structures are known as inclusions. The elementary body undergoes reorganization into a larger, more metabolically active form known as the **reticulate body.** Reticulate bodies grow and multiply by binary fission to create larger intracellular inclusions. Reticulate bodies transform back into elementary bodies, which are released from the epithelial cell by exocytosis and which can then infect other cells. The life cycle of *Chlamydia trachomatis* lasts only 48 hours. Table 5-1 lists in sequential order are the stages of the life cycle.

    C. trachomatis appears to be an **obligate human pathogen** with approximately 15 serotypes. It is the most common bacterial cause of sexually transmitted diseases in humans and also causes **conjunctivitis, lymphogranuloma venereum, and ocular trachoma.** Infection of the conjunctiva by *C. trachomatis* results in scarring and inflammation. This fibrosis pulls the eyelid inward causing the eyelashes to rub against the cornea. Because the eyelid is rolled inward, the individual is unable to completely close the eye resulting in the inability to maintain moisture on the surface of the eye. It is the combination of the lack of surface moisture and constant abrasion by the eyelashes that causes corneal scarring and blindness.

    C. trachomatis also causes other diseases including **pneumonia, urethritis, epididymitis, lymphogranuloma venereum, cervicitis, and pelvic inflammatory disease. Lymphogranuloma venereum** presents with a **painless papule on the genitalia that heals spontaneously.** The infection is then local-

Table 5-1
LIFE CYCLE OF *CHLAMYDIA TRACHOMATIS*

1. Elementary body attaches to host cell.

2. Host cell phagocytizes the elementary body residing in a vacuole, inhibiting phagosome-lysome fusion.

3. The elementary body reorganizes to form a reticulate body.

4. The reticulate body divides by binary fusion.

5. Some reticulate bodies convert back into elementary bodies; elementary bodies are released into host cell.

ized to **regional lymph nodes** where it resides for about two months. As time progresses, the lymph nodes begin to swell, causing pain, and may rupture and expel an exudate. Men with **epididymitis** present with fever, unilateral scrotal swelling, and pain. Women with **cervicitis** present with a swollen, inflamed cervix. There may also be a yellow purulent discharge present. PID occurs when the infection spreads to the uterus, fallopian tubes, and ovaries. PID presents with lower abdominal pain, dyspareunia, vaginal discharge, uterine bleeding, nausea, vomiting, and fever. **Cervical motion tenderness** during the bimanual exam is known as the "chandelier sign." Recurrent PID may scar the fallopian tubes, resulting in infertility or ectopic pregnancy. Children may acquire chlamydial disease during birth via passage through an infected birth canal. **Inflammation of the infant's conjunctiva** may occur with a yellow discharge and swelling of the eyelids within two weeks after birth. The presence of **basophilic intracytoplasmic inclusion bodies** from the conjunctiva is a helpful diagnostic clue. Neonatal **pneumonia** may also occur from passage through an infected birth canal. An infected child may present 4–11 weeks after birth with respiratory distress, cough, and tachypnea.

Other *Chlamydial* species are known to cause disease in humans. **Atypical pneumonia** is caused by *Chlamydia pneumoniae,* and presents with fever, headache, and a dry hacking cough. Additionally, **psittacosis** is another atypical pneumonia caused by *Chlamydia psittaci.* This organism is acquired by inhalation of feces from **infected birds,** which serve as the reservoir.

Diagnosis

Infection with *C. trachomatis* can be rapidly diagnosed by detection of the bacterial nucleic acid in patient samples, collected using a cotton swab, from the vagina, urethra, or conjunctiva. Diagnostic tests for nucleic acid detection include PCR amplification or direct DNA hybridization assays.

Treatment and Prevention

Currently, the best method of preventing chlamydial infection is education and proper sanitation. Ocular infection of *Chlamydia trachomatis* can sometimes but not always be prevented by administration of topical tetracycline drops. It is the lack of this antibiotic in underdeveloped countries that makes *Chlamydia trachomatis* prevalent in these areas. *C. trachomatis, C. psittaci,* and *C. pneumonia* are all treated with tetracycline or erythromycin. **Azithromycin** is effective for cervicitis and urethritis. Pelvic inflammatory disease is treated with ceftriaxone and 2 weeks of doxycycline.

Comprehension Questions

[5.1]   A 32-year-old immigrant woman from Tanzania delivers a healthy baby boy. Because this woman had no regular doctor, no preliminary tests were performed prior to delivery. Thirteen days after delivery, the child develops swelling of both eyes with the presence of a yellow discharge. The presence of intracytoplasmic inclusion bodies is detected. Which antibiotic would be most appropriate in this situation?

A. Tetracycline
B. Ceftriaxone
C. Penicillin G
D. Doxycycline
E. Erythromycin

[5.2]   What diagnostic test is best to identify an infection with *Chlamydia trachomatis?*

A. Aerobic and anaerobic blood cultures
B. Stool culture
C. DNA probe
D. Urine culture
E. Culture and darkfield microscopy

[5.3]   A 29-year-old bird collector presents to the local clinic with what he describes as flu-like symptoms. He doesn't look ill, and has a slight fever, headache, and a dry hacking cough. He denies the production of sputum or hemoptysis. There are no crackles heard on auscultation, and a radiograph shows small streaks of infiltrate. It is determined that he has pneumonia. What is the most likely organism causing his disease?

A. *Streptococcus pneumoniae*
B. *Chlamydia psittaci*
C. *Haemophilus influenzae*
D. *Staphylococcus aureus*
E. *Chlamydia pneumonia*

Answers

[5.1]   **E.** The symptoms described are classic for inclusion conjunctivitis caused by *Chlamydia trachomatis*. The infection was most likely passed from the mother to child during vaginal delivery. The infection usually presents 2 weeks after delivery and is characterized by swollen eyes and a yellow discharge. The drug of choice for this infection is erythromycin eyedrops. Most children are given erythromycin eye drops prophylactically postbirth. Tetracyclines are not given to young children due to staining of teeth.

[5.2]   **C.** The most specific test used to detect a chlamydial infection is a DNA probe. ***Chlamydia trachomatis*** is a gram-negative obligate intracellular parasite, and any blood or urine culture would not be helpful for diagnosis. *C. trachomatis* is not present in stool. Darkfield microscopy is used to view spirochetes, which *C. trachomatis* is not.

[5.3]   **B.** Although all of the organisms listed above cause pneumonia, only two of them are atypical. Atypical pneumonia is characterized by a dry hacking cough, fever, and headache. These include *Chlamydia psittaci* and *Chlamydia pneumoniae*. The mention of birds should point you in the direction of *C. psittaci,* because they are the reservoir for the organism that is inhaled through dry feces. Typical pneumonias are characterized by hemoptysis of pus-laden sputum, and patients appear very sick. The typical pneumonias include streptococcal infections.

MICROBIOLOGY PEARLS

❖ Chlamydial disease is the most common STD in the United States.
❖ Cervical motion tenderness and adnexal tenderness are common findings of pelvic inflammatory disease.
❖ The elementary body is the infectious stage in *Chlamydia trachomatis*.
❖ *Chlamydia trachomatis* is the most common preventable cause of worldwide blindness.

REFERENCES

Murray PR, Rosenthal KS, Kobayashi GS, Pfaller MA. Medical microbiology, 4th ed. St. Louis: Mosby, 2002:412–420.
Schneider AS, Szanto PA. Pathology board review series, 2nd ed. Philadelphia: Lippincott Williams & Wilkins, 2001:272, 280.

A 52-year-old man presents for the evaluation of diarrhea and abdominal pain, which have been worsening over the past week. He is now having 8–10 watery stools a day and mild cramping pain. He denies vomiting, fever, ill contacts, or having had blood in his stool. He has no history of gastrointestinal diseases. He states that about 10 days ago he completed a course of amoxicillin/clavulanate for pneumonia. On examination he is mildly ill appearing, but his vital signs are normal. His abdomen is soft, has hyperactive bowel sounds, and is diffusely, mildly tender. A stool sample is negative for blood but positive for leukocytes. A stool culture is negative, but a specific toxin assay is positive.

◆ **What is the most likely etiologic agent of this disease?**

◆ **Which condition predisposes this organism to cause disease in humans?**

ANSWERS TO CASE 6: *Clostridia*

Summary: A 52-year-old man who recently took oral antibiotics, and now has diarrhea. Fecal leukocytes are present in the stool, and a toxin test is positive.

◆ **Most likely etiologic agent:** *Clostridium difficile.*

◆ **Condition predisposing disease in humans:** Recent antibiotic exposure.

CLINICAL CORRELATION

There are approximately 90 bacterial species of *Clostridium,* about 20 of which are known to cause disease in humans. They are found widely in soil, decaying vegetation, and the intestinal tracts of humans and other vertebrates. Infection occurs in patients with predisposing factors including trauma, surgery, immunosuppression, and prior treatment with antibiotics. *C. perfringens* is the most common *Clostridium* species isolated from human infections and is a cause of wound infections including gas gangrene. *C. tetani* is associated with the toxin mediated disease, tetanus, which occurs in unvaccinated persons who come in contact with the organism. The spores of the organism survive for long periods of time in the soil and are introduced into the person following deep puncture wounds. Tetanus is characterized by tonic spasms usually involving the muscles of the neck, jaw (lockjaw), and trunk. *C. botulinum* is the causative agent of botulism. Botulism occurs when spores are consumed usually from improperly canned vegetables. Symptoms of nausea, blurred vision, and weakness of the upper extremities spreading downward occur within 12–36 hours after ingestion of the toxin.

    C. difficile can be isolated in the stool of fewer than 5 percent of healthy adults; however, up to 70 percent of healthy infants have the organism in their stool. Most cases of *C. difficile* colitis occur during or after a course of antibiotics, particularly clindamycin. Antibiotics alter the intestinal flora allowing for an overgrowth of *C. difficile,* which either already exists in the intestinal tract or is introduced from an environmental source. Disease can range from asymptomatic carriage of the organism to mild diarrhea to pseudomembranous colitis, which can be further complicated by toxic megacolon and bowel perforation.

Approach to Suspected *C. Difficile* Infection

Definitions

Antibiotic-associated colitis: Gastroenteritis caused by *C. difficile.*

Pseudomembranous colitis: Presence of nodules or plaques on erythematous (red) colonic mucosa seen by sigmoidoscopy, associated with *C. difficile* colitis.

Objectives

1. Know the characteristics of the *Clostridium* species.
2. Know the virulence factors and diseases associated with *Clostridium* bacteria.

Discussion

Characteristics of C. Difficile

C. difficile is an **anaerobic, spore-forming, toxigenic gram-positive rod.** Some strains have a thin capsule and some have fimbriae, although the significance of these is uncertain. *C. difficile,* so named because of the initial difficulty in isolating and culturing the organism, requires a selective medium for growth which also inhibits normal stool flora.

The **virulence factors** of *C. difficile* include **toxin production** as well as production of other enzymes, such as **hyaluronidase. Toxin A is an enterotoxin,** and **Toxin B,** the more biologically active toxin in humans, is a **cytotoxin.** The specific role each component plays in disease in humans is unknown. The enterotoxin is chemotactic and initiates the release of cytokines, hypersecretion of fluids in the intestinal tract, and hemorrhagic necrosis. Depolarization of actin microfilaments occurs, which leads to destruction of the cellular cytoskeleton disruption of tight junctions between epithelial cells. Formation of spores allows the organism to survive under stressful situations in the environment for extended periods of time. Spore formation also allows the organisms to survive in the hospital environment and can be transferred from patient to patient on fomites.

Diagnosis

Antibiotic-associated diarrhea is the most common cause of diarrhea that develops in patients who have been hospitalized for three or more days. Clinical diagnosis can be made by visualization of the **pseudomembrane** (fibrin, bacteria, cell debris, white blood cells).

The **gold standard for laboratory diagnosis** of antibiotic-associated diarrhea caused by *C. difficile* is **detection of toxin production in the stool** using a tissue culture assay, where a specific antibody neutralizes the toxin. However, this assay requires tissue culture facilities as well as approximately three days for completion. Culture of *C. difficile* can be performed on selective media, cycloserine, cefoxitin, and fructose agar in an egg-yolk agar base (CCFA medium), in an anaerobic environment. Colonies in 24–48 hours will fluoresce chartreuse on CCFA and have a barnyard odor. Specific identification can be made using commercially available rapid methods that detect fatty acids produced by the organism or by gas liquid chromatography. Growth of the organism would have to be followed up by detection of toxin for a specific diagnosis of disease.

Commercially available membrane or microwell based **enzyme immuno-assays** are available for rapid detection of Toxin A or Toxin A and B in a stool specimen. For optimal recovery testing of three stools on three days is recommended.

Treatment and Prevention

Treatment is with **oral vancomycin or metronidazole.** Unfortunately, relapse can occur in 20–30 percent of adequately treated patients because of the resistance of the spores to treatment. A second round of treatment is usually successful. Failure is not usually attributed to resistance of the organism to vancomycin or metronidazole. Prevention of *C. difficile* in hospitalized patients involves good infection control procedures that include isolation of the patient.

Comprehension Questions

[6.1] Which organism listed below may cause a life-threatening gastroen-teritis as a result of use of a broad spectrum antimicrobial agent?

A. *Bacillus anthracis*
B. *Bacillus cereus*
C. *Clostridium botulinum*
D. *Clostridium difficile*
E. *Clostridium tetani*

[6.2] *Clostridium difficile,* as the causative agent in antibiotic-associated diarrhea, can best be detected using which of the following gold standard laboratory tests?

A. Gas liquid chromatography
B. Pseudomembranous visualization
C. Rapid fatty acid detection assays
D. Tissue culture toxin detection assay

[6.3] A hospitalized patient developed severe diarrhea and pseudomembra-nous colitis within five days after antibiotic therapy was initiated. The severe diarrhea and pseudomembranous colitis occurred as a result of which of the following?

A. Collagenase
B. Fibrinolysin
C. Hyaluronidase
D. Lecithinase
E. Mucinase
F. Toxin A and B

Answers

[6.1] **D.** The use of broad spectrum antibiotics such as ampicillin and clindamycin has been associated with pseudomembranous colitis. Antibiotic administration results in the proliferation of drug-resistant *Clostridium difficile* that produces Toxin A (a potent enterotoxin with cytotoxic activity) and Toxin B (a potent cytotoxin). This disease is best treated by discontinuing the use of the offending antibiotic and administering oral doses of metronidazole or vancomycin. Administration of antibiotics may also lead to a milder form of diarrhea, called antibiotic-associated diarrhea. This form is associated with *C. difficile* about 25 percent of the time.

[6.2] **D.** All of the above tests may be used as detection assays for *C. difficile*. However, only the tissue culture toxin detection assay is the gold standard laboratory test. This test involves a specific toxin neutralizing antibody that detects toxin (Toxin A and B) production in the stool using a tissue culture detection assay. Not all *C. difficile* strains produce toxins, and the tox genes are not carried on either plasmids or phages.

[6.3] **F.** *Clostridium difficile* produces two toxins, toxin A and B. Both toxins are present in stool samples. Toxin A is enterotoxic causing the severe diarrhea, whereas toxin B is cytotoxic leading to the destruction of enterocytes resulting in pseudomembranous colitis. For additional information please refer to the discussions for Questions 6.1 and 6.2.

MICROBIOLOGY PEARLS

 The most common cause of diarrhea in a patient who has been hospitalized for 3 or more days is *C. difficile.*

 The best treatment for pseudomembranous colitis is oral vancomycin or oral metronidazole.

 Detection of toxins in the stool is the method of diagnosis of *C. difficile* colitis.

REFERENCES

Allen SD, Emery CL, Lyerly DM. In: Murray PR, Baron EJ, Jorgensen JH, Pfaller MA, Yolken RH, eds. Manual of clinical microbiology, 8th ed. Washington, DC: ASM Press, 2003:835–56.

Murray PR, Rosenthal KS, Kobayashi GS, Pfaller MA. Clostridium. In: Murray PR, Rosenthal KS, Kobayashi GS, Pfaller MA. Medical microbiology, 4th ed. St. Louis: Mosby, 2002:340–53.

A 6-year-old girl is brought into the office for evaluation of a sore throat and fever, which she has had for about 4 days. She is the daughter of parents who immigrated to the United States from Russia about 6 months ago. She has not had much medical care in her life, and her immunization status is unknown. On examination the child is anxious, tachypneic, and ill appearing. Her temperature is 38.6°C (101.5°F), and her voice is hoarse. Examination of her pharynx reveals tonsillar and pharyngeal edema with the presence of a gray membrane coating of the tonsil, which extends over the uvula and soft palate. She has prominent cervical adenopathy. Her lungs are clear. You immediately transfer her to the local children's hospital with the presumptive diagnosis of pharyngeal diphtheria and order confirmatory tests.

◆ **What Gram stain characteristics does *C. diphtheriae* have on microscopy?**

◆ **What factor is required for the expression of diphtheria toxin?**

ANSWERS TO CASE 7: *Corynebacterium diphtheriae*

Summary: A 6-year-old girl who recently arrived from Russia is diagnosed with pharyngeal diphtheria.

◆ **Characteristics of *C. diphtheriae* on Gram stain:** the club-shaped appearance of the gram-positive bacillus, often characterized as "Chinese letters" because of adherence of cells following division.

◆ **Factor required for the expression of diphtheria toxin:** Lysogenic bacteriophage.

CLINICAL CORRELATION

Corynebacteria are ubiquitous in nature and are part of the normal flora of the human respiratory tract and skin. Although most species of *Corynebacterium* can be opportunistic pathogens, only a few species are commonly associated with human disease. One of those species is *C. jeikeium,* which is most commonly associated with **bacteremia** and line-related infection in immunocompromised patients. This organism is one of the few species of *Corynebacterium* that tends to be multidrug resistant. *C. diphtheriae,* the cause of diphtheria, is one of the most pathogenic of the species. Humans are the only known reservoir and transmission is thought to occur by contact with aerosolized droplets, respiratory secretions, or infected skin lesions. Respiratory diphtheria occurs 2 to 6 days after inhalation of infected droplets. Patients develop nonspecific signs and symptoms of an upper respiratory infection as the organisms multiply locally with in epithelial cells in the respiratory tract. Toxin is then produced eliciting systemic symptoms including fever. An exudate containing organisms, fibrin, and white and red blood cells, is formed which is called a **pseudomembrane.** This grayish membrane covers the tonsils, uvula, and palate and can extend as far as the nasopharynx or larynx. Complications of membrane formation can be respiratory compromise by aspiration of the pseudomembrane, which is a common cause of death in this disease. Symptoms include fever and cervical lymphadenopathy (bull neck).

Cutaneous diphtheria, although rare in the United States, occurs from invasion of the organism from the patient's skin into the subcutaneous tissue. A papule develops at the site of contact that later becomes covered by a grayish membrane. As in respiratory diphtheria, toxin production by the organism elicits a systemic response with fever. Diphtheria toxin can also have effects on the heart (myocarditis) and nervous system (dysphagia, paralysis).

Approach to Suspected Diphtheria Infection

Definitions

Lysogenic bacteriophage: Virus that infects bacteria.

Elek Test: An immunodiffusion test to detect the production of diphtheria toxin in a strain of *C. diphtheria.*

Pseudomembrane: membrane formed in diphtheria, which consists of dead cells, leukocytes, and fibrin.

Objectives

1. Know the characteristics and virulence factors of *Corynebacterium diphtheriae.*
2. Know the factors involved with the expression of and the mechanism of action of the *C. diphtheriae* exotoxin.

Discussion

Characteristics of *C. diphtheriae*

C. diphtheriae is a **non-encapsulated gram-positive bacillus.** It is **nonmotile, non–spore-forming, and club shaped.** The cells often remain attached after division and form sharp angles, giving a **characteristic "Chinese letter" appearance** on microscopy.

C. diphtheriae is divided into **three subtypes—gravis, intermedius, and mitis**—based on colony morphology and biochemical testing.

In the presence of a lysogenic beta-phage, *C. diphtheriae* can produce a highly potent **exotoxin.** The toxin, which is the **major virulence factor** of this organism, consists of two components. The **B segment binds to specific receptors on susceptible cells.** Following proteolytic cleavage, the **A segment** is released into the host cell, where it can **inhibit protein synthesis.** The exotoxin targets a factor present in mammalian cells but not in bacterial cells, thus causing host tissue damage without affecting bacterial replication. Toxin-related tissue necrosis causes the characteristic pseudomembrane seen in clinical diphtheria.

Diagnosis

The **differential diagnosis** with the presence of sore throat, fever, and cervical lymphadenopathy would include streptococcal pharyngitis and infectious mononucleosis.

Clinical diagnosis of diphtheria can be made by visualization of the characteristic **pseudomembrane** formation. The **membrane should not be removed** because of the tight adherence to the epithelial surface and the chance for subsequent bleeding. Cultures should be collected from the throat or nasopharynx. A Gram stain would reveal the characteristic **gram-positive club-shaped bacilli.**

Corynebacterium with the exception of a few lipophilic species will grow well on most nonselective media with in 24 hours. Colonies are usually **nonpigmented and small, without hemolysis on blood agar.** However,

C. diphtheriae is more fastidious and specimens should be plated on a selective medium such as Tellurite in addition to the nonselective media. Colonies of *C. diphtheriae* will appear black on Tellurite media. Colonies growing on Loeffler's media can be stained with methylene blue to observe the characteristic metachromatic granules. Definitive identification is made by biochemical tests usually performed at a reference or state public health laboratory, where the isolate will be further tested for toxin production. The Elek test is an immunodiffusion assay for detection of production of *C. diphtheria* toxin by the isolate.

Treatment and Prevention

Therapy for diphtheria is a combination of **antimicrobial therapy** (erythromycin) and **antitoxin**. The **antitoxin must be administered rapidly**, before the toxin binds to epithelial cells. Diphtheria can be prevented by **vaccination** with diphtheria toxoid (DPT). Infected patients should be isolated from other susceptible persons to prevent secondary spread of the disease. Prophylaxis with erythromycin can also be given to close contacts who are at risk.

Comprehension Questions

[7.1]   The mechanism of action of the exotoxin produced by *Corynebacterium diphtheriae* can be characterized by which of the following?

A. Acting as a superantigen that binds to MHC class II protein and the T-cell receptor.

B. Blocking the release of acetylcholine causing anticholinergic symptoms.

C. Blocking the release of glycine (inhibitory neurotransmitter).

D. Inhibits protein synthesis via EF-2 adenosine diphosphate (ADP) ribosylation.

E. Stimulation of adenylate cyclase by ADP ribosylation of G-protein.

[7.2]   Which of the following most accurately describes the therapy available for the prevention and treatment of *Corynebacterium diphtheriae?*

A. Antimicrobial therapy for prophylaxis only

B. Antimicrobial therapy and prophylaxis, antitoxin, and toxoid (DPT)

C. Antitoxin only

D. Diphtheria toxoid (DPT) booster vaccination only

Answers

[7.1]   **D.** *C. diphtheriae* produces a potent exotoxin encoded by a lysogenic β-prophage. Following proteolytic cleavage, the A segment is released into the host cell where it inhibits *only* mammalian protein synthesis (ribosomal function) via ADP ribosylation of EF-2. Inhibition of protein synthesis disrupts normal cellular physiologic functions that are believed to be responsible for the necrotizing and neurotoxic effects of diphtheria toxin. An exotoxin with a similar mode of action is produced by some *Pseudomonas aeruginosa* strains. *S. aureus* is responsible for producing the toxic shock syndrome toxin that acts as a superantigen leading to T-cell activation. *Clostridium tetani* blocks the release of glycine, leading to "lock-jaw." *Clostridium botulinum* blocks the release of acetylcholine, causing central nervous system (CNS) paralysis and anticholinergic symptoms. Finally, the heat-labile toxin produced by *E. coli* causes watery diarrhea by stimulating adenylate cyclase.

[7.2]   **B.** Protection against *C. diphtheriae* can be established through both active and passive immunity. Active immunity consists of a toxoid administered in the form of the DPT vaccine. Passive immunity is established by administering diphtheria antitoxin (immunoglobulins). Antimicrobial therapy (erythromycin) can be used to effectively treat patients with clinical diphtheria.

MICROBIOLOGY PEARLS

❖ The club-shaped appearance of the gram-positive bacillus *Corynebacterium diphtheriae* is often characterized as "Chinese letters" as a result of adherence of cells following division.

❖ The typical clinical feature of diphtheria is pseudomembrane formation.

❖ Diphtheria is preventable by administration of DPT vaccine, which provides immunity for diphtheria, pertussis, and tetanus.

REFERENCES

Holmes, RK. Biology and molecular epidemiology of diphtheria toxin and the tox gene. J Infectious Diseases 2000;181(suppl 1):S156–67.

Murray PR, Rosenthal KS, Kobayashi GS, Pfaller MA. Corynebacterium and other gram-positive bacilli. In: Murray PR, Rosenthal KS, Kobayashi GS, Pfaller MA. Medical microbiology, 4th ed. St. Louis: Mosby, 2002:250–55.

A 72-year-old female nursing home resident is transferred to the hospital because of fever and altered mental status. She has advanced Alzheimer disease, is bed bound, and has an indwelling Foley catheter as a consequence of urinary incontinence. Her baseline mental status is awake and talkative, but oriented only to person. In the hospital now, she has a temperature of 38.3°C (101°F) and tachycardia (a rapid heart rate). She mumbles incoherently and is otherwise nonverbal. Her skin is cool, dry, and without ulceration. Her mucous membranes are dry. Her abdomen is soft, has normoactive bowel sounds, and is apparently tender in the suprapubic region. Her urinary catheter is draining cloudy urine. A urinalysis reveals too numerous to count white blood cells and bacteria. Gram stain of the urinary sediment reveals gram-positive cocci. Blood and urine cultures also grow gram-positive cocci.

◆ **What is the most likely cause of this infection?**

◆ **How does this organism acquire antibiotic resistance?**

ANSWERS TO CASE 8: *Enterococcus faecalis*

Summary: A 72-year-old woman with an indwelling urinary catheter has a urinary tract infection and bacteremia. Gram-positive cocci are isolated from the urine and blood cultures.

◆ **Most likely etiology of infection:** *Enterococcus faecalis.*

◆ **Mechanism of development of antibiotic resistance:** DNA mutation, or plasmid or transposon transfer.

CLINICAL CORRELATION

Enterococci are normal flora of the gastrointestinal tract and are therefore more likely to cause infections in patients with a history of preceding abdominal or genital tract procedures. Although a common cause of community acquired urinary tract infections, enterococci are most often associated with nosocomial urinary tract infections (UTIs), particularly in patients with urinary catheters. Bacteremia and rarely endocarditis can result as complications of enterococcal urinary tract or wound infections, with the gastrointestinal (GI) tract the most likely source. Patients at higher risk for enterococcal endocarditis are elderly patients and those with underlying heart disease, particularly the presence of artificial heart valves. *Enterococci* usually are a cause of **subacute left-sided or mitral valve endocarditis.**

Approach to Suspected Enterococcal UTI

Definitions

Tachycardia: Increased heart rate above 100 beats per minute.
Transposons: Small pieces of DNA that can replicate and insert randomly in the chromosome.
Leukocyte esterase: An enzyme present in leukocytes, therefore used as an indirect marker of their presence.

Objectives

1. Know the characteristics of *Enterococcus faecalis.*
2. Know the nature of the intrinsic and acquired antibiotic resistances of *E. faecalis.*

Discussion

Characteristics of *Enterococcus* Species

E. faecalis is an **aerobic gram-positive coccus** commonly found as **normal fecal flora** of healthy humans and other animals. It is capable of growing in extreme conditions, including a wide range of temperatures, high pH, the presence of high concentrations of bile salts, and saline concentrations of up to 6.5 percent. *Enterococci* have also been isolated from soil, food, and water. *Enterococci* are difficult to distinguish morphologically from *Streptococci,* and for years were considered a member of the Streptococcus family. They **possess the group D streptococcal carbohydrate antigen on their cell surface.** Like *Streptococci, Enterococci* are often seen **singly, in pairs or short chains on microscopy.** Little is known about the virulence factors associated with *E. faecalis.* Some strains of enterococcus produce factors, not totally elucidated, which allow their adherence to both heart valves and urinary epithelial cells. One of its other major virulence factors is an **intrinsic resistance to multiple antibiotics,** including ampicillin, penicillin, and aminoglycosides, which are effective against other gram-positive bacteria. There is also evidence for acquired antibiotic resistance, either by **mutation** of **native DNA** or **acquisition of new DNA** from **plasmid or transposon transfer.** It is capable of acquiring resistance both from other enterococci and from other bacterial species and has recently been shown to transfer the gene for vancomycin resistance to *Staphylococcus aureus.*

Diagnosis

Clinical diagnosis of urinary tract infections is made by typical clinical symptoms of urgency and/or dysuria followed by a urinalysis and bacterial culture. The presence of white blood cells (positive leukocyte esterase) and bacteria in the urine are indicative of cystitis. The specific etiologic agent can only be determined by culturing the urine in a quantitative manner. The presence of greater than 10^5 colony-forming units (CFUs) per ml of clean catch urine or 10^4 CFU/ml of catheterized urine is considered significant for a urinary tract infection. Colonies of *Enterococcus* appear **nonhemolytic** or, in rare cases, alpha hemolytic on blood agar and can be specifically identified using a **rapid PYR** (L-pyrrolidonyl-β-naphthylamide) test. **Conventional, overnight identification includes growth in 6.5% sodium chloride and esculin hydrolysis in the presence of bile.** Further identification of *Enterococci* to the species level is not commonly done in routine clinical laboratories. Although most commercially available identification methods can speciate *Enterococci* difficulties in accurate speciation occurs without the use of DNA sequence analysis. Most clinically significant *Enterococci* are either *E. faecalis* or *E. faecium. E. faecium* tends to be more resistant to antibiotics particularly ampicillin and vancomycin.

Treatment and Prevention

Although *Enterococci* are intrinsically resistant to low concentrations of beta-lactam antibiotics, such as **ampicillin,** these agents are still the first choice for uncomplicated enterococcal urinary tract infections in cases in which the affecting strain is not highly resistant. For complicated urinary tract infections or endocarditis, bactericidal therapy is necessary and includes **ampicillin or vancomycin plus an aminoglycoside,** assuming that the infecting strain is susceptible to ampicillin or vancomycin and high levels of aminoglycosides. An alternative would be vancomycin if it is susceptible; or if resistant, alternative agents such as linezolid or quinupristin/dalfopristin might be appropriate.

Although there is no specific prevention for *Enterococci* because they are able to survive for extended periods of time on inanimate objects, nosocomial outbreaks have been associated with antibiotic-resistant strains of *Enterococci* and proper disinfection and infection control measures are necessary to prevent further spread.

Comprehension Questions

[8.1]   Testing of blood culture isolates from a hospitalized patient revealed gram-positive cocci, β-lactamase positive, vancomycin-resistant, PYR-positive, and the presence of Lancefield group D antigen. Which of the following is the most likely isolate identification?

A. *Enterococcus faecalis*
B. *Streptococcus agalactiae*
C. *Streptococcus bovis*
D. *Streptococcus pneumoniae*

[8.2]   Which of the following is the most serious condition that can result as complications of enterococcal urinary tract or wound infections?

A. Cellulitis
B. Gastroenteritis
C. Scarlet fever
D. Subacute endocarditis
E. Toxic shock syndrome

[8.3]   After an abdominal surgery for removal of ovarian cysts, this 56-year-old woman has had low-grade fever for the past two weeks. She has a history of rheumatic fever as a child. Three of the blood cultures grew gram-positive cocci. Which of the following is the most likely etiologic agent?

A. Group A *Streptococci*
B. Group B *Streptococci*
C. Group C *Streptococci*
D. Group D *Streptococci*
E. *Streptococcus viridans*

Answers

[8.1]   **A.** All bacteria listed are gram-positive cocci. *S. pneumoniae* does not have a Lancefield grouping, whereas *S. agalactiae* has a group B classification. *S. bovis* is PYR-negative. Thus, only *E. faecalis* fulfills all laboratory test results in the above question.

[8.2]   **D.** In patients, the most common sites of *Enterococci* infection are the urinary tract, wounds, biliary tract, and blood. In neonates, *Enterococci* can cause bacteremia and meningitis. In adults, *enterococci* may cause endocarditis. Thus, bacteremia and/or endocarditis are rare and very serious complications that can result from enterococcal urinary tract infections. Cellulitis and toxic shock syndrome are typically associated with both *Staphylococci* and *Streptococci,* whereas scarlet fever is associated only with *Streptococci.* Finally, gastroenteritis can be associated with a number of organisms such as *Clostridium difficile.*

[8.3]   **D.** *Streptococcus bovis* is among the nonenterococcal group D *Streptococci.* They are part of the enteric flora and have the ability to cause endocarditis.

MICROBIOLOGY PEARLS

 Enterococci, gram-positive cocci, are normal flora of the human and animal GI tract.

 Enterococci are a common cause of wound infections following procedures involving the GI or genitourinary (GU) tracts.

 Bacteremia and/or endocarditis are rare complications of enterococcal urinary tract infections.

 Enterococcal UTIs are often nosocomial infections, especially in elderly patients with urinary catheters.

 Ampicillin and vancomycin are the principal antibiotics used to treat enterococcal infections.

REFERENCES

Moellering, RC. Enterococcus species, streptococcus bovis, and leuconostoc species. In: Mandell GL, Bennett JE, Dolin R, eds. Principles and practice of infectious diseases, 5th ed. Philadelphia: Churchill Livingstone, 2000:2147–56.

Murray PR, Rosenthal KS, Kobayashi GS, Pfaller MA. Enterococcus and other gram-positive cocci. In: Murray PR, Rosenthal KS, Kobayashi GS, Pfaller MA. Medical microbiology, 4th ed. St. Louis: Mosby, 2002:236–39.

A 21-year-old woman presents to the office with a 3-day duration of discomfort with urination and increased urinary frequency. She has noted that her urine has a strong odor as well. She denies fever, abdominal pain, back pain, vaginal discharge, or skin rash. She is sexually active and takes oral contraceptive pills. On examination, she is comfortable appearing and afebrile. She has no costovertebral angle tenderness. Abdominal exam is notable only for suprapubic tenderness. Microscopic examination of the sediment of a centrifuged urine sample reveals 10–15 white blood cells per high power field and numerous bacteria.

◆ **What type of organism would a Gram stain of the urine most likely show?**

◆ **What is the most common etiologic agent of this infection?**

◆ **What is the most likely reservoir of this infection?**

◆ **What is the most likely mechanism by which this organism infects the urinary tract?**

ANSWERS TO CASE 9: *Escherichia coli*

Summary: A 21-year-old woman has urinary frequency and dysuria. The urinalysis shows numerous white blood cells.

◆ **Organism most likely to be seen on Gram stain:** Gram-negative rod.

◆ **Most common etiologic agent:** *Escherichia coli (E. coli).*

◆ **Most likely reservoir for the organism:** Patient's own gastrointestinal (GI) tract.

◆ **Most likely mechanism of introduction of organism into the urinary tract:** Urethral contamination by colonic bacteria followed by ascension of the infection into the bladder.

CLINICAL CORRELATION

E. coli is the most commonly found aerobic, gram-negative bacilli in the GI tract of humans. *E. coli* is responsible for over 80 percent of all urinary tract infections (UTIs), along with other clinical diseases including gastroenteritis, sepsis, and neonatal meningitis. The *E. coli* that causes diarrhea is usually acquired from the environment, whereas most other infections caused by *E. coli* are acquired endogenously. Much of the diarrhea resulting from *E. coli* is acquired in developing countries particularly in travelers to these countries. The serotypes that are associated with travelers' diarrhea can be grouped based on their method of pathogenesis: enterotoxigenic, enterohemorrhagic, enteroaggregative, and enteroinvasive strains. These strains produce toxins, which account for their invasiveness as well as decreased absorption in the GI tract. Most of these cause a self limited diarrhea with the exception of enterohemorrhagic *E. coli,* frequently known as *E. coli* serotype O157:H7, which is usually acquired from eating poorly cook meat from an infected cow. Complications of infection with this organism include hemolytic uremic syndrome (HUS), which is a triad of hemolytic anemia, thrombocytopenia, and anemia. HUS is a significant cause of acute renal failure in children.

Urinary tract infections caused by *E. coli* are associated with organisms from the GI tract or vagina ascending up to the bladder. These organisms can colonize the vagina and be introduced into the bladder during instrumentation or sexual intercourse. Those serotypes that produce adhesions, which mediate adherence of the organisms to epithelial cells in the urinary tract are more likely to cause infections. The majority of cases of uncomplicated and complicated pyelonephritis are caused by *E. coli,* a complication of a UTI, where the organisms continue to ascend from the bladder to the kidney.

Approach to Suspected *E. coli* UTI

Definitions

Pyelonephritis: Infection of the kidney.
Cystitis: Infection of the bladder.
Hemolytic uremic syndrome (HUS): A syndrome characterized by hemolytic anemia, thrombocytopenia (low platelets), and acute renal failure.

Objectives

1. Know the structure, characteristics, and virulence factors of *E. coli.*
2. Know the pathogenic groups and toxins involved in diarrhea caused by *E. coli.*

Discussion

Characteristics of *E. coli*

E. coli is a member of the family **Enterobacteriaceae (see Table 9-1 for an abbreviated list).** All members of this family have in common the fact that they **ferment glucose, are oxidase negative, and reduce nitrates to nitrites.** Many members of the family Enterobacteriaceae, like *E. coli,* are normal flora of the GI tract.

E. coli produces numerous **adhesins,** which allow the organism to attach to cells in the urinary and gastrointestinal tracts. This prevents the bacteria from being flushed from these organs by the normal passage of urine or intestinal motility. *E. coli* also can produce several **exotoxins,** involved in the pathogenesis of diarrhea, including shiga toxins, heat-stable toxins, heat-labile toxins, and hemolysins. **Hemolysin HlyA** is particularly important in producing an **inflammatory response in the urinary tract,** whereas most of the other exotoxins are more pathogenic in the GI tract.

E. coli are divided into **serogroups** based on the **O antigen** found on the **lipopolysaccharide (LPS)** of the cell membrane and the **H antigen found on the flagella (Figure 9-1).**

Table 9-1
ABBREVIATED LISTING OF ENTEROBACTERIACIAE

Shigella
Salmonella
Escherichia
Enterobacter
Klebsiella
Serratia
Proteus

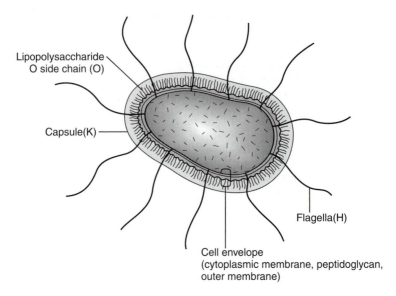

Figure 9-1. Structures used for antigenic identification in Enterobacteriaceae.

Diagnosis

The diagnosis of a UTI is made by urinalysis and urine culture. Complications such as pyelonephritis would be indicated by fever and flank pain. On urinalysis, the presence of white blood cells or leukocyte esterase and bacteria are suggestive of a true infection. Definitive diagnosis of the etiology is made by culture of the urine. *E. coli* is easily grown on most culture media. A quantitative urine culture from a symptomatic patient should demonstrate greater than **10^5 colony-forming units (CFUs) bacteria/ml urine** to be considered significant. *E. coli* would appear as **pink colonies on MacConkey agar** indicating **fermentation of lactose.** A rapid spot **indole** test would give a preliminary identification of *E. coli,* which would be confirmed by biochemical analysis.

Treatment and Prevention

Treatment of UTIs is based on the affecting organism and its susceptibility to antibiotics. Common antimicrobials chosen include trimethoprim sulfamethoxazole, or a fluoroquinolone. Most *E. coli* are resistant to ampicillin and penicillin. Recurrent UTIs are quite common, particularly in young women. Prevention can include consumption of large amounts of liquid and attention to totally emptying the bladder during urination. Fluid and electrolyte replacement should be administered to patients with *E. coli* diarrhea; however, antimicrobial treatment should not be administered. *E. coli* diarrhea is best prevented by improved hygiene.

Comprehension Questions

[9.1] *Escherichia coli* can be classified by their characteristic virulence properties and different mechanisms that cause disease. To which group does the verotoxin producing *E. coli* 0157:H7 serotype belong?

 A. Enteroaggregative *E. coli* (EAEC)
 B. Enterohemorrhagic *E. coli* (EHEC)
 C. Enteroinvasive *E. coli* (EIEC)
 D. Enteropathogenic *E. coli* (EPEC)
 E. Enterotoxigenic *E. coli* (ETEC)

[9.2] Several children are hospitalized with bloody diarrhea and severe hematological abnormalities. A 4-year-old girl dies of kidney failure shortly after admittance. An epidemiological investigation establishes that all of the patients developed symptoms following consumption of hamburgers from the same fast-food restaurant chain. Which of the following organisms is most likely to be responsible for the outbreak?

 A. *Campylobacter jejuni*
 B. non-O1 serogroup of *Vibrio cholerae*
 C. O157:H7 serotype of *E. coli*
 D. *Shigella dysenteriae*
 E. *Salmonella typhimurium*

[9.3] A Gram stain of an isolate from voided urine in a patient with a UTI reveals the presence of pink rods. Further biochemical analysis reveals that these bacteria ferment glucose, reduce nitrates to nitrites and are unable to synthesize the following reaction:
$$2H^+ + 2e^- + \tfrac{1}{2}O_2 \rightarrow H_2O$$
Which of the following characterize the above test results?

 A. *Escherichia coli*
 B. *Neisseria gonorrhoeae*
 C. *Proteus vulgaris*
 D. *Pseudomonas aeruginosa*
 E. *Staphylococcus aureus*
 F. *Streptococcus pyogenes*

[9.4] A 7-year-old child with bloody diarrhea is admitted after lab results indicating anemia and abnormal kidney function. After testing, it is determined that the etiologic agent is an *E. coli* that is most likely to produce which of the following?

 A. Endotoxin
 B. Exotoxin
 C. LT toxin
 D. ST toxin
 E. Verotoxin

[9.5] Several days after an appendectomy a patient develops a high fever, dangerously low blood pressure, and disseminated intravascular coagulation (DIC). Based on these and other findings, a diagnosis of septicemia as a result of an enteric gram-negative rod is made. Which of the following cytokines is most likely to be responsible for the fever, low blood pressure, and DIC?

    A. IFN-gamma
    B. IL-2
    C. IL-10
    D. TGF-beta
    E. TNF-alpha

Answers

[9.1] **B.** All of the above classes of *E. coli* cause diarrhea. However, only EHEC produce a verotoxin that has many properties that are similar to Shiga toxin. EHEC has been associated with hemorrhagic colitis, a severe form of diarrhea, and with hemolytic uremic syndrome (HUS). HUS is a disease resulting in acute renal failure, microangiopathic hemolytic anemia, and thrombocytopenia.

[9.2] **C.** *Escherichia coli* 0157:H7 strains are classically associated with outbreaks of diarrhea after ingestion of undercooked hamburger at fast-food restaurants. Many cases of hemorrhagic colitis and its associated complications can be prevented by thoroughly cooking ground beef. The other organisms listed can cause gastrointestinal disturbances; however, *E. coli* is the classic disturbing pathogen in this case. *Shigella dysenteriae* produces a heat-labile enterotoxin that affects the gut and central nervous system and is a human disease that is transmitted via a fecal-oral route. *Salmonella* and *Campylobacter* are associated with poultry and eggs primarily, whereas *Vibrio* is associated mainly with seafood.

[9.3] **A.** The biochemical reaction described above is catalyzed by the enzyme oxidase. Thus, *E. coli* is the only bacteria listed that is a gram-negative rod (pink), ferments glucose, converts nitrates to nitrites, and is oxidase negative.

[9.4] **E.** The verotoxin produced by *E. coli* is similar to Shiga toxin, causing bloody diarrhea. Please refer to the discussion for Question 9.1.

[9.5]   **E.** The acute phase response involves the increase in the levels of various plasma proteins (C-reactive protein and mannose-binding proteins) and is part of innate immunity. These proteins are synthesized and secreted by the liver in response to certain cytokines such as IL-1, IL-6, and TNF-alpha (produced after exposure to microorganisms) as nonspecific responses to microorganisms and other forms of tissue injury. Specifically, endotoxin (LPS) from gram-negative bacteria has the ability to activate macrophages that, in turn, synthesize TNF-alpha. TNF-alpha then functions to cause fever and hemorrhagic tissue necrosis (inflammatory reaction/immune response).

MICROBIOLOGY PEARLS

 E. coli is the most common cause of UTIs in otherwise healthy patients

 E. coli can easily be identified following growth of a flat lactose fermenter on MacConkey agar that is indole positive.

❖ Many serotypes of *E. coli* are associated with traveler's diarrhea.

REFERENCES

Murray PR, Rosenthal KS, Kobayashi GS, Pfaller MA. Enterobacteriaceae. In: Murray PR, Rosenthal KS, Kobayashi GS, Pfaller MA. Medical microbiology, 4th ed. St. Louis: Mosby, 2002:266–80.

A 48-year-old man presents for the evaluation of a 2-month history of upper abdominal pain associated with nausea. It is made worse when he drinks coffee, soda, or alcohol. He has taken multiple over-the-counter antacid medications that provide temporary relief. He admits to a 20-pack-year smoking history and drinking one or two alcoholic beverages a week but denies significant use of nonsteroidal antiinflammatory drugs (NSAIDs). His general physical examination and vital signs are normal. His abdominal examination is notable for epigastric tenderness without the presence of masses, rebound tenderness, or guarding. A rectal examination reveals his stool to be heme positive. A CBC shows a mild hypochromic, microcytic anemia. He is referred to a gastroenterologist for an upper GI endoscopy, which shows diffuse gastritis and a gastric ulcer.

◆ **What organism is most likely to be visualized on histologic evaluation of a gastric biopsy specimen?**

◆ **Besides microscopic evaluation, what other clinical test may provide a rapid detection of this organism?**

◆ **What two factors facilitate this organism's ability to colonize the stomach?**

ANSWERS TO CASE 10: *Helicobacter pylori*

Summary: A 48-year-old man has diffuse gastritis and a gastric ulcer on endo-scopic examination.

◆ **Organism on histologic evaluation of a gastric biopsy:** The organism likely to be visualized on biopsy specimen is *Helicobacter pylori.*

◆ **Other clinical test for rapid detection of this organism:** The urease test.

◆ **Factors facilitating this organism's ability to colonize the stomach:** Blockage of acid production by a bacterial acid-inhibitory protein and neutralization of acid by ammonia produced by urease activity.

CLINICAL CORRELATION

Helicobacter pylori has been implicated in the development of multiple gas-trointestinal diseases, including gastritis, ulcers, and gastric cancers. Humans are the primary reservoir of the infection and human-to-human transfer, via fecal-oral contact, is likely to be an important mode of transfer. *H. pylori* is a curved gram-negative bacillus with motility facilitated by corkscrew motion and polar flagella. Culture of this organism requires a complex medium and microaerophilic environment. *H. pylori* that colonize the stomach produce ure-ase, an enzyme that has many effects. Urease activity produces ammonia, which neutralizes gastric acid. This, along with a specific acid-inhibitory pro-tein that directly blocks gastric acid production, facilitates the colonization of the acidic stomach environment. Urease byproducts also cause local tissue damage and stimulate an inflammatory response. Urease activity is enhanced by the presence of a heat shock protein, HspB, which exists on the surface of *H. pylori.* The identification of urease activity in a gastric biopsy sample is highly specific for the presence of an active *H. pylori* infection, making it the basis for a widely used clinical test for the rapid detection of *H. pylori* infections.

Approach to Suspected *H. pylori* Infection

Definitions

Urease: *H. pylori* uses this enzyme to convert urea into ammonia and car-bon dioxide. This chemical reaction is the basis of the rapid urea breath test for diagnosis of *H. pylori.* The increased ammonia produced by this reaction neutralizes gastric acid, which allows the organism to survive the normally harsh gastric environment and damages the gastric mucosa.

Type B gastritis: Type B gastritis is gastritis of the antrum caused by *H. pylori* infection (compare with Type A of the fundus, caused by autoimmune disorders).

Corkscrew motility: *H. pylori* is highly motile because of 5–6 polar flagella.

Microaerophilic organisms: Organisms that require reduced oxygen concentration (5%) to grow optimally (include: *H. pylori* and *C. jejuni*).

Upper endoscopy: Visual examination of the mucosa of the esophagus, stomach, and duodenum using a flexible fiberoptic system introduced through the mouth.

Objectives

1. Be able to describe the characteristics of *Helicobacter* bacteria.
2. Understand the role of *H. pylori* in causing gastric ulcers.

Discussion

Characteristics of *H. pylori* Impacting Transmission

H. pylori is a **curved gram-negative bacilli** that requires **microaerophilic** environments to grow. Discovered in 1983, the organism was originally classified under the *Campylobacter* genus, but eventually was reclassified under a new and separate genus, *Helicobacter,* as understanding of the organism has evolved. **Urease production** is the most important enzyme that distinguishes *H. pylori* from *Campylobacter* species and other various *Helicobacter* species, and **allows the organism to survive the harsh gastric environment.** *H. pylori* also has **oxidase, catalase, mucinase, phospholipase enzymes, and vacuolating cytotoxin,** which aid in the virulence and pathogenesis of the organism. Infections of *H. pylori* are ubiquitous, worldwide, and extremely common in developing nations and among lower socioeconomic groups. Humans are the primary reservoir, and no animal reservoir has been identified at the present time. The primary mode of transmission is person to person (usually by the fecal-oral route), and the infection commonly is clustered in families or among close contacts. Some speculation has been made that contaminated water or food sources may be a reservoir, but at the present time there are no data to support this.

Diagnosis

H. pylori has been clearly associated with **Type B gastritis, gastric ulcers, gastric adenocarcinoma of the body and antrum, and gastric MALT lymphomas.** Diagnosis of *H. pylori* should be reserved for patients with symptoms of these diseases. The most rapid test to detect *H. pylori* is the **urease test or urea breath test** that detects byproducts of the **urease reaction cleaving urea into ammonia and carbon dioxide. Microscopy** is both extremely sensitive and specific for diagnosis of *H. pylori* in gastric biopsy specimens when stained with **Warthin-Starry silver stain, hematoxylin-eosin, or Gram stain.** Culture is a more challenging and time-consuming way to diagnose *H. pylori,* because it must be grown in a microaerophilic atmosphere on an enriched medium containing charcoal, blood, and hemin. **Serology** is another way to diagnose exposure to *H. pylori* as a result of the humoral immune response, but it cannot distinguish between past and present infections.

Treatment and Prevention

Because *H. pylori* is primarily **transmitted person to person via fecal-oral route,** the best prevention is improving hygiene by **frequent hand washing,** especially before meals. In symptomatic patients who are positive for infection with *H. pylori,* combination therapy is needed. This therapy includes (1) a **proton pump inhibitor** (omeprazole), (2) one or more **antibiotics** (amoxicillin, metronidazole), and (3) **bismuth.**

Comprehension Questions

[10.1] A 45-year-old man presents to the hospital vomiting blood. He is diagnosed with a perforated peptic ulcer. The causative agent discovered by gastric biopsy is a spiral gram-negative bacillus. What other long-term complications could this organism cause if not treated?

A. Skin ulcers
B. Esophageal varices
C. Gastric MALT lymphomas
D. Colon cancer

[10.2] Which of the following is an important distinguishing characteristic of *H. pylori* as compared to *Campylobacter* species?

A. Oxidase production
B. Catalase production
C. Urease production
D. Curved shape
E. Polar flagellum

[10.3] A 58-year-old man presents to the clinic with decreased appetite, nausea, vomiting, and upper abdominal pain. If the causative agent is a curved gram-negative rod with urease production, what treatment should be given to this patient?

A. Proton pump inhibitor and antibiotic
B. Proton pump inhibitor, antibiotic, and bismuth
C. Over-the-counter antacids and antibiotics
D. Nonsteroidal antiinflammatory drugs (NSAIDs)

Answers

[10.1]   **C.** *H. pylori* is the causative agent that can cause Type B gastritis, peptic ulcers, gastric adenocarcinoma, and gastric MALT B cell lymphomas.

[10.2]   **C.** Both *Campylobacter* species and *H. pylori* have a curved shape, are oxidase and catalase positive, with polar flagellum. Urease production is the distinguishing factor of *H. pylori,* and it is the basis of the rapid urease breath test that diagnoses *H. pylori* infection.

[10.3]   **B.** The combination therapy of proton pump inhibitor, antibiotic, and bismuth is required to eradicate an infection with *H. pylori.*

MICROBIOLOGY PEARLS

❖ *Helicobacter pylori* are *characterized by* curved gram-negative bacilli, multiple polar flagella, microaerophilic, and urease activity.

❖ Clinical manifestations include Type B gastritis, gastric ulcers, gastric adenocarcinoma, gastric MALT lymphomas conjunctivitis, or gastroenteritis.

❖ It is transmitted via fecal-oral route.

❖ Antimicrobial treatment include a proton pump inhibitor (such as omeprazole), antibiotics, and bismuth.

REFERENCES

Johnson AG, Hawley LB, Lukasewycz OA, Jiegler RJ. Microbiology and immunobiology, 4th ed. Baltimore: Lippincott Williams & Wilkins, 2002.

Levinson W, Jawetz E. Medical microbiology and immunology, 7th ed. New York: McGraw-Hill, 2002.

Murray PR, Rosenthal KS, Kobayashi GS, Pfaller MA. Medical microbiology, 4th ed. St. Louis: Mosby, 2002:291–295.

A 19-month-old child is brought to the emergency room following a seizure. His mother says that he had a cold for 2 or 3 days with a cough, congestion, and low-grade fever, but today he became much worse. He has been fussy and inconsolable, he would not eat and has slept most of the morning. He then had two grand-mal seizures. He has no history of seizures in the past. His mother reports that he has not received all of his immunizations. She is not sure which ones he's had, but he's only had two or three shots in his life. On examination his temperature is 38.1°C (100.5°F), his pulse is 110 beats per minute, and he appears very ill. He does not respond to your voice but does withdraw his extremities from painful stimuli. He grimaces when you try to bend his neck. His skin is without rash and his HEENT (head, neck, ear, nose, throat), cardiovascular, lung, and abdominal examinations are normal. His white blood cell count is elevated, and a CT scan of his head is normal. You perform a lumbar puncture, which reveals numerous small gram-negative coccobacilli.

◆ **What organism is the most likely etiology of this illness?**

◆ **What component of this organism is the target of vaccine-induced immunity?**

ANSWERS TO CASE 11: *Haemophilus influenzae*

Summary: A 19-month-old boy who has not received many immunizations presents with meningitis. The lumbar puncture shows multiple gram-negative coccobacilli.

◆ **Organism most likely causing this infection:** *H. influenzae* type B.

◆ **Component of this organism that is the target of vaccine-induced immunity:** Purified polyribitol phosphate, a component of the *H. influenzae* type B polysaccharide capsule.

CLINICAL CORRELATION

Haemophilus species, particularly *H. parainfluenzae* and *H. influenzae* non-type B are normal flora in the human upper respiratory tract. These strains can, however, be associated with respiratory infections such as otitis media and bronchitis. *H. influenzae* type B was the most common cause of pediatric meningitis (ages 2 months to 2 years of age) until the introduction of routine childhood immunization against this bacterium.

Transmission of *H. influenzae* occurs by close contact with respiratory tract secretions from a patient colonized or infected with the organism. Prior viral infection promotes colonization of the respiratory tract with *H. influenzae.* Invasive infections such as meningitis occur when the colonizing organisms invade the bloodstream and subsequently the meninges. Usually as a result of *H. influenzae* type B, the capsule aids in adherence of the organism and evasion of phagocytosis. Neurological sequelae can occur in up to 20 percent of cases of meningitis. *H. influenzae* B can also be a cause of epiglottitis in young children, which can result in respiratory obstruction requiring intubation.

H. aphrophilus and *H. paraphrophilus* are causes of culture negative endocarditis named thus because of the fastidious nature and difficulty in recovering these organisms from the blood of infected patients. *H. ducreyi* is a cause of an uncommon sexually transmitted disease **chancroid.** Chancroid is characterized by genital skin lesions and lymphadenopathy, leading to abscess formation if remains untreated.

Approach to Suspected *H. influenza* Meningitis Patient

Definitions

Epiglottitis: Inflammation of the epiglottis usually caused by *H. influenzae,* which presents as sore throat, fever, and difficulty breathing.

Meningitis: Inflammation of the meninges leads to headache, stiff neck, and fever with increase in cells in the cerebrospinal fluid.

Grand–mal seizure: Seizure that results in loss of consciousness and generalized muscle contractions.

Objectives
1. Know the structure and physiology of *Haemophilus*.
2. Know the significance of the capsule of *Haemophilus* in the virulence, infection, and development of protective immunity.

Discussion

Characteristics of *Haemophilus* Species

Haemophilus are **small, pleomorphic, gram-negative bacilli or coccobacilli.** Humans are the only known reservoir. They are **facultative anaerobes** and grow on media that contain growth-stimulating factors known as X factor (hematin) and V factor (NAD). **Heated sheep blood agar, chocolate agar,** contains both of these factors and is used to grow *Haemophilus*. Many strains of *Haemophilus* have a **polysaccharide capsule,** and specific capsular antigens are used to identify strains of *H. influenzae*. Six types, *A* through *F,* have been identified. The **polysaccharide capsule of *H. influenzae* type B** is and represents its major virulence **antiphagocytic** factor. The **capsule** contains **ribose, ribitol, and phosphate, known collectively as polyribitol phosphate (PRP).** Phagocytosis and complement-mediated activity are stimulated in the presence of antibodies directed at the *H. influenzae* type B capsule. This represents the **basis for the *H. influenzae* type B vaccine,** which contains **purified PRP antigens** conjugated to specific protein carriers.

Diagnosis

Acute meningitis typically involves the rapid onset (over several days) of **headache, fever, and stiff neck,** although in young children only fever and irritability may be evident. Rash may also be present in some forms of meningitis. Without treatment, progression of the disease includes loss of consciousness and/or seizures and coma. Specific diagnosis is based on culture of the etiologic organism from the cerebrospinal fluid (CSF). Prior to culture a rapid presumptive diagnosis of bacterial meningitis is based on increased number of polymorphonuclear leukocytes (PMNs) in the CSF as well as an elevated protein and a decreased glucose. **Gram stain** of the CSF may reveal the presence of bacteria if the number of organisms is high enough. In the case of *H. influenzae* meningitis, the presence of tiny gram-negative coccobacilli are seen in a Gram-stained smear of the CSF.

Haemophilus influenzae **require both X and V factors for growth;** therefore no growth would be seen on blood agar unless growth of *S. aureus* on the agar allowed for lysis of the blood and release of the required factors into the media. Good growth would be evident on chocolate agar as grayish colonies after 24 hours incubation at 35°C (95°F) and 5% CO_2. Identification of *Haemophilus* to the species level can be made by requirement for X or V for growth. More specifically, a commercially available identification system could be used that is based on the presence of preformed enzymes and can be made within 4 hours. *Haemophilus* species other than *H. influenzae* grow much more slowly, particularly *H. ducreyi,* which may require 5–7 days of incubation after culture of an infected lymph node or genital abscess.

Treatment and Prevention

Up to 50 percent of strains of *H. influenzae* produce a β-lactamase, rendering them resistant to ampicillin. Treatment for *H. influenzae* meningitis involves the use of a **third-generation cephalosporin (cefotaxime, ceftriaxone).** Respiratory infections caused by *H. influenzae* may be treated with antibiotics such as **amoxicillin-clavulanate or a macrolide** (such as azithromycin.). Routine pediatric immunization with the vaccine against *H. influenzae* B has reduced the incidence of invasive disease by approximately 90 percent and has also reduced respiratory colonization. *H. ducreyi* is usually treated with **erythromycin** or a newer macrolide antibiotic. An alternative for therapy of chancroid includes a **fluoroquinolone.**

Comprehension Questions

[11.1] A 2-year-old child has high fever, is irritable, and has a stiff neck. Gram-stain smear of spinal fluid reveals gram-negative, small pleomorphic coccobacillary organisms. Which of the following is the most appropriate procedure to follow to reach an etiological diagnosis?

A. Culture the spinal fluid in chocolate blood agar and identify the organism by growth factors.

B. Culture the spinal fluid in mannitol salt agar.

C. Perform a catalase test of the isolated organism.

D. Perform a coagulase test with the isolate.

E. Perform a latex agglutination test to detect the specific antibody in the spinal fluid.

[11.2] *Haemophilus influenzae* synthesizes immunoglobulin A (IgA) protease, which enables the bacterium to penetrate and invade the host's respiratory epithelium. This is an example of a bacterium's ability to evade the host:

A. Cellular or cell-mediated immunity (CMI) against *Haemophilus influenzae.*

B. Nonspecific humoral immunity

C. Nonspecific innate immunity

D. Phagocytic function and intracellular killing of bacteria

E. Specific humoral immunity against *Haemophilus influenzae*

[11.3] An 18-month-old baby girl is suspected to have *Haemophilus influenzae* meningitis. She has not been immunized with the HIB vaccine. A rapid latex agglutination test is performed with the spinal fluid to make a definitive diagnosis. What chemical component in the spinal fluid are we detecting with this assay?

A. IgG antibody
B. IgM antibody
C. Lipopolysaccharide (LPS)
D. Polypeptide
E. Polysaccharide capsule

[11.4] The *Haemophilus influenzae* vaccine contains which of the following?

A. Lipopolysaccharide (LPS)
B. Live attenuated *H. influenzae*
C. Polypeptide antigens containing D-glutamate
D. Polyribitol phosphate antigens
E. Teichoic acid
F. Toxoids

[11.5] Cerebrospinal fluid from a spinal tap of a patient complaining of a severe headache, fever, and nuchal rigidity revealed the presence of gram-negative coccobacilli. Further testing revealed growth of the organism on growth factor X and V supplemented chocolate agar, and no hemolysis when grown on blood agar. Which of the following organisms represents the above description?

A. *Bordetella pertussis*
B. *Haemophilus ducreyi*
C. *Haemophilus haemolyticus*
D. *Haemophilus influenzae*
E. *Haemophilus parainfluenzae*

Answers

[11.1] **A.** The organism in the above description is *Haemophilus influenzae.* This organism is differentiated from other related gram-negative bacilli by its requirements of a chocolate media supplemented with growth factors, such as X and V factors, and by its lack of hemolysis on blood agar.

[11.2] **E.** Immunoglobulin A (IgA) is associated with immunological protection of the host at the epithelial boundary. An IgA protease has the ability to breakdown IgA and thereby act as a virulence mechanism enabling the bacterium to invade the host through an unprotected epithelial boundary. Because IgA is an antibody associated with the humoral (specific) arm of the immune system, IgA protease allows the bacterium the ability to evade the specific humoral immunity of the host.

[11.3]   **E.** The latex agglutination test involves the use of latex beads coated with specific antibody that become agglutinated in the presence of homologous bacteria or antigen. This test is used to determine the presence of the capsular polysaccharide antigen of *Haemophilus influenzae* in serum or spinal fluid.

[11.4]   **D.** Encapsulated *H. influenzae* contains capsular polysaccharides of one of six types (A–F). *H. influenzae* type B is an important human pathogen with its polyribose phosphate capsule being its major virulence factor. As a result, active immunity is built using polyribitol phosphate antigens (capsular polysaccharide) of *H. influenzae*.

[11.5]   **D.** *H. haemolyticus* and *H. influenzae* are the only organisms listed above that require both growth factors X and V for growth; however, they can be distinguished from each other in that *H. influenzae* is hemolysis negative on blood agar, whereas *H. haemolyticus* is hemolysis positive.

MICROBIOLOGY PEARLS

 Haemophilus species other than *H. influenzae* B are still a significant cause of systemic infections.

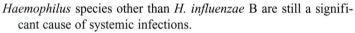 The widespread use of *H. influenzae* vaccines in developed countries has decreased the incidence of *H. influenzae* meningitis.

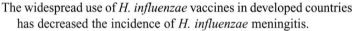 *H. influenzae* meningitis is treated with cefotaxime or ceftriaxone.

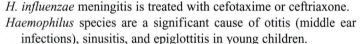 *Haemophilus* species are a significant cause of otitis (middle ear infections), sinusitis, and epiglottitis in young children.

REFERENCES

Murray PR, Rosenthal KS, Kobayashi GS, Pfaller MA. Pasteurellaceae. In: Murray PR, Rosenthal KS, Kobayashi GS, Pfaller MA. Medical microbiology, 4th ed. St. Louis: Mosby, 2002:317–24.

Slack MPE. Gram-negative coccobacilli. In: Infectious diseases. Philadelphia: Mosby, 1999;8(20):1–18.

A 45-year-old homeless alcoholic man presents to the emergency room with fever and cough of 4 days duration. The cough is productive of thick, bloody phlegm. He complains of pain in the right side of his chest with coughing or taking a deep breath. He denies any other medical history and says he can't remember the last time he saw a doctor. He doesn't smoke cigarettes, drinks a pint of whiskey whenever he can get it, and denies drug use. On examination, he is dirty, disheveled, and appears malnourished. His temperature is 38.9°C (102°F), pulse 105 beats per minute, and respiratory rate is 30 breaths per minute. The lung examination is notable for decreased breath sounds and crackles in the right lower, posterior field. His white blood cell count is elevated. A chest x-ray reveals a dense right lower lobe infiltrate with evidence of a pulmonary abscess. Sputum samples are collected for Gram stain and culture, and a blood culture is sent. A bacterial etiology is suspected.

◆ **What is the most likely organism to be isolated in the sputum and blood cultures?**

◆ **By what mechanism does this organism commonly develop antibiotic resistance?**

ANSWERS TO CASE 12: *Klebsiella pneumoniae*

Summary: A 45-year-old alcoholic man has developed a bacterial cavitary pneumonia with evidence of a pulmonary abscess.

◆ **Most likely organism to be isolated:** *Klebsiella pneumoniae.*

◆ **Mechanism whereby *Klebsiella* commonly develops antibiotic resistance:** plasmid acquisition.

CLINICAL CORRELATION

Klebsiella causes lower respiratory infections, wound soft tissue infections and is a common cause of hospital-acquired urinary tract infections (UTIs). *K. pneumoniae* is also associated with lobar pneumonia in a person with an underlying debilitating condition such as alcoholism or diabetes. Pneumonia caused by this organism tends to be necrotic, inflammatory, and hemorrhagic and has a high propensity for cavitation or abscess formation. Patients often produce thick, bloody sputum. Because of the destructive nature of the infection and the underlying debility of the patient, pneumonia caused by *K. pneumoniae* carries a high mortality.

Community-acquired pneumonia is usually the result of spread of organisms that normally reside in the upper respiratory tract into the lower respiratory tract. Organisms that have virulence factors that allow them to survive the host response in the lung can establish an infection. Patients with disruption of their immune defenses are at greater risk of infection. *K. pneumoniae* pneumonia is therefore considered an opportunistic infection because it is not a common cause of pneumonia in normally healthy patients. Symptoms of bacterial pneumonia are usually nonspecific and include malaise, anorexia, headache, myalgia, arthralgia, and fever. *K. pneumoniae* produces a severe acute, necrotic, and hemorrhagic pneumonia, which is evidenced by cavitary lung lesions on chest x-ray, pleural effusions, and possible abscess formation or empyema. Because of the hemorrhagic nature of the pneumonia, patients tend to have blood-tinged sputum.

Two uncommon species of *Klebsiella* are also causes of respiratory disease. *K. rhinoscleroma* is associated with chronic granulomatous disease of the upper respiratory mucosa (predominantly outside the United States), and *K. ozaenae* is associated with chronic atrophic rhinitis.

Approach to Suspected *K. pneumoniae* Pneumonia

Definitions

Chronic obstructive pulmonary disease (COPD): A progressive lung disease that commonly results from heavy smoking and is evident by difficulty breathing, wheezing, and a chronic cough.

Empyema: Accumulation of pus in the pleural space around the lung.

Objectives

1. Know the structure, physiology, and virulence factors of *K. pneumoniae.*
2. Know the nature of the native and acquired antibiotic resistance of *K. pneumoniae.*

Discussion

Characteristics of *Klebsiella* Species

The genus *Klebsiella,* which belongs to the family **Enterobacteriaceae** includes five species, with the most clinically significant being *K. pneumoniae. Klebsiella pneumoniae* is a **large, nonmotile, gram-negative rod** with a **prominent polysaccharide capsule.** The **capsule is antiphagocytic** and retards leukocyte migration into an infected area.

Another virulence factor of *K. pneumoniae* is its propensity to develop **resistance** to multiple antibiotics. All strains of *K. pneumoniae* are innately **resistant to ampicillin,** because of the production of **β-lactamase.** Acquisition of resistance to other antibiotics usually occurs by **transfer of plasmids** from other organisms. Recently strains of nosocomially acquired *K. pneumoniae* have been isolated that produce an extended spectrum β-lactamase and therefore are resistant to all β-lactam antibiotics.

Diagnosis

Diagnosis of community-acquired pneumonia is made clinically based on symptoms of cough, especially with blood, and chest x-ray indicating infiltrates, cavitary lesions, or pleural effusions. Specific diagnosis of pneumonia is made by culture of expectorated sputum. Sputum samples must be of good quality (many white blood cells and rare squamous epithelial cells) represent the flora of the lower respiratory tract and not mouth flora. In a small percentage of cases of community-acquired pneumonia blood cultures will also be positive for the affecting organism.

K. pneumoniae will **grow rapidly producing large mucoid colonies** on routine laboratory media. Colonies are often extremely mucoid and will tend to **drip into the lid of the plate** while incubating in an inverted position. **Pink colonies** will be evident on MacConkey agar indicating their fermentation of lactose. Confirmatory identification is made for other members of the family Enterobacteriaceae by commercially available identification systems using a combination of **sugar fermentation and enzyme production.** Both *K. oxytoca* and especially *K. rhinoscleromatis* are slower growing than *K. pneumoniae* and the other Enterobacteriaceae. All *Klebsiella* species are very closely related with nearly identical biochemical reactions, except for the fact that *K. pneumoniae* is indole negative, and *K. oxytoca* is indole positive. Commercial identification systems have a difficult time differentiating these species.

Treatment and Prevention

Treatment of *K. pneumoniae* pneumonia would be based on the susceptibility of the isolate. Treatment can be complicated by the presence of multidrug-resistant strains. Most strains are susceptible to **extended spectrum cephalosporins** such as cefepime as well as **fluoroquinolones** such as gatifloxacin. In cases of strains that produce an extended spectrum β-lactamase, the treatment of choice would be imipenem.

Prevention of community-acquired pneumonia would involve avoidance of high-risk activities such as smoking or drinking in excess. Prevention of spread in the hospital would involve appropriate infection control procedures to isolate patients with multidrug-resistant organisms. *K. oxytoca* has similar susceptibility patterns as *K. pneumoniae* and can also produce extended spectrum β-lactamases.

Comprehension Questions

[12.1] The most common mechanism by which *Klebsiella pneumoniae* attains its antibiotic resistance is by plasmid acquisition. Which of the following best describes the direct transfer of a plasmid between two bacteria?

A. Competence
B. Conjugation
C. Recombination
D. Transduction
E. Transformation

[12.2] A specimen of thick, bloody sputum from a hospitalized 80-year-old patient with diabetes mellitus and difficulty in breathing is sent for laboratory analyses. The tests yield heavy growth of a lactose-positive, non-motile, gram-negative rod with a large capsule. Which of the following bacteria is most likely to be the cause of the pulmonary problems?

A. *Enterobacter aerogenes*
B. *Escherichia coli*
C. *Klebsiella pneumoniae*
D. *Pseudomonas aeruginosa*
E. *Yersinia pseudotuberculosis*

[12.3] A 65-year-old diabetic man presents to the emergency room with a severe productive cough producing thick bloody sputum resembling a "currant-jelly" like appearance. Culture using MacConkey agar reveals pink colonies, with large mucoid colonies on routine laboratory media. Which of the following organisms is most likely responsible for this patient's pneumonia?

A. *Enterobacter cloacae*
B. *Escherichia coli*
C. *Klebsiella pneumoniae*
D. *Pseudomonas aeruginosa*
E. *Serratia marcescens*

[12.4] The O antigens that are used to help characterize members of the Enterobacteriaceae family are found on which of the following?

A. Capsules
B. Endotoxins
C. Exotoxins
D. Fimbriae
E. Flagella

Answers

[12.1] **B.** The three important processes by which DNA is transferred between bacteria are via transformation, transduction, and conjugation. Transformation is defined as the uptake of soluble DNA by a recipient cell. Transduction refers to the transfer of DNA by a virus from one cell to another. Conjugation refers to the direct transfer of soluble DNA (plasmids) between cells. Examples of such plasmids are the sex factors and the resistance (R) factors.

[12.2] **C.** Whereas all of the above listed organisms are gram-negative rods, only *Klebsiella pneumoniae* fulfill all of the laboratory criteria listed in the question, such as the presence of a very large capsule, which gives a striking mucoid appearance to its colonies.

[12.3] **C.** Patients with *K. pneumoniae* infections usually have predisposing conditions such as alcoholism, advanced age, chronic respiratory disease, and diabetes. The "currant-jelly" sputum distinguishes *K. pneumoniae* from the other organisms. Infections can lead to necrosis and abscess formation. Please refer to the discussion for Question 12.2.

[12.4]   **B.** There are three surface antigens associated with several members of the Enterobacteriaceae. The cell wall antigen (somatic or O antigen) is the outer polysaccharide portion of the lipopolysaccharide (LPS/ endotoxin). The H antigen is on the flagellar proteins (*Escherichia* and *Salmonella*). The capsular or K polysaccharide antigen is particularly prominent in heavily encapsulated organisms such as *Klebsiella*.

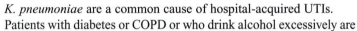

MICROBIOLOGY PEARLS

❖   *K. pneumoniae* are a common cause of hospital-acquired UTIs.
❖   Patients with diabetes or COPD or who drink alcohol excessively are predisposed to pneumonia with *K. pneumoniae*.
❖   *K. pneumoniae* produces a large mucoid colonies on agar plates as a result of the presence of a polysaccharide capsule that also acts to allow the organism to avoid phagocytosis.

REFERENCES

Baldwin DR, MacFarlane JT. Community acquired pneumonia: In: Infectious diseases. Philadelphia: Mosby, 1999;2(27):1–10.

Eisenstein BI, Zaleznik DF. Enterobacteriaceae. In: Mandell GL, Bennett JE, Dolin R, eds. Principles and practice of infectious diseases, 5th ed. Philadelphia: Churchill Livingstone, 2000:2294–310.

Murray PR, Rosenthal KS, Kobayashi GS, Pfaller MA. Enterobacteriaceae. In: Murray PR, Rosenthal KS, Kobayashi GS, Pfaller MA. Medical microbiology, 4th ed. St. Louis: Mosby, 2002:266–80.

An 18-day-old female infant is brought to the pediatric emergency room by her panicked mother. The child has developed a fever and has been crying nonstop for the past 4 hours. She has fed only once today and vomited all of the ingested formula. The baby was born by vaginal delivery after an uncomplicated, full-term pregnancy to a healthy 22-year-old gravida$_1$ para$_1$ (one pregnancy, one delivery) woman. The mother has no history of any infectious diseases and tested negative for group B *Streptococcus* prior to delivery. The immediate postpartum course was routine. The baby had a routine check-up in the pediatrician's office 3 days ago, and no problems were identified. On exam, the child has a temperature of 38.3°C (100.9°F), pulse of 140 beats per minute, and respiratory rate of 32 breaths per minute. She is not crying at the moment. She has poor muscle tone, will not regard your face or respond to loud stimuli. Her anterior fontanelle is bulging. Her mucous membranes are moist, and her skin is without rash. Her heart is tachycardic but regular, and her lungs are clear. Her white blood count is elevated, a urinalysis is normal, and a chest x-ray is clear. A Gram stain of her cerebrospinal fluid (CSF) from a lumbar puncture shows gram-positive coccobacilli.

◆ **What organism is responsible for this infection?**

◆ **How does this organism avoid antibody-mediated host defenses?**

ANSWERS TO CASE 13: *Listeria monocytogenes*

Summary: An 18-day-old infant presents with meningitis and Gram stain of the CSF reveals gram-positive coccobacilli.

◆ **Organism responsible for this infection:** *Listeria monocytogenes.*

◆ **Mechanism of avoidance of antibody-mediated defenses:** intracellular replication and spread from cell to cell by phagocytosis.

CLINICAL CORRELATION

Listeria is found in the environment but is not normal fecal flora in humans. Infection with *Listeria* is more common in the summer months. Disease is often the result of ingestion of the organism from infected foods such as milk, soft cheese, undercooked meat, or unwashed vegetables. *Listeria monocytogenes* causes asymptomatic or mild gastrointestinal infections in persons with intact immune systems and severe disease, most commonly meningitis, in those with impaired cellular immunity, such as pregnant women, neonates, AIDS patients, and posttransplant patients on immunosuppressive medications. Two types of neonatal disease have been described. Early-onset disease, which occurs with in the first two days of life, is the result of transplacental infection. Initial signs and symptoms include difficulty breathing and pneumonia. This infection is also called granulomatosis infantiseptica, because severe disease can be associated with a granulomatous rash with abscesses. Late-onset disease, which usually occurs 2–3 weeks after birth, is thought to result from exposure to *Listeria* either during or shortly after delivery. This infection most commonly presents as meningitis. Clinically these syndromes can be difficult to distinguish from that seen with group B streptococci.

Approach to Suspected *Listeria Monocytogenes*

Definitions

Cold enrichment: Used to enhance growth of *Listeria,* particularly from food.

Granulomatosis infantiseptica: Severe form of *Listeria* infection of neonates in which granulomatous skin lesions are evident.

Anterior fontanelle: An opening of the neonatal skull between the sutures.

Gravida: Number of total pregnancies.

Para: Number of deliveries (usually after 20 weeks gestation); a pregnancy that ends prior to 20 weeks gestation is an abortus.

Objectives

1. Know the structure and physiology of *L. monocytogenes.*
2. Know the life cycle, virulence factors, and diseases associated with *L. monocytogenes.*

Discussion

Characteristics of *Listeria*

L. monocytogenes is a **small, facultative anaerobic, gram-positive bacillus.** It may appear as **coccobacilli in pairs or chains,** so it can be mistaken for *Streptococcus pneumoniae* or *Enterococcus* on Gram stain. *L. monocytogenes* is an **intracellular** pathogen, which allows it to avoid antibody-mediated defenses of the host. It initially **enters host cells via the action of a protein, internalin,** which induces phagocytosis of the bacteria. *Listeria* produces a **toxin,** which then lyses the phagosome, releasing the bacteria into the host cell's cytoplasm. It replicates in the host cytoplasm and moves to the host membrane. By pushing against the membrane, a protrusion, known as a **filopod,** is produced, which can be phagocytized by adjacent cells.

This cycle is then repeated in the new host cell, allowing *Listeria* to spread without being exposed to antibodies or other humoral immunity factors. For this reason, host cellular immunity factors protect against infection and those with impaired cellular immunity are vulnerable.

Diagnosis

Clinical diagnosis is difficult based on the nonspecific signs and symptoms. Clinically *Listeria meningitis* in neonates resembles group B *Streptococci,* both are a significant cause of bacteria meningitis in that age group. Definitive diagnosis of *Listeria* is made by **culture of cerebrospinal fluid (CSF) and/or blood.** Gram stain of the CSF would demonstrate **small gram-positive bacilli,** appearing similar to corynebacteria or *Streptococcus pneumoniae.*

Listeria will grow on routine agar media within 24–48 hours. On blood agar media *Listeria* demonstrate **β-hemolysis,** which differentiates it from *Corynebacterium,* but adds to the difficulty in distinguishing them from *Streptococci.* Specific identification is made in part by observation of characteristic tumbling motility on a wet preparation after room temperature incubation. A reaction of **catalase positive** helps to distinguish *Listeria* from *Streptococci.*

Culture of *Listeria* from food may require cold enrichment, which would enhance the growth of *Listeria.* Food samples would be sent to a public health laboratory where some of the food would be enriched in a selective broth media at room temperature or lower.

Treatment and Prevention

Treatment of *Listeria* septicemia or meningitis is with **ampicillin** plus or minus gentamicin. Of significance is the inherent resistance of *Listeria* to cephalosporins, which are commonly chosen as empiric therapy for meningitis in adults and would be appropriate for treatment of streptococcal meningitis in children. Prevention involves the avoidance of the consumption of **undercooked foods,** especially in high-risk patients.

Comprehension Questions

[13.1] A 22-year-old medical student suffers diarrhea for more than a week since his return from a short vacation in Mexico. While in Mexico, he consumed a large quantity of raw cheeses almost every day. Which of the following is the most likely organism causing his diarrhea?

A. *Bacillus cereus*
B. *Escherichia coli*
C. *Listeria monocytogenes*
D. *Salmonella enteritidis*
E. *Shigella dysenteriae*

[13.2] A premature neonate suffers pneumonia and sepsis. Sputum culture on blood agar plate yields pinpointed beta-hemolytic colonies. Which of the following is a simple test to determine whether the organism is *Streptococcus agalactiae* or *Listeria monocytogenes* (these two organisms are important neonatal pathogens)?

A. Bacitracin test
B. Catalase test
C. Coagulase test
D. Polymerase chain reaction
E. Sugar fermentation test

[13.3] The most frequent source of infection with *Listeria monocytogenes* is through which of the following?

A. Human feces
B. Livestock
C. Raw milk
D. Soil
E. Ticks

Answers

[13.1] **C.** Outbreaks of gastroenteritis, as a consequence of *Listeria monocytogenes,* are related to the ingestion of unpasteurized milk products, for example, cheese. *Bacillus cereus,* causing food poisoning, is associated with spore survival and germination when rice is held at warm temperatures. *Escherichia coli* is usually associated with the enterohemorrhagic *Escherichia coli* (EHEC) form (verotoxin) that causes a bloody diarrhea and is associated with improperly cooked hamburger. *Salmonella* causes a diarrhea associated with contaminated chicken consumption. Finally, *Shigella* is usually associated with enterocolitis outbreaks among children in mental institutions and daycare centers.

[13.2]   **B.** *Streptococcus agalactiae* (group B streptococci) is the leading cause of neonatal sepsis and meningitis. All streptococci (including *Streptococcus agalactiae*) are catalase-negative, whereas Staphylococci are catalase-positive. *Listeria monocytogenes* is also catalase-positive.

[13.3]   **C.** Unpasteurized milk is a common vector for transmission of *Listeria.* See answer to question [13.1].

MICROBIOLOGY PEARLS

 Listeria meningitis clinically resembles group B streptococcal meningitis and needs to be distinguished because of the resistance of *Listeria* to cephalosporins.

 Listeria grown on blood agar media will be β-hemolytic and resemble streptococci; however, by Gram stain *Listeria* are small bacilli and not chains of cocci.

 Listeria infection is commonly associated with consumption of undercooked food or unpasteurized milk or cheese products.

REFERENCES

Bortolussi R, Schlech WF. Listeriosis. In: Infectious diseases of the fetus and new-born infant, 4th ed. Philadelphia: W.B. Saunders, 1995:1055–73.

Murray PR, Rosenthal KS, Kobayashi GS, Pfaller MA . Listeria and erysipelothrix. In: Murray PR, Rosenthal KS, Kobayashi GS, Pfaller MA. Medical microbiology, 4th ed. St. Louis: Mosby, 2002:245–49.

A 50-year-old man, a recent immigrant from Vietnam, is brought to the emergency room with a cough productive of bloody sputum. He first noticed a cough about 2 months ago, but there was not much sputum. In the past several days his sputum production has increased and become mixed with blood. He reports having lost approximately 15 lb in this time frame as well. He also notes that he's had drenching night sweats 2 or 3 nights a week for the past month. He has a 50-pack-year smoking history but no other medical history. He came to the United States from Vietnam 7 months ago. On examination, he is a thin, frail-appearing male. His vital signs are normal. His head and neck exam is normal. He has no palpable adenopathy in his neck or axilla. His lung exam is notable only for decreased breath sounds diffusely. A chest x-ray shows a cavitary infiltrate of the left upper lobe.

◆ **What type of organism is likely to be seen on Gram stain of a sputum sample?**

◆ **What technique of staining is most commonly used to identify this organism?**

◆ **What is the histologic characteristic of Langhans' cells?**

ANSWERS TO CASE 14: *Mycobacteria*

Summary: A 50-year-old Vietnamese man presents with a chronic bloody sputum, weight loss, and a cavitary lesion on chest radiograph, all consistent with tuberculosis.

◆ **Likely Gram stain findings of sputum sample:** *M. tuberculosis* appear as colorless ("ghost") cells.

◆ **Most commonly used staining technique for *M. tuberculosis:*** acid-fast staining.

◆ **Histologic characteristics of Langhans' cells:** multinucleated giant cells of fused macrophages.

CLINICAL CORRELATION

It is estimated that *M. tuberculosis* infects approximately one-third of the world's population. *M. tuberculosis* is spread from **person to person via aerosolized respiratory droplets** that travel to the terminal airways. The bacteria are phagocytized by alveolar macrophages but inhibit destruction by the phagosome and proceed to replicate. Circulating macrophages are attracted to the site of infection and create **multinucleated giant cells, composed of fused macrophages called Langhans cells.** Extrapulmonary sites are infected through the spread of infected macrophages via lymphatic or hematogenous dissemination. Because of the **intracellular** nature of *M. tuberculosis* infections, **antibody mediated defenses are relatively ineffective.** Persons with conditions of reduced cellular immunity, such as AIDS, alcoholism, or drug abuse, or persons living in crowded, close quarters, such as prisoners, are at increased risk for infection. Organisms can remain **dormant in granulomas** for many years and reactivate following immunosuppression at a later date. At that time the organisms usually infect extrapulmonary sites.

M. avium intracellulare is found in the environment and is an opportunistic pathogen that causes disease in **AIDS patients.** Disease can range from pneumonia to gastroenteritis to disseminated disease.

M. kansasii can clinically mimic pulmonary tuberculosis, but it is most often seen in middle-aged men with prior lung damage such as **silicosis or asbestosis.** *M. leprae* is acquired by contact with the **nine-banded armadillo.** Most infections are seen in the southern United States including Texas and Louisiana. Thought to be lepers (skin lesions and deformation of the features of the face), these patients were contained in sanitariums and left to die. Infection can be either of the lepromatous or tuberculous type. Most infections caused by rapidly growing *Mycobacteria* are chronic wound infections, because this organism is found in the soil.

Approach to Suspected *Mycobacterial* Infection

Definitions

Langhans cells: Multinucleated giant cells composed of fused macrophages.
Granuloma: Chronic inflammatory response to either *Mycobacterium* or fungi, composed of macrophages and multinucleated giant cells.
PPD: Purified protein derivative, prepared from *Mycobacterium tuberculosis* antigens inoculated intradermally and a positive reaction is indicative of exposure to *M. tuberculosis.*

Objectives

1. Know the structure and physiology of *Mycobacteria.*
2. Know the reservoirs, transmission, and diseases caused by *Mycobacteria.*
3. Know the mechanisms of host defenses and treatments for *Mycobacterial* diseases.

Discussion

Characteristics of *Mycobacteria* Species

Mycobacterium are **small rod-shaped bacilli that stain as ghost cells with Gram stain,** but because of the presence of **mycolic acids in their cell wall** stain with an **"acid-fast stain"** such as Kinyon or Ziehl-Neelsen. This complex, lipid-rich cell wall also makes the organisms resistant to many commonly used laboratory stains and is responsible for the resistance of this organism to many common detergents and antibiotics.

In general, *Mycobacterium* species are **slow-growing organisms,** with a generation time of 15–20 hours, compared to about 1 hour for most bacteria. *Mycobacterium* can be divided into groups as characterized by **Runyon,** based on their growth characteristics, particularly **pigment production.** The **photochromogens,** which are pigmented only in the presence of light, include *M. kansasii,* as well as other saprophytic *Mycobacteria.* The **scotochromogens,** which are **pigmented even without the presence of light,** include *M. szulgai,* as well as the nonpathogenic *M. gordonae,* which has an orange pigment. The **nonchromogens** are **not pigmented in the light or dark** including *M. avium-intracellulare,* as well as *M. haemophilum.* The fourth runyon group is composed of the **rapidly growing *Mycobacteria*** such as *M. fortuitum, M. chelonae,* and *M. abscessus.* The *M. tuberculosis* complex includes *M. tuberculosis, M. africanum, M. ulcerans,* and *M. bovis,* as well as other rarely identified *Mycobacterium.* These colonies appear buff or tan color and are dry when growing on Lowenstein-Jensen agar. *M. leprae* is not considered in that classification because it cannot be cultured in the laboratory.

One of the virulence factors of *M. tuberculosis* is **cord factor.** This can be visualized microscopically as organisms grown in broth culture will demonstrate a **ropelike pattern** indicating cording. The rapid growing *Mycobacterium* include *M. fortuitum* complex, *M. chelonae* complex, and *M. abscessus,* as well as other uncommonly isolated nonpathogenic *Mycobacteria*. These organisms by definition will grow within seven days of subculture onto routine microbiological media such as a blood agar plate

Diagnosis

Diagnosis of tuberculosis is initially made based on a history (exposure to patient with tuberculosis, immigration, a stay in a jail or homeless shelter) and physical exam in patients with a productive cough, night sweats, and fever. A **positive PPD test** would indicate exposure to *M. tuberculosis* and warrant further testing with chest x-ray. Patients with the characteristic upper lobe cavitary lesion would have sputum collected and cultured for *Mycobacterium*.

A **fluorescent, direct smear, of the respiratory specimen** after decontamination to remove bacterial flora is reported within 24 hours of receipt of the respiratory specimen in the laboratory. Several first early morning deep cough specimens should be collected. Growth of *M. tuberculosis* on Lowenstein-Jensen (LJ) agar can take 3–8 weeks because of the slow dividing time of the organism; however, with the use of broth medium growth time has been decreased to as short as 1 week. Newly designed automated broth systems read bottles for growth based on CO_2 production of the organisms on a daily basis for up to eight weeks. Bottles which are determined to be positive are stained by Kinyoun stain to visualize the presence of *Mycobacteria*. Positive bottles can be tested directly for *M. tuberculosis, M. kansasii, M. avium-intracellulare,* or *M. gordonae* using **DNA probes.** Other *Mycobacteria* species are identified either by routine biochemical tests, which require several weeks, or by high-pressure liquid chromatography, which can speciate *Mycobacterium* based on mycolic acids extracted from their cell surface. Optimal growth temperature for *Mycobacterium* species is 35°C (95°F); however, the *Mycobacterium* that infect the skin such as *M. haemophilum* grow best at lower temperatures, and organisms such as *M. szulgai* prefer 42°C (107.6°F). Growth on solid media is also enhanced in the presence of 5–10% CO_2.

Treatment and Prevention

Prophylaxis for tuberculosis consists of oral **isoniazid** for 6–9 months and is given to all patients with a recent conversion of their PPD to positive and a negative chest x-ray. Treatment for tuberculosis based on **culture** of *M. tuberculosis* from any patient specimen is initially (first 2 months) with a **multiagent regimen** based on likely resistance patterns; one such combination is isoniazid, rifampin, ethambutol, and pyrazinamide. Once the results indicate susceptibility to all of the four firstline drugs, treatment can continue with two drugs (usually isoniazid and rifampin) for the remaining 4–6 months. Because of the interaction of rifampin with other drugs, particularly HIV drugs and antifungals, this therapy may need to be individualized.

Prevention of tuberculosis besides prophylactic isoniazid includes isolation of patients in the hospital to prevent spread. Patients with a positive acid-fast smear must remain in isolation until a diagnosis of tuberculosis is ruled out, until they leave the hospital, or following several weeks of appropriate antituberculous therapy with obvious clinical improvement. All known close contacts (family members) of the index case should have a PPD test to determine if they should be given therapy and/or worked up for disease.

Vaccination with BCG, (an attenuated strain of *M. bovis*) is not routinely performed in the United States because of the comparatively low incidence of tuberculosis. Protection from tuberculosis is not 100 percent with the vaccine and can confuse the results of the PPD for screening of recent converters.

Treatment of the other atypical *Mycobacteria* varies based on the species. *M. avium-intracellulare* is usually treated with clarithromycin or azithromycin and ethambutol plus or minus amikacin. Current treatment for leprosy is dapsone and rifampin for at least 6 months.

Comprehension Questions

[14.1] An emaciated prisoner in a New York prison began coughing up sputum streaked with blood. Examination of the sputum revealed the presence of acid-fast bacilli. Which of the following would confirm a diagnosis of tuberculosis?

A. Inclusion bodies of the nuclei of macrophages
B. Presence of gram-positive pleomorphic organisms
C. Rough, nonpigmented colonies
D. Rapid growth on Lowenstein-Jensen medium

[14.2] A 45-year-old traveler discovers that he has converted from negative to positive on the tuberculin (PPD) skin test. This indicates which of the following?

A. He has active tuberculosis.
B. He has delayed-type hypersensitivity against *Mycobacterium tuberculosis*.
C. He is most likely to be infected with an "atypical" *Mycobacterium*.
D. He needs to immediately isolated to prevent spread of *M. tuberculosis*.
E. He will eventually develop tuberculosis.

[14.3] A 60-year-old man with a chronic cough, bloody sputum, and marked weight loss is diagnosed as having tuberculosis. A "serpentine-like" colonial morphology is noted on Lowenstein-Jensen agar. This latter finding is caused by which of the following factors?

A. A large "slimy" capsule
B. An endotoxin
C. Coagulase
D. Cord factor
E. Wax D

[14.4] A 25-year-old man known to have AIDS experiences a gradual onset of malaise and anorexia, proceeding within a few weeks to photophobia, impaired consciousness, and oculofacial palsy. An acid-fast bacterium with trehalose-6,6'-dimycolate is isolated. The identity of this organism is which of the following?

A. *Mycobacterium fortuitum-chelonei*
B. *Mycobacterium kansasii*
C. *Mycobacterium marinum*
D. *Mycobacterium scrofulaceum*
E. *Mycobacterium tuberculosis*

Answers

[14.1] **C.** To mount a protective immune response against a specific microorganism requires that the appropriate population of cells play a role in the response. A lipoprotein of *Mycobacterium tuberculosis* stimulates a specific "toll-like receptor" on the macrophage. Activated macrophages then synthesize IL-12, which causes differentiation of naïve helper T cells into the Th-1 type of helper T cells that participates in the cell-mediated (delayed hypersensitivity) response. In addition, delayed hypersensitivity (not humoral) reactions are produced against antigens of intracellular pathogens such as *M. tuberculosis*. Thus, humoral immunity is not protective against *M. tuberculosis,* and the patient will suffer severe tuberculosis if cell-mediated immunity is not functional. Therefore, an agglutination test for antibodies is useless as *M. tuberculosis* is an intracellular pathogen and will not elicit a humoral (antibody-formation) immune response that will protect the patient against *M. tuberculosis*. The growth is usually slow, and the colonies are rough and nonpigmented.

[14.2] **B.** The purified protein derivative (PPD) skin test, or tuberculin skin test, contains several proteins from *M. tuberculosis,* which when combined with waxes elicits a delayed hypersensitivity. It does not assess for the status of infection, but only speaks about prior exposure. The clinical presentation and/or chest radiograph would be the next steps in evaluation.

[14.3]   **D.** Virulent strains of *M. tuberculosis* grow in a characteristic "serpentine" cordlike pattern, whereas avirulent strains do not. Virulence of the organism is correlated with cord factor (trehalose dimycolate).

[14.4]   **E.** *Mycobacterium tuberculosis* commonly has the trehalose dimycolate factor (see answer to Question 14.3).

MICROBIOLOGY PEARLS

- *Mycobacterium tuberculosis* is a slow growing organism that causes pulmonary infection after close contact with an infected individual.
- A positive skin test (PPD) indicates exposure to the organism and not necessarily disease.
- *Mycobacterium* species stain positive with an acid-fast stain because of components in their cell wall.
- Initial therapy for tuberculosis requires multiple agents to avoid resistance, and culture susceptibilities will dictate which agents should be continued.

REFERENCES

Haas DW. Mycobacterium tuberculosis. In: Mandell GL, Bennett JE, Dolin R, eds. Principles and practice of infectious diseases, 5th ed. Philadelphia: Churchill Livingstone, 2000:2576–607.

Murray PR, Rosenthal KS, Kobayashi GS, Pfaller MA. Mycobacterium. In: Murray PR, Rosenthal KS, Kobayashi GS, Pfaller MA. Medical microbiology, 4th ed. St. Louis: Mosby, 2002:366–77.

A 15-year-old teenager is brought to the office for evaluation of a cough and fever. His illness began several days ago with low-grade fever, headache, myalgias, and fatigue, and has slowly worsened. He now has a persistent cough. He has tried multiple over-the-counter cold and cough medications without relief. He has no significant medical or family history. No family members have been ill recently, but one of his good friends missed several days of school about 2 weeks ago with "walking pneumonia." On examination he is coughing frequently but is not particularly ill-appearing. His temperature is 38.1°C (100.5°F), pulse 90 is beats per minute, and respiratory rate is 22 breaths per minute. His pharynx is injected; otherwise, a head and neck exam is normal. His lung exam is notable only for some scattered rhonchi. The remainder of his examination is normal. A chest x-ray shows some patchy infiltration. A sputum Gram stain shows white blood cells but no organisms.

◆ **What is the most likely etiology of this infection?**

◆ **What is the explanation for no organisms being seen on Gram stain?**

◆ **What rapid, although nonspecific, blood test can provide presumptive evidence of infection by this organism?**

ANSWERS TO CASE 15: *Mycoplasma*

Summary: A 15-year-old adolescent presents with a persistent cough, patchy infiltrate on chest x-ray, and exposure to a friend with "walking pneumonia."

◆ **Most likely infectious agent:** *Mycoplasma pneumoniae.*

◆ **Reasons no organisms are seen on Gram stain:** *M. pneumoniae* does not stain because it does not have a cell wall.

◆ **Rapid blood test for presumptive evidence of *M. pneumoniae:*** Cold agglutinins.

CLINICAL CORRELATION

M. pneumoniae is transmitted from person to person by aerosolized respiratory droplets and close association with an index case is usually required. There is usually a 1–3 week incubation period before the onset of clinical disease. Although it can infect those of all ages, disease more commonly occurs in children and young adults. Disease caused by *M. pneumonia* usually has an insidious onset and can progress to tracheobronchitis or pneumonia, which is often patchy or diffuse, as opposed to lobar. Because of the inability to diagnose this on microscopy, and the difficulty and length of time required for culture, serologic testing is often used to identify this organism. One useful test is the titer of cold agglutinins. *M. pneumonia* infection often results in the stimulation of an IgM antibody against the I-antigen on erythrocytes. This antigen/antibody complex binds at 4°C, causing clumping of erythrocytes. Although this response can be triggered by other organisms, titers of these antibodies of 1:128 or greater, or a fourfold increase, in the presence of an appropriated clinical presentation are considered presumptive evidence of *M. pneumonia* disease.

Objectives
1. Know the structure and physiology of *M. pneumoniae* and other *Mycoplasma* organisms.
2. Know the clinical diseases associated with and tests for identification of *M. pneumoniae.*

Discussion

Characteristics of *Mycoplasma pneumoniae* that Impact Transmission

M. pneumoniae is a **short, strictly aerobic rod.** It has a trilamellar, sterol-containing cell membrane but **no cell wall,** therefore it is **not identifiable with Gram or other stains.** The lack of a cell wall also confers resistance against **β-lactams** and other antibiotics that act on the cell walls of bacteria. It is the

smallest free-living bacterium, even during infection, it remains extracellular. It divides by binary fission and has a doubling time of about 6 hours, much slower than most bacteria. This contributes to the difficulty in isolating this organism by culture, as up to 6 weeks of incubation are required. *Mycoplasma* has the **adherence protein P1** at one end, which is responsible for its attachment to a protein on target cells and may confer its preference for respiratory epithelium. When attached to ciliated respiratory epithelial cells, first the cilia and then the cell is destroyed. This interferes with normal mucociliary clearance and allows the lower airways to be irritated and contaminated with infectious agents.

M. pneumoniae is **transmitted from person to person by aerosolized respiratory droplets and secretions,** and close association with an index case is usually required. No seasonal peak is observed. There is usually a **1–3 week incubation period** before the onset of clinical disease. Although it can infect those of all ages, disease more commonly occurs in children and young adults. Disease caused by *M. pneumoniae* usually has an insidious onset and can progress to tracheobronchitis or **pneumonia,** which is often **patchy or diffuse, as opposed to lobar.** *M. pneumoniae* is responsible for 15–20 percent of community-acquired pneumonias. Clinical presentation consists of a low-grade fever, headache, malaise, and later a nonproductive cough, with a slow resolution.

Diagnosis

Diagnosis is primarily made from clinical presentation. Because of the inability to diagnose the infection with microscopy and the difficulty and length of time required for culture, serologic testing is often used to confirm a clinical diagnosis. Antibody-directed enzyme immunoassays and immunofluorescence tests or complement fixation tests are used in diagnosis. Another useful test is to analyze the titer of **cold agglutinins.** *M. pneumoniae* infection often results in the stimulation of **an IgM antibody against the I-antigen on erythrocytes.** This antigen-antibody complex binds at 4°C causing the clumping of erythrocytes. Although this response can be triggered by other organisms, titers of these antibodies of 1:128 or greater, or a fourfold increase with the presence of an appropriated clinical presentation are considered presumptive evidence of *M. pneumoniae* disease.

Another *Mycoplasma, M. hominis,* causes **pelvic inflammatory disease (PID), nongonococcal urethritis (NGU), pyelonephritis, and postpartum fever.** Another cause of NGU and an organism that is detected with cold agglutinins is *Ureaplasma urealyticum,* a facultative anaerobic rod. Although this organism can also be a commensal, it can also lead to the sexually transmitted disease NGU and infertility. It is diagnosed via serology, by both cold agglutinins and specific serology with complement fixation and ELISA (enzyme-linked immunosorbent assay) for IgM. Like *Mycoplasma,* culture is not reliable and takes many weeks. PCR probes are also used for diagnosis. The clinical picture of NGU consists of urethral discharge, pruritus, and dysuria. Typically, systemic symptoms are absent. The onset of symptoms in NGU can often be subacute. There are 3 million new cases of NGU (including *M. hominis, U. urealyticum, Chlamydia trachomatis,* and *Trichomonas vaginalis*) a year, and 10–40 percent of women suffer PID as a result, compared to only 1–2 percent of males, with morbidity from NGU because of stricture or stenosis. NGU occurs equally in men and women, though can be asymptomatic in 50 percent of women.

Treatment and Prevention

M. pneumoniae-related pneumonia, as well as other *Mycoplasma* infections resulting in NGU, can be effectively treated with **tetracycline** and **erythromycin.** Tetracyclines can be used to treat most *mycoplasmas,* as well as *Chlamydia;* whereas erythromycin can be used to treat *Ureaplasma* infections, which are resistant to tetracycline. *M. pneumoniae* infections are difficult to prevent because patients are infectious for extended periods of time, even during treatment. Several attempts have been made to produce inactivated and attenuated live vaccines without success.

Comprehension Questions

[15.1] A 33-year-old woman is diagnosed with "walking pneumonia" caused by *Mycoplasma.* Which of the following best describes the characteristics of the etiologic organism?

    A. Absence of a cell wall
    B. Belonging to the class of Eukaryotes
    C. Often evoke an IgM autoantibody response leading to human erythrocyte agglutination
    D. Typically colonize the gastrointestinal tract

[15.2] Which of the following antibiotics is the best treatment for the above patient?

    A. Ampicillin
    B. Ceftriaxone
    C. Erythromycin
    D. Gentamicin
    E. Vancomycin

[15.3] *Mycoplasma* organisms may also cause disease in nonpulmonary sites. Which of the following is the most commonly affected nonpulmonary site?

    A. Meningitis
    B. Prosthetic heart valve
    C. Septic arthritis
    D. Urethritis

[15.4] A 20-year-old man presents to the clinic with a history of fever and nonproductive cough. The patient's chest x-ray shows consolidation of the right lower lobe. An infection with *Mycoplasma pneumoniae* is considered as the cause of the patient's pneumonia. Which of the following methods would confirm this diagnosis?

A. Culture of sputum specimen on solid medium
B. Detection of organism by microscopy
C. Complement fixation test of acute and convalescent sera
D. PCR amplification of patient's sputum specimen
E. Enzyme immunoassay to detect cell wall antigens

Answers

[15.1] **A.** *Mycoplasma* are the smallest living organisms, and they do not have cell walls but rather have cell membranes. Thus, they are typically resistant to antibiotics that interfere with cell wall synthesis. Also, because of their absence of a cell wall, they are not usually detected on Gram stain. They have a propensity for attaching to respiratory, urethral, or genital tract epithelium.

[15.2] **C.** Erythromycin, clarithromycin, or azithromycin (macrolides) are effective against mycoplasma species.

[15.3] **D.** *Mycoplasma* and *Ureaplasma* species are commonly isolated from the lower genital tract. They are likely the most common cause of nonchlamydial nongonococcal urethritis.

[15.4] **C.** Answers A, B, D, and E are all incorrect: (A) culturing *M. pneumoniae* is difficult and slow and is not used for diagnosis; (B) *Mycoplasmas* lack a cell wall making microscopy inappropriate; (D) PCR amplification of a sputum specimen is not an appropriate method of diagnosis; (E) *M. pneumoniae* lacks a cell wall and thus, cell wall antigens.

MICROBIOLOGY PEARLS

 Mycoplasmas are small free-living microorganisms that lack a cell wall.

 M. pneumoniae is a common cause of atypical pneumonia in children and adolescents.

 Symptoms include nonproductive cough, fever, headache, and "walking" pneumonia.

 Effective treatment is with erythromycin or tetracycline.

REFERENCES

Baseman JB, Tully JG: Mycoplasmas: sophisticated, reemerging, and burdened by their notoriety. Emerg Infect Dis 1997;3:21. Available online at www.cdc.gov/ncidod/EID/vol3no1/baseman.htm

Murray PR, Rosenthal KS, Kobayashi GS, Pfaller MA. Medical microbiology, 4th ed. St. Louis: Mosby, 2002:395–399.

Ryan JR, Ray CG. Sherris medical microbiology, 4th ed. New York: McGraw-Hill, 2004:409–411.

A 19-year-old woman presents to the office for the evaluation of a swollen knee. She states that for the past week or two she has had some achiness in several of her joints and a low-grade fever, but it seemed to localize to her left knee about 3 days ago. It has been red, hot, and swollen. She has had no injury to the area and has never had anything like this before. Her past medical history is significant for having been treated for *Chlamydia* at the age of 17. She takes oral contraceptive pills regularly. She is sexually active, has been with her most recent boyfriend for about a month, and has had 5 partners in her lifetime. On examination, her vital signs are normal, but you notice that she walks with a limp. Her general examination is normal, and her skin is without rash. Her left knee is erythematous and warm to the touch. There is a visible effusion. Movement is limited because of pain and stiffness from the swelling. She refuses a pelvic examination because she doesn't see what that has to do with her sore knee. However, she does allow you to perform a joint aspiration.

◆ **What are the most likely Gram stain findings of the aspirated joint fluid?**

◆ **What cell surface factors facilitate attachment and penetration of this organism into the host cell?**

ANSWERS TO CASE 16: *Neisseria*

Summary: A 19-year-old woman presents with septic arthritis. She has had an infection previously with Chlamydia.

◆ **Likely findings on Gram stain of the joint fluid aspirate:** Multiple polymorphonuclear leukocytes with intracellular gram-negative diplococci.

◆ **Cell surface factors facilitating attachment and penetration into the host cell:** Pili, which attach to epithelial cells, and Opa protein, which promotes firm attachment and cell penetration.

CLINICAL CORRELATION

Humans are the only known reservoir of *Neisseria* species. *N. gonorrhoeae* is transferred from person to person by sexual contact. Approximately half of infected women have an asymptomatic carrier state. This is much less common in men. *N. gonorrhoeae* causes urethritis in men and cervicitis in women. Complications of genital infections include pelvic inflammatory disease. The organism can also infect the rectum and oropharynx. Newborns passing through an infected birth canal may develop conjunctivitis by direct contact, a disease called ophthalmia neonatorum. Disseminated disease, including bacteremia with resultant joint and/or skin infections is more common in patients with complement deficiencies. Septic arthritis as a complication of disseminated disease may present in two forms, either as a systemic disease with fever, chills, and polyarticular syndrome, or as a monoarticular suppurative infection of a single joint without skin lesions or systemic symptoms. Most cases of disseminated gonococcal disease occur in persons with an asymptomatic genital infection.

Neisseria meningitidis is carried as normal upper respiratory flora in approximately 10 percent of the population. The polysaccharide capsule allows the organism to avoid phagocytosis and under unknown circumstances enter the blood and in some cases the central nervous system. The subsequent inflammatory response induced by the organism causes shock and disseminated intravascular coagulation. This is evidenced by skin lesions, which can mimic those seen in disseminated gonococcal infection. Bacteremia with or without meningitis usually occurs in teenage children. If untreated, the disease has a high mortality rate.

Approach to Suspected Gonorrhoeae Patient

Definitions

Disseminated intravascular coagulation (DIC): A complication of septic shock usually caused by endotoxin produced by the affecting organism.

Ophthalmia neonatorum: Conjunctivitis in the first month of life usually as a result of *Neisseria gonorrhoeae* or *Chlamydia trachomatis.*

Objectives

1. Know the structure and characteristics of *Neisseria* species.
2. Know the factors associated with the development on *Neisseria* infections and diseases.

Discussion

Characteristics of *Neisseria* Species

Neisseria species are **aerobic, nonmotile, nonspore-forming, gram-negative cocci.** They usually are arranged in **pairs** (diplococci) with adjacent sides flattened, resembling **kidney beans.** *Neisseria* are **fastidious organisms** that require a complex medium and an atmosphere supplemented with **carbon dioxide** for optimal growth. *N. gonorrhoeae* has specific cell surface components related to its adherence, cellular penetration, toxicity, and evasion of host defenses. Cellular adherence is conferred by the presence of **pili,** which attach to host epithelial cells and also provide resistance to killing by host neutrophils. The **outer membrane also contains the Opa proteins** (opacity proteins), which promote tight attachment and migration of the bacteria into the host. Then **Por proteins** (porin), which form channels (pores) in the outer membrane, **prevent phagolysosome fusion,** allowing intracellular survival. **Rmp proteins** (reduction-modifiable proteins) stimulate antibodies, which inhibit host bactericidal antibodies, protecting the other surface antigens from host attack.

Plasmid acquisition and transfer appear to play significant roles in the development of **antibiotic resistance** by *N. gonorrhoeae.* Multiple plasmids, which confer **β-lactamase,** have been identified. A conjugative plasmid that causes high-level tetracycline resistance has also been identified. These plasmids are becoming more common, resulting in more antibiotic-resistant gonococcal disease. LOS (lipooligosaccharide), also present in the cell wall, produces the inflammatory response responsible for most of the symptoms associated with gonococcal disease by its release of tumor necrosis factor-α.

Neisseria meningitidis appear the same as *N. gonorrhoeae* on Gram stain. They also produce a polysaccharide capsule that prevents phagocytosis. *N. meningitidis* is divided into 13 serogroups, the most common of which are A,C,Y, W135, and b.

Diagnosis

Septic arthritis must be differentiated from other noninfectious forms of arthritis such as rheumatoid arthritis and gout. **Definitive diagnosis** is made by **analysis of cells and Gram stain from an aspirate of the joint.** Gram stain would reveal **intracellular gram-negative diplococci.** A presumptive diagnosis of gonorrhoeae can be made from a smear from a male urethra; otherwise, culture is required for diagnosis.

Neisseria species are **fastidious organisms** in that they require CO_2 **atmosphere,** and *N. gonorrhoeae* also require **chocolate agar.** *N. gonorrhoeae* also may require at least 48 hours for production of small grey colonies. **Selective media** such as **Thayer Martin** or **Martin Lewis** is usually needed to isolate *N. gonorrhoeae* from nonsterile sites such as the cervix or urethra. *Neisseria gonorrhoeae* are quite sensitive to drying, so plates must be placed in a warm environment quickly to maintain viability. If a delay in transit to the laboratory is expected to be longer than several hours, a transport media such as Jembec is required. Rapid identification can be made from gram-negative diplococci, growing on selective media that are **oxidase positive.** Isolates are specifically identified by acid production from select sugars. *N. gonorrhoeae* ferments glucose only, and *N. meningitidis* ferments both glucose and maltose. Because of the fastidious nature of *N. gonorrhoeae,* genital infections are identified using DNA probes, which detect both *N. gonorrhoeae* and *Chlamydia trachomatis,* which commonly occur together and don't require live organisms for detection.

Treatment and Prevention

Penicillin is the treatment of choice for meningococcemia. Approximately 30 percent of *N. gonorrhoeae* **produce β-lactamase and are therefore resistant to penicillin.** Treatment with **ceftriaxone** or a quinolones is usually recommended, although increase in **resistance to quinolones** has been demonstrated in some geographic locations. **Prevention of meningococcal disease is by vaccination** of susceptible persons such as military personnel and teenagers in dormitories as well as asplenic patients. Prophylaxis of close contacts is also recommended to prevent spread of the disease. Prevention of *N. gonorrhoeae* includes practicing safe sex and use of a condom, as well as screening sexually active persons. Screening of pregnant women for congenitally transmitted infections with appropriate treatment would prevent infection of the neonate with *N. gonorrhoeae,* as well as other congenitally transmitted infections.

Comprehension Questions

[16.1] The source of *Neisseria meningitidis* is the nasopharynx of human carriers who exhibit no symptoms. The ability of this bacterium to colonize the respiratory mucosa is associated with its ability to synthesize which of the following?

   A. Coagulase
   B. Collagenase
   C. Hyaluronidase
   D. Lipases
   E. Pili

[16.2] Several *Neisseria* species are a part of the normal flora (commensals) of the human upper respiratory tract. Which of the following statements accurately describes the significance of these bacteria?

   A. As a part of the normal flora, *Neisseriae* provide a natural immunity in local host defense.
   B. As a part of the respiratory flora, they are the most common cause of acute bronchitis and pneumonia.
   C. Commensal bacteria stimulate a cell-mediated immunity (CMI).
   D. Commensal *Neisseriae* in the upper respiratory tract impede phagocytosis by means of lipoteichoic acid.
   E. Normal flora such as nonpathogenic *Neisseriae* provide effective nonspecific B-cell–mediated humoral immunity.

[16.3] A 22-year-old man presents to the STD clinic with a 5-day history of burning on urination and a 3-day history of a nonpurulent urethral discharge. He is sexually active with many female partners and does not use condoms. There is no history of prior sexually transmitted diseases. Laboratory findings from endourethral exudate are most likely to show which of the following?

   A. A negative gonorrhea culture
   B. Abundant intracellular diplococci in neutrophils
   C. Immunofluorescence using monoclonal antibodies to serotypes A–C
   D. Intracellular elementary bodies

[16.4] The two pathogenic *Neisseria* species, *N. meningitidis* and *N. gonorrhoeae,* differ from the nonpathogenic *Neisseria* species in that:

   A. The former are less resistant to certain antibiotics than the nonpathogenic species.
   B. The pathogenic species are oxidase positive.
   C. The pathogenic species grow well in enriched chocolate agar.
   D. The pathogenic species do not grow well at room temperature.

Answers

[16.1] **E.** Both *Neisseria gonorrhoeae* and *N. meningitidis* adhere to the mucous membrane tissues by means of pili (short protein appendages from the membrane through the cell wall). Coagulase and lipase are products of *Streptococci,* whereas collagenase and hyaluronidase are enzyme products of *Streptococci.*

[16.2] **A.** The normal or usual flora seldom cause disease in humans, except the several species that may be opportunistic in the right circumstances. One mechanism that has been suggested as to how the normal flora help to protect humans from pathogenic strains of bacteria is to stimulate the immune system to produce antibodies (or CMI) that would recognize related pathogens and inhibit their growth. An unexplained component of this mechanism is how the normal flora continue to exist as part of the body flora in spite of these immune mechanisms.

[16.3] **B.** This presentation is classic for gonorrhea infection and symptoms. Abundant gram-negative diplococci will be found both intracellularly and outside of the phagocytic cells. Interestingly, gonococci may even divide within the phagocytic cell. This evidence (Gram stain of the exudate) is presumptive evidence of gonococcal infection, and treatment should be made immediately. Such a specimen should be positive for culture with the correct medium (e.g., Thayer-Martin) and incubation conditions (37°C, increased CO_2 atmosphere). Serotypes A–C refers to *N. meningitidis,* and elementary bodies would indicate *Chlamydia* microorganisms.

[16.4] **D.** *Neisseria gonorrhoeae* and *N. meningitidis* are true human pathogens, surviving best in the human host. They are more fastidious in their nutritional requirement, requiring an enriched selective medium for growth. All *Neisseria* are oxidase positive. Normal flora (nonpathogenic) *Neisseria* will grow at room temperature on simple medium. Because of beta-lactamase production, sensitivities should be done to ensure proper antimicrobial selection for treatment.

MICROBIOLOGY PEARLS

❖ *Neisseria meningitidis* is a highly contagious organism, which can cause meningitis in otherwise healthy young people.

❖ *Neisseria meningitidis* can be successfully prevented with the use of the vaccine for high-risk individuals.

❖ *Neisseria gonorrhoeae* is a treatable sexually transmitted disease and should be ruled out in high-risk patients to prevent further complications including disseminated disease.

REFERENCES

Apicella, MA. Neisseria meningitidis. In: Mandell GL, Bennett JE, Dolin R, eds. Principles and practice of infectious diseases, 5th ed. Philadelphia: Churchill Livingstone, 2000:2228–41.

Murray PR, Rosenthal KS, Kobayashi GS, Pfaller MA. Neisseria. In: Murray PR, Rosenthal KS, Kobayashi GS, Pfaller MA. Medical microbiology, 4th ed. St. Louis: Mosby, 2002:256–65.

Sparling, PF, Handsfield, HH. Neisseria gonorrhoeae. In: Mandell GL, Bennett JE, Dolin R, eds. Principles and practice of infectious diseases, 5th ed. Philadelphia: Churchill Livingstone, 2000:2242–58.

A 35-year-old woman presents to the emergency department with right flank pain. She reports that she had a few days of urinary urgency, frequency, and burning which she tried to treat herself by drinking cranberry juice. Earlier today she started having a severe, colicky pain on her whole right side. She has had a fever, and when she urinated this morning she noticed that it appeared to have blood. She's had a few urinary tract infections (UTIs) in the past but nothing like this. She is on no medications regularly and has no other significant medical history. On examination, she has a temperature of 37.5°C (99.5°F), her other vital signs are normal, and she appears to be in pain. Notable on examination is some tenderness on the right flank but no masses, rebound tenderness, or guarding on palpation of her abdomen. She has costovertebral angle tenderness on the right side but not the left. Her peripheral white blood cell count is elevated. A urinalysis shows the presence of leukocyte esterase, blood, and a high pH. An abdominal CT scan reveals an obstructing stone in the right ureter causing hydronephrosis of the right kidney.

◆ **What organism is likely to be responsible for this infection?**

◆ **What is the cause of the high pH of this patient's urine?**

ANSWERS TO CASE 17: *Proteus mirabilis*

Summary: A 35-year-old woman presents with a UTI and nephrolithiasis (kidney stones). The urine has a high pH.

◆ **Organism most likely to be responsible for this infection:** *Proteus mirabilis.*

◆ **Mechanism of high pH in urine:** *Proteus* produces urease, which splits urea into CO_2 and ammonia, raising the urinary pH.

CLINICAL CORRELATION

Proteus species are normal flora of the gastrointestinal tract and predominantly associated with hospital-acquired urinary tract infections as well as bacteremia, osteomyelitis, empyema, and neonatal encephalitis. *Proteus* causes UTIs after urethral contamination with fecal bacteria followed by ascension into the bladder. Most infections occur in patients with structural abnormalities or long-term catheters of the urinary tract. *Proteus* infections can result in significant renal damage by several mechanisms. *Proteus* produces large amounts of urease, which breaks down urea into carbon dioxide and ammonia and results in elevated urinary pH levels. High urinary pH can contribute to direct renal toxicity and also can result in increased urinary stone formation. Urinary stones can result in further renal damage by obstructing urine flow and serving as a focus of ongoing infection. Crystalline material tends to build up inside of a long-term catheter leading to biofilm formation. This can essentially block flow through the catheter. *Proteus* is also among the most common causes of bacteremia in the family Enterobacteriaceae often associated with underlying disease such as diabetes, malignancy, or heart or lung disease. Bacteremia is usually secondary to a primary UTI. Pediatric meningitis with *Proteus* species, especially in the first week of life, has a high mortality rate and a predilection for abscess formation when the organism gains access to the brain. It is hypothesized that the organisms gain entry into the blood through the umbilicus and from the blood they disseminated into the brain.

Definitions

Nephrolithiasis: The presence of calculi (solid, crystalline) that develop in the kidney and pass through the genitourinary tract.

Hydronephrosis: Enlargement of the kidney because of an abnormality such as the presence of stones.

Objectives

1. Know the structure and characteristics of *Proteus mirabilis.*
2. Know the mechanisms by which *P. mirabilis* produces renal damage.

Discussion

Characteristics of *Proteus* Species

The genus *Proteus* includes five species, the most common of which are *P. mirabilis* and *P. vulgaris*. *Proteus* species are commonly found in the environment and as normal flora in the intestinal tract of humans and other animals. *Proteus mirabilis,* like other members of the Enterobacteriaceae family, is a **nonspore-forming, facultative anaerobic, gram-negative bacillus.** *Proteus* has **fimbriae,** which facilitate attachment to uroepithelium, and **flagellae,** which provide the **motility** required for ascending infection. *Proteus* also has the ability to transform from a **single cell form to a multicell elongated (swarmer)** form. The swarmer cells are more likely to be associated with cellular adherence in the kidney as demonstrated in an animal model of infection. **Hemolysin,** which induces cell damage by forming pores, may also play a role in establishment of pyelonephritis.

Diagnosis

Diagnosis of a UTI is initially by the urinalysis followed by a culture. The presence of **leukocyte esterase,** which is an indicator of the presence of white blood cells, in this patient indicated a presumptive UTI. The **increased urinary pH** as well as the evidence of a stone by CT indicated an obstructive process. Gram stain of the urine may be helpful if a significantly large number of organisms are present in the urine (greater than 10^5 colonies per mL). Culture of urine would likely be diagnostic after 24 hours. Members of the family Enterobacteriaceae, the most common cause of UTIs in an otherwise healthy young person, should grow rapidly on blood as well as MacConkey agars. The presence of greater than or equal to 10^5 CFU/ml in the urine of a single organism would indicate a significant pathogen. *Proteus* is easily identified on a MacConkey agar plate as a **clear colony (nonlactose fermenter).** The **obvious swarm** seen on blood agar would indicate a *Proteus* species. Definitive confirmation of *Proteus mirabilis* would be made by biochemical tests included in most commercially available identification systems. A quick test to differentiate *P. mirabilis* and *P. vulgaris* would be indole positivity in the latter.

Treatment and Prevention

Proteus species are usually among the most susceptible genera of all of the Enterobacteriaceae, **most susceptible to penicillin,** although it is not uncommon for them to be resistant to tetracyclines. *P. vulgaris,* however, tends to be resistant to more antimicrobials than *P. mirabilis.* As is the case with most bacteria, new resistance mechanisms are being seen in otherwise susceptible organisms.

Comprehension Questions

[17.1] A 78-year-old patient with an episode of acute urinary retention was catheterized. Three days later, he developed fever and suprapubic pain. Culture of the urine revealed a thin film of bacterial growth over the entire blood agar plate, and the urease test was positive. Which of the following is the most likely organism to cause this infection?

    A. *Escherichia coli*
    B. *Helicobacter pylori*
    C. *Morganella morganii*
    D. *Proteus mirabilis*
    E. *Enterococcus faecalis*

[17.2] A urinary tract infection as a result of *Proteus mirabilis* facilitates the formation of kidney stones because the organism:

    A. Destroys blood vessels in the kidney
    B. Exhibits "swarming" motility
    C. Ferments many sugars
    D. Produces a potent urease
    E. Secretes many exotoxins

[17.3] A 55-year-old woman is noted to have pyelonephritis with shaking chills and fever. Blood cultures are obtained, and the Gram stain is read preliminarily as consistent with *Proteus* species. Which of the following bacteria also may be the etiology?

    A. *E. coli*
    B. Group B *Streptococcus*
    C. *Staphylococcus* aureus
    D. *Streptococcus* pyogenes

Answers

[17.1]   **D.** *Proteus* species produce infections in humans only when the bacteria leave the intestinal tract. They are found in urinary tract infections and produce bacteremia, pneumonia, and focal lesions in debilitated patients or those receiving intravenous infusions. *P. mirabilis* is a common cause of urinary tract infections. *Proteus* species produce urease, making urine alkaline and promoting stone formation. The rapid motility of these organisms is evidenced by "swarming," a thin film of organisms over the entire agar plate.

[17.2]   **D.** *Proteus* species produce a urease, which hydrolyzes urea leading to ammonia, which alkalinizes the urine (leading to a higher pH).

[17.3]   **A.** Both proteus and *E. coli* are gram-negative rod bacilli. *E. coli* is the most common isolate in UTIs.

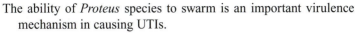

MICROBIOLOGY PEARLS

❖ The ability of *Proteus* species to swarm is an important virulence mechanism in causing UTIs.

❖ The swarming nature of *Proteus* also is an early diagnostic indicator as to the organism's identity.

❖ *Proteus* species have the ability to produce obstructive stones because of the presence of the urease enzyme.

❖ *Proteus mirabilis* is the most common cause of *Proteus* infections.

REFERENCES

Mobley HLT, Belas R. Swarming and pathogenicity of proteus mirabilis in the urinary tract. Trends in Microbiology 1995;3:280–84.

Murray PR, Rosenthal KS, Kobayashi GS, Pfaller MA. Enterobacteriaceae. In: Murray PR, Rosenthal KS, Kobayashi GS, Pfaller MA. Medical microbiology, 4th ed. St. Louis: Mosby, 2002:266–80.

O'Hara CM, Brenner FW, Miller JM. Classification, identification, and clinical significance of proteus, providencia and morganella 2000;13:534–46.

A 73-year-old man with a history of hypertension and type II diabetes mellitus presents to the office with excruciating left ear pain for the past three days. He also has noticed today that his speech seems a bit slurred, and his wife says that the left side of his face looks "droopy." He has had so much pain and swelling that he hasn't been able to put his hearing aid in for several days. He has had "swimmer's ear" in the past, which responded to treatment with ear drops, but has not had any ear problems in several years. He cleans his ears daily with cotton swabs prior to putting in his hearing aid. He denies having a fever, but says that his blood sugars have been higher than usual for the past two days. On examination, his vital signs are normal, and he is in obvious pain. He has a prominent left-sided facial droop. His left ear is diffusely swollen, and he is tender on the pinna, the entire periauricular area, and mastoid. There is purulent drainage from the ear canal. You are unable to insert a speculum into the canal because of the swelling and pain. He has evidence of facial nerve palsy on the left side. Blood tests show an elevated white blood cell count and a markedly elevated erythrocyte sedimentation rate (ESR). Your diagnosis is malignant external otitis infection.

◆ **What organism is the most likely cause of this infection?**

◆ **Which two toxins contribute to most of the systemic toxicity of this organism?**

ANSWERS TO CASE 18: *Pseudomonas aeruginosa*

Summary: A 73-year-old man is diagnosed with malignant otitis externa.

◆ **Organism most likely to cause this infection:** *Pseudomonas aeruginosa.*

◆ **Which two toxins contribute to most of the systemic signs of infection:** Lipopolysaccharide endotoxin and exotoxin A.

CLINICAL CORRELATION

Pseudomonas causes numerous types of infections, with the common factor being that they are usually in a debilitated host. *P. aeruginosa* is an opportunistic pathogen that is most commonly associated with nosocomial pneumonia. Pulmonary infections primarily occur in patients with underlying disease such as cystic fibrosis or chronic lung or heart disease, who have immune suppression, or who are on ventilators. Skin infections occur in patients whose skin has been disrupted either by burn or trauma. Skin lesions can also be a secondary effect of disseminated disease and are known as ecthyma gangrenosum. Other common infections include urinary tract infection in catheterized patients and chronic otitis. Malignant otitis externa, a severe external ear infection, which can potentially invade through the cranial bones and nerves, is seen primarily in the elderly and in diabetics. Other complications are uncommonly a result of *Pseudomonas* bacteremia, such as endocarditis, meningitis, and bone and joint infections.

Approach to Suspected *Pseudomonas* Patient

Definitions

Periauricular: Around the external ear.

Erythrocyte sedimentation rate (ESR): A measure of the time it takes for red blood cells to settle, which is a nonspecific measure of inflammation.

Ecthyma gangrenosum: Pustular skin lesions that later become necrotic ulcers and can lead to gangrene.

Objectives

1. Know the structural and physiologic characteristics of *Pseudomonas aeruginosa.*
2. Know the virulence factors associated with *Pseudomonas aeruginosa.*

Discussion

Characteristics of *Pseudomonas* Species

Pseudomonas species is a **ubiquitous, aerobic gram-negative bacillus.** At least 10 species are included in the genus that can cause disease in humans. Some of the closely related organisms have been transferred to their own genus, such as *Burkholderia cepacia,* formerly *Pseudomonas cepacia. P. aeruginosa* **is the most common cause of human infections.** It is motile as a result of the presence of **polar flagellae.** It is found commonly in the environment and has a predilection for **moist areas.** Reservoirs in nature include soil, vegetation, and water. **Reservoirs in a hospital include sinks, toilets, mops, respiratory therapy, and dialysis equipment.** It exhibits **intrinsic resistance** to many **antibiotics and disinfectants.** It has minimal growth requirements and can be easily cultured on many media in a wide range of temperatures. It has multiple virulence factors. *Pseudomonas* adheres to host cells by pili and non-pili adhesins. It produces a **polysaccharide capsule** that allows the organism to adhere to epithelial cells, inhibits phagocytosis, and confers protection against antibiotic activity. Patients with **cystic fibrosis** are more likely to be infected with a strain whose colony appears **mucoid** because of the presence of the **capsule.**

Pseudomonas produces **multiple toxins and enzymes,** which contribute to its virulence.

Its **lipopolysaccharide endotoxin and exotoxin A** appear to cause most of the systemic manifestations of *Pseudomonas* disease. **Exotoxin A blocks protein synthesis** in host cells, causing direct **cytotoxicity.** It mediates systemic toxic effects as well. It is similar in function to diphtheria toxin but is structurally and immunologically distinct. **Endotoxin** contributes to the development of many of the symptoms and signs of **sepsis,** including fever, leukocytosis, and hypotension.

Antibiotic resistance is another important aspect of its virulence. It is **intrinsically resistant to numerous antibiotics** and has acquired resistance to others through various means. The **polysaccharide capsule prevents the penetration of many antibiotics** into *Pseudomonas.* Penetration of antibiotic into the *Pseudomonas* cell is usually through pores in the outer membrane. **Mutation of these porin proteins** appears to be a primary mechanism of its antibiotic resistance. **Multidrug efflux pumps and β-lactamase production** also contribute to the antibiotic resistance that so frequently complicates the treatment of *Pseudomonas* infections.

Some *P. aeruginosa* strains produce a diffusable pigment: **pyocyanin,** which gives the colonies **a blue color;** fluorescein, which gives them a **yellow color; or pyorubin,** which gives them a red-brown color. **Pyocyanin** also seems to aid in the virulence of the organism by stimulating an inflammatory response and by producing toxic oxygen radicals.

Diagnosis

Diagnosis of malignant otitis externa is by the common clinical features of otorrhea, painful edematous ear canal with a purulent discharge. Culture of the discharge from the internal ear grows *P. aeruginosa* in most cases. *P. aeruginosa* grows readily on routine laboratory media. Preliminary identification can be made by **colony morphology** particularly if **typical green pigment** is produced. *P. aeruginosa* appears as a clear to dark colony on MacConkey agar, indicating that it **does not ferment lactose.** Colonies of *P. aeruginosa* are β-hemolytic and dark colored, as a result of pigment production and blood agar media. The organisms are motile, and therefore colonies appear spread. It does not ferment glucose, is oxidase positive, and is therefore not a part of the Enterobacteriaceae family, but is considered a **nonfermenter.** *P. aeruginosa* can be distinguished from some of the other closely related species by its ability to grow at a wide range of temperatures, up to as high as 42°C. The colonies also have a distinct odor, sometimes considered a grape-like odor. Confirmatory identification can be made by numerous commercially available identification systems.

Treatment and Prevention

Treatment of malignant otitis externa includes **surgery** to remove necrotic tissue and pus **and appropriate antibiotics. Treatment with two antibiotics** to which the organism is susceptible is optimal. *P. aeruginosa* is usually inherently resistant to multiple antibiotics. Most are susceptible to the **antipseudomonal penicillins,** such as piperacillin and ticarcillin and to the newer **fluoroquinolones** as well as the **aminoglycosides.** Imipenem is often reserved for treatment of infections caused by drug-resistant strains.

Comprehension Questions

[18.1] A severely burned firefighter develops a rapidly disseminating bacterial infection while hospitalized. "Green pus" is noted in the burned tissue and cultures of both the tissue and blood yield small oxidase-positive gram-negative rods. Which of the following statements most accurately conveys information about this organism?

    A. Endotoxin is the only virulence factor known to be produced by these bacteria.

    B. Humans are the only known reservoir hosts for these bacteria.

    C. The bacteria are difficult to culture because they have numerous growth requirements.

    D. These are among the most antibiotic resistant of all clinically relevant bacteria.

    E. These highly motile bacteria can "swarm" over the surface of culture media.

[18.2] The fluoroquinolone resistance seen with increasing frequency in *Pseudomonas aeruginosa* infections is best explained by which of the following mechanisms?

A. Changes in the structure or composition of the cell envelope that make it more difficult for the antibiotic to gain entrance
B. Enzymatic cleavage of the antibiotic molecule
C. Inactivation of the antibiotic by enzymatic acetylation
D. Overproduction of the cellular target that the antibiotic attacks
E. Removal of the antibiotic from the cell interior by a membrane pump

[18.3] An aerobic, oxidase positive organism is isolated from the sputum of a 12-year-old cystic fibrosis patient with pneumonia and lung abscesses. On culture the organisms have a "fruity" odor and form greenish colonies. The etiologic agent of the respiratory tract infection is most likely to be which of the following?

A. *Chlamydia pneumoniae*
B. *Klebsiella pneumoniae*
C. *Pseudomonas aeruginosa*
D. *Serratia marcescens*
E. *Streptococcus pneumoniae*

Answers

[18.1]   **D.** *Pseudomonas aeruginosa* is an obligate aerobe that grows on many types of culture media, sometimes producing a sweet or grape-like odor. It often produces a nonfluorescent bluish pigment (pyocyanin) which diffuses into agar or pus fluids. Many strains also produce a fluorescent pigment (pyoverdin), which gives a greenish color. One of the most significant problems with *Pseudomonas* infections is the high level of natural resistance to many antimicrobials that this widespread environmental opportunist exhibits.

[18.2]   **E.** Clinically significant infections with *P. aeruginosa* should not be treated with single-drug therapy, because the bacteria can develop resistance when single drugs are employed. The newer quinolones, including ciprofloxacin, are active against *Pseudomonas.* Quinolones inhibit bacterial DNA synthesis by blocking DNA gyrase. The fluorinated forms of ciprofloxacin and norfloxacin have low toxicity and greater antibacterial activity than the earlier forms. Plasmids code for enzymes that determine the active transport of various antimicrobials across the cell membrane.

[18.3]   **C.** All of the options are potential etiological agents for pneumonias in humans. The laboratory descriptions of the organism best fits *Pseudomonas aeruginosa* (also see the answer for Question 18.1).

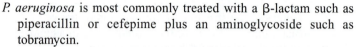

MICROBIOLOGY PEARLS

 ❖ *P. aeruginosa* is most commonly treated with a β-lactam such as piperacillin or cefepime plus an aminoglycoside such as tobramycin.

 ❖ *P. aeruginosa* is an opportunistic pathogen that is most often found in hospital environments as a source of nosocomial infection.

 ❖ *P. aeruginosa* is a nonfermentative gram-negative bacilli that is oxidase positive.

REFERENCES

Murray PR, Rosenthal KS, Kobayashi GS, Pfaller MA. Pseudomonas and related organisms. In: Murray PR, Rosenthal KS, Kobayashi GS, Pfaller MA. Medical microbiology, 4th ed. St. Louis: Mosby, 2002:297–304.

Sparling PF, Handsfield HH. Pseudomonas aeruginosa. In: Mandell GL, Bennett JE, Dolin R, eds. Principles and practice of infectious diseases, 5th ed. Philadelphia: Churchill Livingstone, 2000:2310–27.

A 48-year-old man presents to the emergency room with two days of crampy abdominal pain, nausea, vomiting, diarrhea, and fever. He has not had any blood in his stool. He denies contact with anyone with similar symptoms recently. He has not eaten any raw or unprocessed foods recently. The only food that he did not prepare himself in the past week was a breakfast of eggs "sunny-side up" and bacon that he had at a diner the day before his symptoms started. On examination, he is tired appearing; his temperature is 37.7°C (99.9°F); and his heart rate is 95 beats per minute (BPM) while he is lying down, but it increases to 120 BPM when he sits up. His blood pressure is 145/85 mm Hg while lying down and 110/60 mmHg when sitting. The physician interprets this as a positive "tilt test," indicating significant volume depletion. His mucous membranes appear dry. His abdominal exam is notable for diffuse tenderness but no palpable masses, rebound, or guarding. A rectal exam reveals only heme-negative watery stool.

◆ **What is the most likely etiologic agent of this infection?**

◆ **What are the most common sources of human infections with this organism?**

ANSWERS TO CASE 19: *Salmonella* and *Shigella*

Summary: A 48-year-old man with acute gastroenteritis has fever, a positive tilt test, abdominal pain, and diarrhea after eating eggs 1 day before.

◆ **Most likely etiology of infection:** *Salmonella.*

◆ **Most common sources of infection:** undercooked poultry, eggs, dairy products, or foods prepared on contaminated work surfaces.

CLINICAL CORRELATION

This individual has the acute onset of diarrhea and vomiting. The first priorities as with any patient are the ABC's: airway, breathing, circulation. Circulatory status is assessed by monitoring the pulse rate and blood pressure, which may be normal at rest, but abnormal on changing of position. This patient had a rise in 10 BPM heart rate from the lying to the sitting position, and a fall of 10 mmHg of blood pressure. This constitutes a **positive tilt test** and may indicate a volume depletion of 10–25 percent. Thus, the first therapeutic goal would be volume repletion, such as with intravenous normal saline.

In humans, most cases of nontyphoidal *Salmonella* result from ingesting contaminated food products. Poultry, eggs, dairy products, or other foods prepared on contaminated work surfaces are the most common sources. Fecal-oral spread is common among children. Live animals, especially exotic pets such as reptiles, have also been identified as sources of infection. Host gastric acid is a primary defense against the organism, and conditions or medications that reduce gastric acidity may predispose to infection. The primary site of invasion of *Salmonella* is the M (microfold) cells in the Peyer's patches of the distal ileum. M cells internalize and transfer foreign antigens from the intestinal lumen to macrophages and leukocyte. The infection can then spread to adjacent cells and lymphoid tissue. Host inflammatory responses usually limit the infection to the gastrointestinal (GI) tract, but bacteremia can occur. Bacteremia is more common in the children, elderly patients, or those with immune deficiencies, such as AIDS. Gastroenteritis is the most common clinical manifestation of *Salmonella* infection. Nausea, vomiting, nonbloody diarrhea, fever, and abdominal cramps starting 8–48 hours after ingestion of contaminated food are typical. The illness is generally self-limited and will last from 2 to 7 days.

Enteric fever, or typhoid fever, is a more severe form of gastroenteritis with systemic symptoms that are caused by either *S. typhi* or *S. paratyphi.* Symptoms include chills, headache, anorexia, weakness, and muscle aches; and later fever, lymphadenopathy, and hepatosplenomegaly; and in a third of patients a maculopapular rash (rose spots). Symptoms persist for a longer period of time than nontyphoidal gastroenteritis as does the carrier state in a small percentage of infected patients.

Gastroenteritis caused by *Salmonella* can mimic the signs and symptoms of other forms of infections such as *Shigella*. Infection with *Shigella* produces predominantly diarrhea, sometimes grossly bloody as a result of invasion of the mucosa. The infection is also usually self-limited; however, dehydration can occur if diarrhea is severe.

Approach to Suspected *Salmonella* & *Shigella* Infection

Definitions

Rose spots: Papular rash usually on the lower trunk leaving a darkening of the skin, characteristic of typhoid fever.

Fecal leukocytes: White blood cells found in the stool, nonspecific finding of an invasive process.

Hepatosplenomegaly: Enlargement of both the liver and the spleen which can be a feature of many diseases, including typhoid fever.

Objectives

1. Know the structure, characteristics, and clinical diseases associated with *Salmonella*.
2. Know the virulence, epidemiology, and pathogenesis of *Salmonella* infections.
3. Know the structure, characteristics, and clinical diseases associated with *Shigella*.
4. Know the virulence, epidemiology, and pathogenesis of *Shigella* infections.

Discussion

Characteristics of *Salmonella* and *Shigella*

Salmonella are **motile, facultative anaerobic, nonspore-forming, gram-negative bacilli** that are part of the family Enterobacteriaceae. The genus *Salmonella* consists of more than 2400 serotypes capable of infecting almost all animal species. However, *S. typhi* and *S. paratyphi* only colonize humans. *Salmonella* is **protected from phagocytic destruction** by two mechanisms: an **acid tolerance response gene,** which protects it both from gastric acid and from the acidic pH of the phagosome, and *Salmonella*-**secreted invasion proteins (Sips or Ssps).** These rearrange M cell actin, resulting in membranes that surround and engulf the *Salmonella* and enable intracellular replication of the pathogen with subsequent host cell death.

Shigella is a **nonmotile gram-negative bacilli** that is also part of the family Enterobacteriaceae. There are 40 serotypes of *Shigella* that are divided into four groups or species, based on biochemical reactivity. *S. dysenteriae* is group A, *S. flexneri* is group B, *S. boydii* is group C, and *S. sonnei* is group D. Virulence mechanisms of *Shigella* include their ability to **invade the intestinal mucosa**

and production of shiga toxin, which acts to destroy the intestinal mucosa once the organism has invaded the tissue. Some strains of *E. coli* are closely related to *Shigella* species and are also capable of producing shiga toxin.

Diagnosis

The diagnosis of gastroenteritis is based on the patient's age, risk factors, exposures, and symptoms. **Collection of stool and blood cultures,** if fever and other systemic symptoms are present, is necessary for the definitive diagnosis. A direct exam for **fecal leukocytes and occult blood** may initially help narrow down the differential diagnosis. For example, blood in the stools usually indicates invasive bacterial infection. In cases of bacterial gastroenteritis, final diagnosis is made by culture of the stool for enteric pathogens such as *Campylobacter, Shigella,* and *Salmonella.* Although culture of *Campylobacter* requires specialized media and incubation conditions, both *Salmonella* and *Shigella* grow rapidly on routine microbiological media. Because of the fact that stool contains many organisms that are normal flora, stools are also cultured onto selective media to aid in more rapid diagnosis.

Both *Salmonella* and *Shigella* are nonlactose fermenters that appear as clear colonies on MacConkey agar. The use of a medium that contains an indicator for production of H_2S helps differentiate the two genera. *Shigella* **does not produce H_2S and appears as clear or green colonies on a media such as Hektoen enteric (HE) agar,** whereas *Salmonella* appears black as a result of production of H_2S. This is only presumptive and further biochemical testing needs to be performed because other organisms also produce black colonies on HE agar. The diagnosis of *Shigella* can also be made by **testing for Shiga toxin** directly in the stool. This cannot differentiate *Shigella* from the **enterohemorrhagic *E. coli*** that also produce **shiga toxin** and are associated with **hemolytic uremic syndrome.**

Treatment and Prevention

Nontyphoid *Salmonella* gastroenteritis is usually not treated because it is a self-limited disease, and antibiotics have not been shown to alter the course of the infection. Primary treatment should be supportive including fluid replacement if necessary. **Antibiotic treatment is recommended for treatment of bacteremia, long-term carriers, or typhoid fever.** Amoxicillin, sulfamethoxazole and trimethoprim (SMX-TMP), or, in areas where antibiotic resistant strains are prevalent (India, Asia and Africa), quinolones can be used. The specific choice of antimicrobial agent should be based on susceptibility testing of the patient's isolate.

In the case of infection caused by *Shigella,* **antibiotic therapy has been shown to be useful,** especially in the prevention of person-to-person spread of the disease. **Quinolones** can also be used to treat, although *Shigella* therapy should be based on antimicrobial susceptibility testing of the isolate.

Prevention of disease caused by enteric pathogens is based on control of the contaminated source in the environment and good personal hygiene. The thorough cooking of poultry and cooking eggs until the yolk is hard can kill *Salmonella* and prevent infection. A vaccine does exist for prevention of typhoid fever, which is useful for travelers to endemic areas of the world. The efficacy of the vaccine is thought to be between 50 and 80 percent.

Comprehension Questions

[19.1] In which of the following sites is *Salmonella typhi* most likely to be found during the carrier state?

A. Blood
B. Gallbladder
C. Kidney
D. Liver
E. Spleen

[19.2] A 4-year-old has fever and diarrhea. Blood culture grows a gram-negative rod. This is most likely to be which of the following?

A. Group B *Streptococcus*
B. *Listeria* species
C. *Salmonella*
D. *Shigella*

[19.3] Which of the following is a frequent cause of osteomyelitis in patients with sickle cell anemia?

A. Group A *Streptococcus*
B. Group B *Streptococcus*
C. *Salmonella* species
D. *Streptococcus pneumoniae*

[19.4] Which of the following is mismatched?

A. Ecthyma gangrenosum – *Pseudomonas aeruginosa*
B. Halophilic – *Salmonella typhi*
C. K1 antigen – neonatal meningitis caused by *E. coli*
D. Red pigment – *Serratia marcescens*
E. Severe dehydration – *Vibrio cholerae*

Answers

[19.1] **B.** The feces of persons who have unsuspected subclinical disease or are carriers is a more important source of contamination than frank clinical cases that are promptly isolated. The high incidence of *Salmonellae* in commercially prepared chickens has been widely publicized, possibly related to the use of animal feeds containing antimicrobial drugs that favor the proliferation of drug-resistant *Salmonellae* and their potential transmission to humans. Permanent carriers usually harbor the organisms in the gallbladder or biliary tract and, rarely, in the intestine or urinary tract.

[19.2] **C.** Enterocolitis is the most common manifestation of *Salmonella* infection. In the United States, *S. typhimurium* and *S. enteritidis* are prominent, but enterocolitis may be caused by more than 1400 strains of *Salmonella*. Bacteremia is rare (2–4%) except in immunodeficient persons. Stool cultures may remain positive for *Salmonella* weeks after clinical recovery. *Streptococci* and *Listeria* stain gram-positive, and *Shigella* organisms rarely, if ever, enter the blood stream from the intestines.

[19.3] **C.** Hematogenous infections account for about 20 percent of cases of osteomyelitis and primarily affect children, in whom the long bones are infected. More than 95 percent of these cases are caused by a single organism, with *S. aureus* accounting for 50 percent of the isolates. Group B *Streptococci* and *E. coli* are common during the newborn period and group A *Streptococci* and *Haemophilus influenzae* in early childhood. *Salmonella* species and *S. aureus* are major causes of long-bone osteomyelitis complicating sickle-cell anemia and other hemoglobinopathies. Septic arthritis may be encountered in sickle cell disease with multiple joints infected. Joint infection may result from spread of contiguous osteomyelitis areas. *Salmonella* infection is seen more often in osteomyelitis than in septic arthritis.

[19.4] **B.** Organisms requiring high salt concentrations are called halophilic. Usually, this refers to microorganisms that are capable of living or surviving in an ocean or salt water area. *Vibrios* are especially well known for this ability. *Salmonella typhi* (typhoid fever) multiply in intestinal lymphoid tissue and are excreted in stools. They are hardy survivors in water sources, but they do not survive in halophilic conditions as well as *Vibrios*.

MICROBIOLOGY PEARLS

❖ *Shigella* is a common cause of gastroenteritis, which can be bloody as a result of the ability of the organism to invade the mucosa. Because of the low inoculum required for infection, person-to-person transmission may occur in close contacts.

❖ *Salmonella* nontyphi is associated with a self-limited diarrhea associated with ingestion of contaminated food products such as undercooked eggs.

❖ *Salmonella* and *Shigella* are nonlactose fermenters that are differentiated in the laboratory by production of H_2S; the appearance of black colonies on Hektoen enteric agar result from *Salmonella* species.

REFERENCES

Dupont HL. Shigella species (bacillary dysentery) In: Mandell GL, Bennett JE, Dolin R, eds. Principles and practice of infectious diseases, 5th ed. Philadelphia: Churchill Livingstone, 2000:2363–69.

Mandell GL, Bennett, JE, Dolin, R eds. Principles and Practice of Infectious Disease. 5th ed. Philadelphia: Churchill Livingstone, 2000:2344–63.

Miller SI, Pegues DA. *Salmonella species,* including *salmonella typhi.* In: Mandell GL, Bennett JE, Dolin R, eds. Principles and practice of infectious diseases, 5th ed. Philadelphia: Churchill Livingstone, 2000.

Murray PR, Rosenthal KS, Kobayashi GS, Pfaller MA. Enterobacteriaceae. In: Murray PR, Rosenthal KS, Kobayashi GS, Pfaller MA. Medical microbiology, 4th ed. St. Louis: Mosby, 2002:266–80.

A 59-year-old man with emphysema secondary to a 50-pack-year smoking history presents with a fever, chills, chest pain, and cough. He had a "cold" with mild cough and congestion for about 3 days but then had the abrupt onset of more severe symptoms. His temperature has been as high as 39.4°C (103°F), and he's had shaking chills. His cough is productive of sputum that looks like "rust." When he coughs or takes a deep breath, he gets a sharp, stabbing pain in his left lower chest. He has been taking numerous over-the-counter cold medications without relief and has had to use his ipratropium inhaler more often than usual. On examination, he is quite ill appearing. His temperature is 38.8°C (101.9°F), pulse is 110 beats per minute, blood pressure 110/60 mmHg, and respiratory rate is 28 breaths per minute. His pulmonary examination is significant for the presence of crackles and rhonchi in the left lower fields and expiratory wheezing heard in all other fields. His heart is tachycardic but otherwise normal on auscultation. The remainder of his examination is normal. His white blood cell count is markedly elevated. An electrocardiogram is normal. A chest x-ray shows a dense infiltration of the left lower lobe along with a pleural effusion on the left side.

◆ **What would you expect to see on Gram stain of a sputum sample?**

◆ **What is the likely reservoir from which this patient's pneumonia occurred?**

ANSWERS TO CASE 20: *Streptococcus*

Summary: A 59-year-old male complains of fever and cough, with "rust" colored sputum. A chest x-ray shows a dense infiltration of the left lower lobe and a left pleural effusion.

◆ **Most likely Gram stain findings:** multiple polymorphonuclear leukocytes (PMNs) and encapsulated gram-positive cocci in pairs and short chains.

◆ **Likely reservoir of this infection:** colonization of the upper airway (naso- or oropharynx) and aspiration into the lower airways.

CLINICAL CORRELATION

Streptococci cause a wide range of diseases from localized skin and soft tissue infections to systemic infections such as necrotizing fasciitis, endocarditis, and arthritis. *Streptococcus pyogenes* is commonly associated with pharyngitis and its sequelae of rheumatic fever and glomerulonephritis, in addition to the skin and soft-tissue infections previously mentioned. *Streptococcus agalactiae* is most well known for its association with neonatal meningitis following vaginal colonization of the pregnant women.

    Streptococcus pneumoniae is a cause of otitis media, sinusitis, bronchitis, pneumonia, and meningitis. *Streptococcus pneumoniae* (pneumococcus) is the most frequent cause of bacterial pneumonia, otitis, and meningitis. It commonly colonizes the upper airways in humans, more frequently in children than adults. Pneumococcal diseases occur when organisms spread from the site of colonization to a distant, susceptible site. Pneumonia occurs when pneumococcus is aspirated into the distal airways and multiplies in the alveoli. Pneumococcal pneumonia typically follows a milder upper respiratory infection. Symptoms of pneumococcal pneumonia include cough, fever, chills, and shortness of breath. Patients may also have increased white blood cells and anemia. A common complication of pneumococcal pneumonia is pleural effusion, which occurs in up to 40 percent of patients. Meningitis either follows sinusitis or otitis or occurs as a result of bacteremic spread of the organisms. Patients that are immunocompromised, elderly, or have underlying heart or lung disease, as well as those that are asplenic, are at higher risk than normal for developing serious disease with *S. pneumoniae.*

Approach to Suspected Pneumococcus Infection

Definitions

Rhonchi: A vibration of the chest wall that can be felt with the hand and sounds like a dull roaring or murmuring.

Cytokines: Proteins that are produced by leukocytes that act as mediators of a further inflammatory response.

Objectives

1. Know the structure and physiologic features common to the genus *Streptococcus*.
2. Know the virulence factors, epidemiology, and diseases associated with specific *Streptococcus* species.

Discussion

Characteristics of *Streptococcus*

The genus *Streptococcus* contains multiple species that are differentiated either by their **cell wall carbohydrate group antigen,** their **hemolysis on blood agar,** or their **biochemical reactivity.** Not all *Streptococci,* including *S. pneumoniae,* possess a carbohydrate cell wall antigen. *Streptococci* are **facultative anaerobes** that require CO_2 for growth. *Streptococci* are **gram-positive cocci that form either pairs or chains, whereas *S. pneumoniae* are elongated, lancet shaped, gram-positive cocci,** and are usually in pairs or short chains.

Virulent strains of pneumococcus are **encapsulated by a polysaccharide capsule.** Strains that are unencapsulated are easily cleared by host defenses. Colonization is facilitated by binding of the pneumococcus to epithelial cells by surface protein adhesins, producing **secretory IgA protease,** which prevents host immunoglobulin A from binding to it and producing **pneumolysin,** which **destroys phagocytic and ciliated epithelial cells** by creating pores in their cell membranes. Phagocytosis is limited by the **antiphagocytic nature of the polysaccharide capsule** and by the pneumolysin's inhibition of the oxidative burst required for intracellular killing. Much of the tissue damage caused by pneumococcal infections is mediated by the inflammatory response of host defense systems. The complement system is activated by teichoic acid, peptidoglycan fragments, and pneumolysin. Cytokine production is stimulated, causing more inflammatory cells to migrate to the site of infection. **Hydrogen peroxide** is produced by pneumococcus, which **causes tissue damage** via reactive oxygen intermediates.

Antibiotic resistance in pneumococcus is an increasing problem. **Penicillin resistance** has developed, primarily via mutations in penicillin-binding proteins in the cell wall. This is a consequence of mutations in the cellular DNA and from acquisition of DNA from both other pneumococci and other bacteria with which pneumococcus comes in contact. **Efflux pumps** also confer some degree of resistance to antibiotics.

Diagnosis

Diagnosis of pneumococcal pneumonia is made based on clinical signs and symptoms, chest x-ray demonstrating infiltration of a single lobe, and sputum Gram stain with many PNMs and gram-positive cocci in pairs and chains. Confirmation of the diagnosis can be made by culturing the organisms from the sputum and/or blood. *S. pneumoniae* grows rapidly on routine laboratory media including blood and chocolate agar. Colonies on blood agar demonstrate **α-hemolysis (green color)** and may be slightly to extremely **mucoid** because of their polysaccharide capsule. Colonies are differentiated from viridans streptococci by **sensitivity to optochin and bile solubility.** Although optochin susceptibility is considered definitive, the addition of bile to a colony will identify the organism as *S. pneumoniae* if the colony lyses and disappears within a few minutes.

More rapid diagnosis of pneumococcal pneumonia can be made using the urinary antigen test.

Treatment and Prevention

Treatment of uncomplicated pneumonia is usually with either a **quinolone** or a **macrolide** such as azithromycin. Complicated or disseminated pneumococcal disease is usually treated with **penicillin or cefotaxime** depending on susceptibility of the isolate to penicillin. Treatment of the other streptococcal species is usually with penicillin, but in serious infections should be based on the individual isolate susceptibility. Adult and pediatric **vaccines directed against pneumococcal capsular antigens** are available, and current guidelines recommend universal vaccination of children, persons over the age of 65, and others at high risk for pneumonia, such as persons with diabetes or chronic lung disease.

Comprehension Questions

[20.1] A newborn has a temperature of 39.4°C (103°F). Blood culture grows gram-positive cocci in chains. This is most likely to be which of the following?

    A. Group A *Streptococci (Streptococcus pyogenes)*
    B. Group B *Streptococci (Streptococcus agalactiae)*
    C. *Salmonella* species
    D. *Streptococcus pneumoniae*

[20.2] A 3-year-old is diagnosed with bacterial meningitis. Cerebrospinal fluid grows out gram-positive cocci in short chains and diplococci. This is most likely to be which of the following?

    A. Group B *Streptococci*
    B. *Salmonella*
    C. *Staphylococcus aureus*
    D. *Streptococcus pneumoniae*

[20.3] Which of the following is the primary virulence factor of *Streptococcus pneumoniae?*

    A. Bile solubility
    B. Optochin production
    C. Pili
    D. Polypeptide capsule
    E. Polysaccharide capsule

[20.4] Which of the following is true regarding meningitis with *Streptococcus pneumoniae?*

    A. Cephalosporins are always effective.
    B. One desires a concentration of antibiotics in the cerebral spinal fluid 10 times the minimal inhibition concentration.
    C. Penicillin is always effective.
    D. Resistance is not increasing in *Streptococcus pneumoniae.*

Answers

[20.1]   **B.** Most human infections caused by *Streptococci* involve the group A organisms *(Streptococcus pyogenes)*. The group B *Streptococci* are members of the female genital tract and are important causes of neonatal sepsis and meningitis. They are usually beta-hemolytic (similar to group A), hydrolyze hippurate and give a positive response in the so-called CAMP test (Christie, Atkins, Munch-Peterson). Detection of the infection and prompt antimicrobial treatment is necessary because the infections may become life-threatening. *Streptococcus pneumoniae* organisms are important in meningitis cases in young children, but are more frequently seen as diplococci forms rather than long chains.

[20.2]   **D.** Streptococcus *pneumoniae* is responsible for 10–20 percent of meningitis cases in children ages 1 month to 15 years. *Neisseria meningitidis* range from 25–40 percent, whereas *Haemophilus influenzae* may be involved in 40–60 percent. Group A and B *Streptococci* appear to be involved only 2–4 percent of the time. Under the conditions described above, *Streptococcus pneumoniae* would be the most likely etiologic agent.

[20.3]   **E.** Bile solubility and optochin sensitivity are presumptive identification tests that identify *Streptococcus pneumoniae* from other alpha-hemolytic *Streptococci*. The polysaccharide capsule occurs in dozens of antigenic types, but types 1–8 are responsible for about 75 percent of the cases of pneumococcal pneumonia. Vaccines are available that give approximately 90 percent protection and usually contain 23 types of carbohydrates for the U.S.-licensed preparation.

[20.4] **B.** Because pneumococci are sensitive to many antimicrobial drugs, early treatment usually results in rapid recovery. Antibody response (host's active immunity) seems to play a diminished role today. Penicillin G is the drug of choice, but 5–10 percent of the isolates in the United States are penicillin resistant (MIC $\geq$ 2 microgram/mL), and 20 percent are moderately resistant (0.1–1 microgram/mL). Resistance to cephalosporins, tetracycline, and erythromycin has been demonstrated, although pneumococci remain susceptible to vancomycin. In reference to penicillin therapy, one rule of thumb is to aim for a concentration of 10 times the MIC in the CSF.

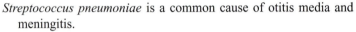

MICROBIOLOGY PEARLS

❖ *Streptococcus pneumoniae* is a common cause of otitis media and meningitis.

❖ Because of the increasing incidence of penicillin resistance of *S. pneumoniae* empiric therapy of disseminated disease is with ceftriaxone.

❖ *S. pneumoniae* is an α-hemolytic streptococci susceptible to optochin.

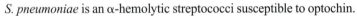

REFERENCES

Murray PR, Rosenthal KS, Kobayashi GS, Pfaller MA. Streptococcus. In: Murray PR, Rosenthal KS, Kobayashi GS, Pfaller MA. Medical microbiology, 4th ed. St. Louis: Mosby, 2002:217–39.

Musher, DM. *Streptococcus pneumoniae.* In: Mandell GL, Bennett JE, Dolin R, eds. Principles and practice of infectious diseases, 5th ed. Philadelphia: Churchill Livingstone, 2000:2128–47.

While on call on a Saturday night in July, you receive a call from the mother of a 15-year-old man who developed the acute onset of nausea, vomiting, and diarrhea shortly after returning from an outdoor party that was held at the home of a friend. At the party, a picnic lunch of hamburgers, hot dogs, potato salad, baked beans, and lemonade was served. The food was served on an outdoor picnic table, and the guests were free to eat at any time during the party. None of the food tasted spoiled or tainted. His symptoms started abruptly about an hour after he returned home, which was about 4 hours after he had eaten. He currently is unable to keep down anything. He does not have a fever and has not passed any blood in his stool or vomitus. Prior to calling you, your patient's mother spoke with the hostess of the party, who said that she had heard from three other guests who became ill with similar symptoms.

◆ **What organism is the most likely cause of this patient's illness?**

◆ **Your patient's mother requests that you call in a prescription for an antibiotic to treat the infection. What is your response?**

ANSWERS TO CASE 21: *Staphylococci*

Summary: A 15-year-old male with gastroenteritis after eating food at an outdoor picnic. Several other participants also developed similar symptoms.

◆   **Most likely organism causing this infection:** *Staphylococcus aureus.*

◆   **Response to request to treat with antibiotic:** No, the gastroenteritis is caused by a preformed toxin, not by the ingested *Staphylococci,* therefore antibiotic therapy would be of no help.

CLINICAL CORRELATION

Staphylococcus aureus is a common colonizer of the human nasopharynx and skin. Infection occurs when the normal skin barrier is disrupted by either surgery or trauma.

    S. aureus causes numerous infections, ranging from simple localized skin and soft tissue infections to disseminated disease, such as bacteremia, endocarditis, osteomyelitis, and septic arthritis. Many of the infections caused by *S. aureus* are toxin mediated, such as toxic shock syndrome, scalded skin syndrome, and gastroenteritis.

    Staphylococcal food poisoning, the second most reported cause of food poisoning in the United States, is a result of the presence of enterotoxin. Food is contaminated by a human carrier, with processed meats, custard-filled baked goods, potato salad, or ice cream being common vectors. The toxin rapidly produces nausea, vomiting, and diarrhea, usually within 2–6 hours of ingestion. Further toxin is not produced by the ingested *S. aureus,* and the disease also rapidly resolves, usually within 12–24 hours.

    Other staphylococcal species also frequently colonize human skin but can cause disease in certain situations. Although there are more than 20 other species, the majority of the species isolated are *S. epidermidis.* The most common predisposing factor for disease with *Staphylococci* not (*S. aureus*) is the presence of artificial devices in the patient such as catheters and replacement joints. *S. epidermidis* produces a slime that allows it to adhere to plastics and form a biofilm that makes it very difficult for antibiotics to penetrate.

Approach to Suspected Staphylococcal Infection

Definitions

Biofilm: Bacteria grow on an artificial surface and form a conglomerate with secreted polysaccharides and glycopeptides.

Superantigens: Antigens, most often bacterial toxins, that recruit a large number of T lymphocytes to an area.

Enterotoxins: Substances produced by bacteria that are toxic to the GI tract that cause diarrhea and/or vomiting.

Objectives

1. Know the structure, physiology, and virulence factors associated with *S. aureus* and the coagulase-negative *Staphylococci*.
2. Know the diseases caused by *Staphylococci* and the mechanisms by which *Staphylococci* develop antibiotic resistance.

Discussion

Characteristics of *Staphylococcus*

Staphylococci belong to the family **Micrococcaceae,** which includes the genus *Micrococcus* in addition to *Staphylococcus. Staphylococci* grow rapidly on multiple culture media, in a wide range of environments, including up to 10 percent sodium chloride, and in a broad range of temperatures. *Staphylococcus aureus* is a **nonmotile, nonspore forming, facultative anaerobic gram-positive coccus** that commonly colonizes healthy humans and is a frequent cause of disease. It is frequently identified as growing in **clusters or clumps.** This is a result of the effect of **bound coagulase** ("clumping factor"), which **binds fibrinogen,** converts it to insoluble fibrin, and results in aggregation. *S. aureus* **is the only *Staphylococcus* found in humans which produces coagulase;** other staphylococcal species are commonly identified as coagulase-negative *Staphylocci.*

S. aureus produces **at least five cytolytic toxins, two exfoliative toxins, eight enterotoxins,** and **toxic shock syndrome toxin.** Some of these toxins act as superantigens, which recruit host defense cells that liberate cytokines and, therefore, produce systemic effects. Heating will kill the *S. aureus* organisms, but not inactivate the **enterotoxins, because they are stable to heating at 100°C for 30 minutes** and are resistant to breakdown by gastric acids.

Of growing public health concern is the rapid spread of antibiotic resistance within *S. aureus* isolates. Almost all *S. aureus* produces penicillinase, a β-lactamase specific for penicillin. Many isolates have also acquired a gene that codes for an **altered penicillin binding protein, PBP2',** providing antibiotic resistance to semisynthetic penicillins and cephalosporins as well, including methicillin and nafcillin. Some of these genes will also be associated with resistance to non-β-lactamase antibiotics, such as quinolones and macrolides. Some *S. aureus* isolates have been identified recently with reduced sensitivity to vancomycin. The mechanism of this resistance is unknown. Genes that confer resistance can be transferred between organisms by plasmid transfer, transduction and cell-to-cell contact.

Diagnosis

The initial diagnosis of staphylococcal infection may be difficult because many of the skin and soft tissue infections mimic those of *Streptococci.* Definitive diagnosis is made by Gram stain and culture of the infected site as well as blood. *Staphylococci* are large **gram-positive cocci grouped in clusters (Figure 21-1).** *Staphylococci* grow rapidly on routine laboratory media. Their colony morphology is different from *Streptococci* in that the colonies are larger, white or yellow instead of grey. They also can be differentiated from *Streptococci* by a **positive catalase test** (reactivity with hydrogen peroxide). *S. aureus* is **β-hemolytic on blood agar medium** and is differentiated from the other *Staphylococcus* species by production of coagulase or positive latex agglutination for *Staphylococcus* **protein A.** Further confirmation of the identification of *S. aureus* is not necessary; however, many commercially available identification systems can identify the organism based on biochemical reactivity. A selective media such as mannitol salts agar, which also differentiates *S. aureus* from other staphylococcal species is available, but not often used in clinical laboratories.

Staphylococcal gastroenteritis is usually self-limited with symptoms disappearing within 12 hours, and therefore diagnosis is made clinically based on incubation period and history of others eating similar foods with same symptoms. *Staphylococcus saprophyticus* is the only other staphylococcal species that is identified as a consequence of its association with **urinary tract**

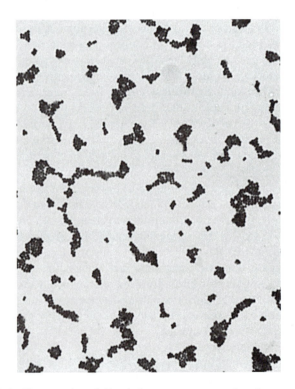

Figure 21-1. Gram stain of *Staphylococcus aureus* showing gram-positive cocci in clusters.

Reproduced, with permission, from Brooks G, Butel J, Morse S. Javetz, Melnick, and Aldelburg's Medical microbiology, 23rd ed. New York: McGraw-Hill, 2004:224.

infections in young women. _S. saprophyticus_ is differentiated from the other coagulase negative _Staphylococci_ by its susceptibility to novobiocin, which is tested by disk diffusion.

Treatment and Prevention

Treatment of local wound infections without systemic symptoms does not usually require treatment with antibiotics; however, in the cases of more complicated infections or presence of fever, antimicrobial therapy is usually warranted. Although **nafcillin** is the drug of choice for staphylococcal infections, because of the high percentage of strains that are resistant to methicillin and nafcillin, initial treatment in hospitalized patients is usually with **vancomycin** until the susceptibility results are available. Oral antibiotics, such as, rifampin and sulfamethoxazole and trimethoprim (SMX-TMP) or clindamycin can also be used dependent on the susceptibility of the isolate. **Treatment of _Staphylococcus_ non-_aureus_ is with vancomycin,** because the majority of isolates are resistant to nafcillin.

Control of _S. aureus_ involves **strict adherence to hand washing** policies, particularly in the hospital setting. The organism can easily be spread from person to person. Colonization with _S. aureus_ is usually transient; however, an attempt can be made in some situations to decolonize the nares by using intranasal mupirocin and/or the skin by using oral antistaphylococcal antibiotics in combination with topical agents.

Comprehension Questions

[21.1] A 12-year-old girl was playing soccer when she began to limp. She has pain in her right leg and right upper thigh. Her temperature is 38.9°C (102°F). X-ray of the femur reveals that the periosteum is eroded, suggestive of osteomyelitis. Blood culture yields gram-positive bacteria. The most likely etiologic agent is which of the following?

    A. _Listeria monocytogenes_
    B. _Salmonella enteritidis_
    C. _Staphylococcus aureus_
    D. _Staphylococcus saprophyticus_
    E. _Streptococcus pneumoniae_

[21.2] An outbreak of staphylococcal infection involving umbilical cords of seven newborn babies was reported in the nursery. Bacteriological survey reveals that two nurses have a large number of _Staphylococcus aureus_ in the nasopharynx. What test should be performed to determine whether these nurses may have been responsible for the outbreak?

    A. Bacteriophage typing
    B. Coagulase testing
    C. Nasopharyngeal culture on mannitol salt agar
    D. Protein A typing
    E. Serological typing

[21.3] Virulence factors of *Staphylococcus aureus* include all of the following except one. Which one is this exception?

A. Beta-lactamases
B. Coagulase
C. Enterotoxins
D. M Protein
E. Protein A

[21.4] Short incubation food poisoning, caused by ingestion of preformed enterotoxin, is caused by which bacteria listed below?

A. *Staphylococcus aureus*
B. *Staphylococcus epidermidis*
C. *Enterococcus faecalis*
D. *Streptococcus pneumoniae*
E. *Streptococcus pyogenes*

Answers

[21.1] **C.** *Staphylococci,* especially *S. epidermidis,* are normal flora of the human skin and respiratory and gastrointestinal tracts. Nasal carriage of *S. aureus,* the pathogen, occurs in 20–50 percent of humans. Abscesses are the typical lesion of *S. aureus.* From any one focus, organisms may enter the bloodstream and lymphatics to spread to other parts of the body. In osteomyelitis, the primary focus is generally in a terminal blood vessel of the metaphysis of a long bone, which may lead to necrosis of bone and chronic suppuration. *S. saprophyticus* is usually a nonpathogenic normal flora organism. *Listeria* is usually transmitted in unpasteurized dairy products, whereas *Salmonella enteritidis* is primarily intestinal. *Streptococcus pneumoniae* is primarily a respiratory pathogen, although it is an important central nervous system (CNS) pathogen in children.

[21.2] **A.** Bacterial viruses (bacteriophages or phages) can attach to separate receptors on the cell walls of various strains of *S. aureus.* Different specific receptors have been identified and used as the basis of epidemiological typing of pathogenic *S. aureus* strains. Typical cultures from the outbreak and strains obtained from personnel can be subjected to a standardized procedure using a series of bacteriophages that attack *S. aureus* strains. This procedure can readily identify the source of the outbreak organism if it came from a medical care worker.

[21.3] **D.** M proteins are virulence factors of group A *Streptococci (Streptococcus pyogenes).* All of the other listed virulence factors may be found routinely in *S. aureus* bacteria.

[21.4] **A.** Of the options given the best answer is *S. aureus,* as a result of enterotoxin production in food. None of the other strains listed produce enterotoxins that result in short-term gastroenteritis.

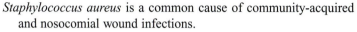

MICROBIOLOGY PEARLS

❖ *Staphylococcus aureus* is a common cause of community-acquired and nosocomial wound infections.

❖ Treatment of *S. aureus* is with nafcillin if the isolate is susceptible, or alternatively with vancomycin.

❖ *S. aureus* is differentiated from the other staphylococcal species by production of coagulase.

REFERENCES

Murray PR, Rosenthal KS, Kobayashi GS, Pfaller MA. Staphylococcus and related organisms In: Murray PR, Rosenthal KS, Kobayashi GS, Pfaller MA. Medical microbiology, 4th ed. St. Louis: Mosby, 2002:202–16.

Waldvogel, FA. *Staphylococcus aureus* (including staphylococcal toxic shock). In: Mandell GL, Bennett JE, Dolin R, eds. Principles and practice of infectious diseases, 5th ed. Philadelphia: Churchill Livingstone, 2000:2069–92.

A 20-year-old man presents for evaluation of a rash that he thinks is an allergic reaction. For the past 4 or 5 days he has had the "flu," with fever, chills headache, and body aches. He has been taking an over-the-counter flu medication without any symptomatic relief. Yesterday he developed a diffuse rash made up of red, slightly raised bumps. It covers his whole body, and he says that it must be an allergic reaction to the flu medication. He has no history of allergies and takes no other medications, and his only medical problem in the past was being treated for gonorrhea about 2 years ago. On further questioning, he denies dysuria or penile discharge. He denies any genital lesions now, but says that he had a "sore" on his penis a few months ago that never really hurt and went away on its own after a few weeks so he didn't think much about it. On exam, his vital signs are all normal. He has palpable cervical, axillary, and inguinal adenopathy. His skin has an erythematous, maculopapular eruption covering his whole body including his palms and soles of his feet. No vesicles are noted. His genital examination is normal.

◆ **What organism is the likely etiology of this disease?**

◆ **What disease and stage does this patient have?**

◆ **What microscopic examination could confirm this diagnosis?**

◆ **Which serologic tests could assist in his diagnosis?**

ANSWERS TO CASE 22: *Treponema pallidum*

Summary: A 20-year-old man has adenopathy and a macular papular rash affecting his soles and palms. He had a painless penile "sore" that spontaneously resolved.

◆ **Most likely causative organism:** *Treponema pallidum.*

◆ **Disease and stage:** The patient has syphilis, more specifically secondary syphilis.

◆ **Microscopic examination to confirm the diagnosis:** Examination by darkfield microscopy of exudates from skin lesion could confirm the diagnosis of *Treponema pallidum* infection and secondary syphilis.

◆ **Serologic tests to assist in the diagnosis:** The following serologic examinations could aid in diagnosis: Venereal Disease Research Laboratory (VDRL) and rapid plasmin reagin (RPA) tests for screening, and the fluorescent treponemal antibody-absorption (FTA-ABS), and the microhemagglutination test for *T. pallidum* (MHA-TP), which are the specific tests.

CLINICAL CORRELATION

Treponema pallidum is a gram-negative, microaerophilic spirochete that causes venereal syphilis, the third most common bacterial sexually transmitted disease in the United States. It is transmitted by contact with fluid from an ulcer containing the infectious agent either through sexual contact by penetrating intact mucous membranes or through nonsexual contact with the agent with skin that is broken or abraded. Studies estimate that transmission occurs in over half of sexual encounters where a lesion is present. *T. pallidum* infection results in multiple disease phases with distinctive clinical manifestations. Primary syphilis usually involves the formation of a painless ulcer at the site of entry of the organism, called a chancre. Chancres are highly contagious by contact and can spontaneously heal after a few weeks to a few months. Secondary syphilis develops 2–12 weeks after the primary stage and is characterized by a flulike illness, followed by a rash that typically starts on the trunk but can spread to any skin or mucous membrane surface. Without treatment, the symptoms generally resolve in 3–12 weeks. This is followed by a relatively asymptomatic period known as latency, which can last for years. Some infected persons have no further symptoms; however, some progress to tertiary syphilis, a diffuse disease with many effects on the dermatologic, musculoskeletal, cardiovascular, and central nervous systems. Currently the population most at risk is heterosexual African Americans living in urban areas.

Approach to Suspected *T. Pallidum* Infection

Definitions

Macule: Flat lesion that is not palpable, of a different color from surrounding skin and smaller than 1cm.

Microaerophilic: Organisms that can tolerate small amounts of oxygen because they contain superoxide dismutase. They use fermentation in the absence of oxygen.

Tabes dorsalis: A condition characterized by diminished vibratory, proprioceptive, pain, and temperature senses, as well as the loss of reflexes.

Argyll Robertson pupil: Constricts during accommodation but does not react to light.

Objectives

1. Be able to describe the natural history of syphilis infection.
2. Know the methods of diagnosis and treatment of syphilis.

Discussion

Characteristics of *Treponema pallidum* that Impact Transmission

Treponema pallidum is a **thin spirochete and an obligate human pathogen.** It consists of three subspecies, each of which causes disease in humans. *T. pallidum* is labile, unable to survive exposure to drying, and is very difficult to grow in culture. *T. pallidum* does not have a capsule and usually contains six axial filaments, located between the outer membrane and the peptidoglycan layer. It produces no toxins that have been currently identified. *T. pallidum* is too thin to be seen with standard microscopy with Gram stain but can be seen with **darkfield microscopy** or by staining with antitreponemal antibodies labeled with **fluorescent dyes.** *T. pallidum* is transmitted by direct contact with an infectious lesion, transfusion of infected blood, or congenital transfer. It attaches by one or both ends to host cells, although it rarely penetrates the cell. The resultant disease of syphilis occurring primarily because of the host immune response to the treponemal infection, with both humoral and cell-mediated immune systems playing a role.

Syphilis disease presents in **three different stages** with characteristics specific to each stage. **Primary syphilis** presents with a **hard, painless, broad-based chancre.** The chancre has a punched-out base and rolled up edges, sometimes expelling a serous exudate. This primary lesion presents 3–6 weeks after the initial contact with the infectious agent. It typically resolves in 4–6 weeks and does not leave scar tissue. **Secondary syphilis** presents with a symmetrical widely distributed macular rash. The rash can infect the mucous membranes including the cervix, throat, and mouth. It may also appear on the **palms and soles** of the patient, an important clinical finding because there are few diseases that present with a rash on palms and soles. Patchy hair loss is also seen, typically causing the eyebrows to fall out. There is usually a low-grade fever, weight loss, and general malaise. **Condyloma latum** is a **painless, wart-like lesion** on the scrotum or vulva that may also be present during this stage (Figure 22-1). **Secondary syphilis** occurs 6 weeks after the lesion of primary syphilis has healed. It is during the secondary stage where syphilis is considered to be most infectious.

After secondary syphilis, there is a **latent period** where the disease is not infectious, although the patient is still seropositive. This stage can range from 2 years to several decades. **Tertiary syphilis** can present with personality

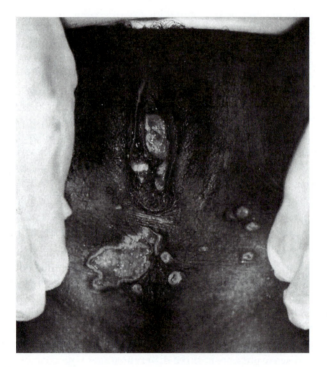

Figure 22-1. Genital condylomata lata of secondary syphilis.

Reproduced, with permission, from Cunningham FG et al. William's Obstetrics, 21st ed. New York: McGraw-Hill, 2001:1487.

changes, blindness, paresis, gummas, **Argyll Robertson pupils** and **tabes dorsalis**. **Gummas** are granulomatous lesions of the skin and bone which are necrotic and fibrotic. Tabes dorsalis is characterized by diminished vibratory, proprioceptive, pain, and temperature sense, as well as the loss of deep tendon reflexes. It is the damage to the dorsal roots and ganglia which cause the loss of reflexes, pain, and temperature sense, while the loss of proprioception and vibratory sense are because of the posterior column involvement. The Argyll Robertson pupil constricts during accommodation but does not react to light.

Diagnosis

The **diagnosis of syphilis** can be made by **identification of spirochetes by darkfield microscopy** from a chancre or skin lesion in the secondary stage; however, most syphilis is diagnosed by serologic studies. The **VDRL** and **RPR** are **nonspecific tests** of host production of anticardiolipin antibody. These will be positive in about 80 percent of cases of primary and all secondary stages of syphilis. More specific tests, the MHA-TP and FTA-ABS, are used for confirmation.

There are several laboratory tests that may be used to detect syphilis. The nontreponemal tests detect the presence of antibodies to cardiolipin and lecithin. These tests include the VDRL and RPR. False positive VDRLs may be encountered in patients with lupus, infectious mononucleosis, hepatitis A, the antiphospholipid antibody syndrome, leprosy, malaria, and occasionally pregnancy. False negative RPR and VDRLs may be obtained early in the disease. The treponemal tests detect the presence of antibodies to *Treponema pallidum*. These tests are the FTA-ABS and the MHA-TP.

Treatment and Prevention

The drug of choice for the treatment of syphilis is **benzathine penicillin.** Patients who are allergic to penicillin are treated with erythromycin and doxycycline. However, doxycycline is contraindicated in patients who are pregnant, because it can cross the placenta and is toxic to the fetus. Universal precautions used in the clinical setting are adequate to prevent the transmission of syphilis. Outside of the clinical setting, safe sex should be practiced to prevent the transmission through sexual contact. Currently, there is no vaccine available for the prevention of *T. pallidum* infection.

Comprehension Questions

[22.1] A 21-year-old Asian woman visits her obstetrician and is later diagnosed with secondary syphilis. On further questioning, it is determined she is allergic to penicillin. Because *Treponema pallidum* is known to cross the placenta, treatment is started immediately. Which antibiotic would be most appropriate in this situation?

A. Tetracycline
B. Ceftriaxone
C. Penicillin G
D. Doxycycline
E. Erythromycin

[22.2] A 27-year-old white man presents to his family doctor complaining of being tired all the time and having a slight fever for the past two weeks. He recently returned from a trip to Las Vegas, where he indulged in some of the infamous nightlife. His physical exam is unremarkable except for a macular rash over his trunk and on the palms of his hands. There are no lesions or ulcers on the penis. What organism is causing this man's illness?

A. *Chlamydia trachomatis*
B. *Neisseria gonorrhea*
C. *Treponema pallidum*
D. *Borrelia burgdorferi*
E. *Rickettsia rickettsii*

[22.3] A sample is taken from a vulvar ulcer in a 25-year-old sexually active African American female. The organism is a weakly staining gram-negative, microaerophilic organism. When attempting to view a smear under a microscope, no organisms are seen. Which method of visualization is most appropriate in this setting?

A. Ziehl-Neelsen stain
B. India ink preparation
C. Congo red stain
D. Darkfield microscopy
E. Giemsa stain

[22.4] A third-year medical student is on his first rotation in internal medicine. His attending physician points out that there are several tests that are used to diagnose syphilis. Which test is most specific for the detection of syphilis?

A. Rapid plasmin reagin (RPR)
B. Fluorescent treponemal antibody-absorption (FTA-ABS)
C. Venereal Disease Research Laboratory (VDRL)
D. Ziehl-Neelsen stain
E. Aerobic and anaerobic blood cultures

[22.5] A 28-year-old sexually active woman presents for her annual well-woman exam. She at times has a low-grade fever and lately has noticed a rash on her face, mainly on the cheeks. She is saddened to learn she has a positive VDRL test for syphilis. However, she is asymptomatic for syphilis and is in a monogamous relationship with her husband who has not had any other sexual contacts. Which of the following is the most likely reason for the positive syphilis test?

A. She has secondary syphilis.
B. She has HIV, altering her immune reaction.
C. She had exposure to syphilis earlier this week.
D. She has systemic lupus erythematosus (SLE).
E. She has chlamydia.

Answers

[22.1] **E.** erythromycin and doxycycline are used when allergy to penicillin is present. Doxycycline is contraindicated in pregnant women because it crosses the placenta and is toxic to the fetus. Ceftriaxone and tetracycline are not used for the treatment of syphilis. Penicillin is contraindicated because of the patient's allergies.

[22.2] **C.** *Treponema pallidum* is usually transmitted through unprotected sexual activity with an infected individual. This man presents with the symptoms of secondary syphilis, which includes malaise, mild fever, and rash on the palms or soles of the feet. The primary lesion (chancre) may go unnoticed because it is painless and subsides in a few weeks. *Neisseria gonorrhea* is associated with a serous exudate. *Chlamydia* is associated with painful urination. *Rickettsia rickettsii* and *Borrelia burgdorferi* are associated with arthropod vectors.

[22.3] **D.** The organism present is *Treponema pallidum,* a spirochete. No organisms are seen under light microscopy because spirochetes are too small to be visualized by this technique. Use of darkfield microscope allows for visualization of the corkscrew morphology. The Ziehl-Neelsen stain is used to detect acid-fast bacteria such as *Mycobacteria.* India ink preparations are used to visualize a capsule that is present in *Cryptococcus neoformans* but that spirochetes do not have. Giemsa stain is used to detect *Borrelia, Plasmodium, Trypanosomes,* and *Chlamydia* species.

[22.4] **B.** There are two classes of test used to detect the presence of an infection. The nontreponemal tests detect the presence of antibodies against lipids present on the organism. The nontreponemal tests include RPR and VDRL. Specific tests that detect antibodies against the organism itself, include MHA-TP and FTA-ABS. Aerobic and anaerobic cultures are not specific tests used to identify syphilis. The Ziehl-Neelsen stain is used to identify acid fast bacteria.

[22.5]   **D.** In the presence of a woman with no known contacts with syphilis and a low-grade fever and rash, it is most likely that she had a false positive reaction to the VDRL test because of lupus (SLE). This is often a common finding in lupus patients, and may be the first sign that they have lupus. In contrast, the VDRL test would be positive in secondary syphilis, often in high titer (greater than 1:32). Her being positive for HIV, while she may also have a false positive reaction to the VDRL test if HIV positive, is not the most likely answer choice for this patient. The presence of the malar rash makes SLE more likely. Recent exposure to syphilis would lead to a false negative test result; antibodies form between 4–8 weeks from exposure. *Chlamydia trachomatis* infection would not lead to a positive test result for syphilis.

MICROBIOLOGY PEARLS

❖ Some of the nontreponemal nonspecific tests are the VDRL and RPR.

❖ The specific treponemal tests include the FTA-ABS and MHA-TP.

❖ Primary syphilis generally consists of a painless chancre.

❖ Secondary syphilis consists of a generalized macular popular rash especially affecting the palms or soles, or condyloma latum.

❖ Tertiary syphilis is typified by gummas, neurosyphilis, tabes dorsalis, Argyll Robertson pupil.

❖ The best treatment for syphilis is penicillin.

REFERENCES

Murray PR, Rosenthal KS, Kobayashi GS, Pfaller MA. Medical microbiology, 4th ed. St. Louis: Mosby, 2002:378–384.

Ryan JR, Ray CG. Sherris medical microbiology, 4th ed. New York: McGraw-Hill, 2004:422–430.

Schneider AS, Szanto PA. Pathology: board review series, 2nd ed. Philadelphia: Lippincott Williams & Wilkins, 2001:272,278,281.

A 35-year-old woman presents to the emergency room with a two-day history of severe diarrhea and vomiting. Her symptoms started shortly after returning from a mission trip that she took with her church to a rural area in central Africa. She recalls eating shrimp that seemed undercooked. Her symptoms started abruptly, with watery diarrhea followed by vomiting. She has not had a fever and denies abdominal pain. On examination, her temperature is 37.2°C (98.9°F), pulse is 115 beats per minute, and blood pressure is 80/50 mmHg. Her mucous membranes are dry, and her eyes appear sunken. Her skin is dry and tents when lightly pinched. Her abdomen has hyperactive bowel sounds but is soft and nontender. Her stool is watery and tests negative for blood. A complete blood count shows an elevated white blood cell count and an elevated hematocrit. A metabolic panel shows hypokalemia, low serum bicarbonate, and prerenal azotemia. You assess this patient to be in hypovolemic shock and metabolic acidosis, and institute appropriate therapy.

◆   **What organism is most likely to be identified on stool culture?**

◆   **What is the cause of this patient's diarrhea?**

ANSWERS TO CASE 23: *Vibrio cholerae*

Summary: A 35-year-old woman recently traveled to Africa and developed diarrhea causing hypovolemic shock and metabolic acidosis. She remembers eating undercooked shrimp.

◆ **Most likely etiologic agent:** *Vibrio cholerae.*

◆ **Cause of the diarrhea:** hypersecretion of water and electrolytes into the intestinal lumen caused by cholera toxin.

CLINICAL CORRELATION

The first priorities as with any patient are the ABCs: airway, breathing, circulation. This patient is in hypovolemic shock, meaning insufficient circulation to maintain tissue perfusion needs. The most important step in intervention is volume repletion, usually with intravenous isotonic saline solution. A likely therapy would be 3 liters of normal saline intravenously.

Vibrio species are found in salt water and infections usually occur in the spring and summer. Transmission is by either consumption of contaminated shellfish or traumatic injury associated with infected water. The disease cholera is caused by toxigenic strains of *V. cholerae* (01 and 0139 serotypes). *V. cholerae* is spread by ingestion of contaminated water or food. The organism is sensitive to gastric acid; therefore, the dose required to cause an infection is high. Conditions that reduce gastric acid, such as antacid medications or achlorhydria, increase the risk of infection.

The hallmark of cholera is severe watery diarrhea with mild to severe dehydration because of production of toxin by the organism. In cases of severe dehydration, patients have a nonpalpable pulse and very low blood pressure. **Fever is usually not present.** Patients may become obtunded with sunken eyes and dry mucous membranes.

V. parahaemolyticus is associated with gastroenteritis that is self-limited even though patients present with explosive watery diarrhea, with abdominal pain and fever. The disease rarely progressed to the severity of dehydration of *V. cholerae. V. vulnificus* is more often associated with wound infections, that is, cellulitis, rather than gastroenteritis. In alcoholic patients or those with other underlying liver disease, the organism can become disseminated and be associated with a high mortality rate.

Approach to Suspected *Vibrio* Infection

Definitions

Azotemia: Buildup in the blood of nitrogenous end-products of protein metabolism.

Obtunded: Loss or dulling of sensations.

Objectives
1. Know the structure, physiology and virulence factors of *V. cholerae*.
2. Know the reservoirs and mechanisms of spread of *V. cholerae* and the mechanism of action of the cholera toxin in causing disease.

Discussion

Characteristics of *Vibrio*

Vibrio species are **motile, curved, gram-negative bacilli with a single polar flagellum.** They are **facultative anaerobic organisms.** Their natural environment is **salt water,** where they can multiply freely, and it has been found in **shellfish and plankton.** The major human pathogens are *V. parahaemolyticus V. vulnificus* and *Vibrio cholerae.*

Over 200 serotypes of *V. cholerae* have been identified, based on their **O antigen** serogroup. Serotype O1 has been responsible for the major cholera pandemics of the past 200 years, but serotype O139 has been identified as contributing to disease since 1992.

The major virulence of this organism is its **enterotoxin.** The toxin consists of five B subunits, which bind to mucosal cell receptors and allow for release of the single A subunit into the cell. **The A subunit activates adenyl cyclase,** resulting in the **hypersecretion of water, sodium, potassium, chloride, and bicarbonate** into the intestinal lumen.

Bacteria that survive transit through the stomach can colonize the upper small intestine. Colonization pili facilitate attachment to the intestinal mucosa. The volume of the secreted fluid and electrolytes can overwhelm the gastrointestinal tract's ability to reabsorb them, resulting in large volumes of watery diarrhea. **The loss of an isotonic, bicarbonate-containing fluid results in dehydration, hypovolemia, metabolic acidosis, hemoconcentration, and hypokalemia.**

Diagnosis

The presumptive diagnosis of *Vibrio* disease can be made after history of association with saltwater, either involving trauma or consumption of **raw shellfish.** The watery diarrhea associated with *V. parahaemolyticus* cannot be easily distinguished clinically from other forms of bacterial gastroenteritis. **Cellulitis** caused by *V. vulnificus* should be diagnosed rapidly to avoid mortality. History of recent exposure to seawater is helpful in making a presumptive diagnosis.

The diagnosis of cholera should be suspected in those with severe diarrheal illness who live in or have traveled to an endemic area. Diagnosis of *Vibrio* infection can be confirmed by culturing stool or wound samples. **Gram stain** of wound or blood cultures may demonstrate a **characteristic curved appearance to the gram-negative bacilli.**

Most of the *Vibrio* species require salt for growth and therefore specialized media, such as thiosulfate citrate bile salts sucrose (TCBS) agar. Most of the *Vibrio* species will grow on blood agar and may appear β-hemolytic, but poor growth is seen on MacConkey agar. *V. cholerae* appear as yellow colonies, and **V. parahaemolyticus and V. vulnificus appear as green colonies** on TCBS agar.

Treatment and Prevention

The **treatment** of cholera involves **volume replacement** with **isotonic, bicarbonate-containing fluids,** either using oral rehydration solutions in mild to moderate dehydration or IV fluids, such as Ringer lactate, in the profoundly dehydrated or those unable to tolerate oral intake. **Oral antibiotics** can be given to kill the bacteria and decrease the duration of the illness, but do not take away the need for appropriate rehydration therapy. Most commonly administered antimicrobial is **doxycycline.**

Treatment with antimicrobials is not usually needed for gastroenteritis caused by *V. parahaemolyticus.* **Wound infections or bacteremia caused by V. vulnificus require rapid administration of antimicrobials such as tetracycline or a quinolones.** Prevention of cholerae includes improvement of hygienic practices including treatment of the potable water supply with either heat or chlorine and ensuring thorough cooking of seafood. Research is ongoing to perfect a vaccine to prevent cholera.

Comprehension Questions

[23.1] An individual experiences diarrhea after eating raw shellfish in San Francisco. What is the most probable cause of the problem?

   A. *Campylobacter jejuni*
   B. *Salmonella choleraesuis*
   C. *Shigella dysenteriae*
   D. *Vibrio parahaemolyticus*
   E. *Yersinia enterocolitica*

[23.2] Which of the following statements is true of cholera enterotoxin?

   A. Appears to produce its effect by stimulating adenyl cyclase activity in mucosal cells
   B. Causes destruction of the intestinal mucosa allowing for invasive infection
   C. Causes a net efflux of ions and water from tissue into the lumen of the large intestine
   D. Is a protein with a molecular weight of about 284,000

[23.3] Fever, leukopenia, disseminated intravascular coagulation, and hypotension caused by members of the Enterobacteriaceae family are most strongly associated with which of the following structures?

A. H antigens
B. K antigens
C. Lipid A
D. Polysaccharides
E. R antigens

[23.4] A 50-year-old man recently visited India and developed diarrhea before returning to the United States. *Vibrio cholerae* O1 (El Tor, Ogawa) was isolated from his stool. Which of the following is the biotype of the *V. cholerae* strain?

A. Classical
B. El Tor
C. 10
D. Ogawa

Answers

[23.1] **D.** *Vibrio parahaemolyticus* is a halophilic bacterium that causes acute gastroenteritis following ingestion of contaminated seafood such as raw fish or shellfish. After 12–24 hours, the patient develops nausea and vomiting, abdominal cramps, fever, and watery to bloody diarrhea. It is usually self-limited in 1–4 days, requiring only restoration of water and electrolytes. All other answer options could produce episodes of gastroenteritis, but the halophilic nature of *V. parahaemolyticus* and seafood is recognized as a classic combination.

[23.2] **A.** The clinical correlation section of this case study summarizes the action of the *V. cholerae* enterotoxin quite well. It can be the cause of 20–30 L/day diarrheal output, resulting in dehydration, shock, acidosis, and death. It is antigenically related to the LT of *E. coli,* has a molecular weight of about 84,000 daltons, does not damage the mucosa, and affects the small intestine.

[23.3] **C.** The lipopolysaccharide (LPS) of gram-negative cell walls consists of a complex lipid, lipid A, to which is attached a polysaccharide made up of a core and a terminal series of repeat units. LPS is attached to the outer membrane by hydrophobic bonds and is required for the function of many outer membrane proteins. LPS is also called endotoxin. All the toxicity resides in the lipid A component. Endotoxin (lipid A) can activate complement, resulting in inflammation and the clinical features referred to in the question.

[23.4]   **B.** The O antigen of *Vibrio* species has been given numbers to indicate biotype, a form of subdivision for strains of cholera organism.
V. cholerae serogroups O1 and O139 have long been recognized as
strains responsible for epidemic and pandemic cholera. There have
been six pandemics from 1817–1923, most likely caused by the O1
subtype. A new pandemic caused by the El Tor biotype started in Asia
in 1961 and spread to Central and South America by 1991. The disease and biotype is rare in North America, but it does have an endemic
focus on the Gulf of Mexico coastal areas (Louisiana and Texas).

MICROBIOLOGY PEARLS

❖   The A subunit of the *Vibrio* enterotoxin activates adenyl cyclase,
resulting in the hypersecretion of water, sodium, potassium, chloride, and bicarbonate into the intestinal lumen.

❖   The predominant clinical presentation of *Vibrio* gastroenteritis is
watery diarrhea.

❖   The *Vibrio* organism appears as gram–negative, curved, motile bacilli.

❖   *Vibrio* gastroenteritis or cholera are associated with consumption of
contaminated seafood or water.

❖   *Vibrio vulnificus* is associated with cellulitis caused by trauma
incurred in a seawater environment and carries a high mortality
rate if not treated rapidly.

❖   *Vibrio* species require salt for growth and can be differentiated from
other organisms by growth on TCBS agar.

REFERENCES

Murray PR, Rosenthal KS, Kobayashi GS, Pfaller MA. Vibrio, Aeromonas, and
Plesiomonas. In: Murray PR, Rosenthal KS, Kobayashi GS, Pfaller MA.
Medical microbiology, 4th ed. St. Louis: Mosby, 2002:281–87.

Neill MA, Carpenter CCJ. Other pathogenic vibrios. In: Mandell GL, Bennett JE,
Dolin R, eds. Principles and practice of infectious diseases, 5th ed. Philadelphia:
Churchill Livingstone, 2000:2272–76.

Seas C, Gotuzzo E. Vibrio cholerae. In: Mandell GL, Bennett JE, Dolin R, eds.
Principles and practice of infectious diseases, 5th ed. Philadelphia: Churchill
Livingstone, 2000:2266–72.

A 5-year-old girl is brought to the office because of "pink eye." She was sent home from kindergarten yesterday by the school nurse because her left eye was red. When she awakened this morning, the right eye was red as well. She has had watery drainage but no purulent discharge. She's had a mild head cold with a runny nose and a mild sore throat but no fever. When her mother called the school this morning, she was told that five of her daughter's classmates were out with pink eye today. On examination, the child has injected conjunctiva bilaterally with clear drainage. No crusting of the lashes is noted, and the corneas are clear. She has mildly tender preauricular adenopathy. The remainder of her examination is unremarkable.

◆ **What organism is the most likely cause of this infection?**

◆ **How does this organism gain entry into host cells?**

ANSWERS TO CASE 24: Adenovirus

Summary: A 5-year-old girl with conjunctivitis of both eyes, with nonpurulent drainage associated with an upper respiratory infection.

◆ **Most likely organism causing the infection:** Adenovirus.

◆ **Method that the organism gains entry into host cells:** Adenoviruses gain entry into host cells by binding to the coxsackie adenovirus receptor (CAR) followed by receptor-mediated endocytosis.

CLINICAL CORRELATION

Conjunctivitis is a normal feature of many childhood infections. However, the most common cause of conjunctivitis is related to infection with adenoviruses. In addition to being the most common cause of viral conjunctivitis, adenoviruses also commonly cause upper respiratory infections and gastrointestinal infections. Most adenoviral diseases are mild and self-limiting in immune-competent persons. Children are infected more frequently than adults.

Approach to Suspected Adenoviral Infection

Definitions

Conjunctivitis: Inflammation of the eye tissue.
Lymphadenopathy: Enlargement of a lymph node occurring singly or in multiple nodes.
Preauricular adenopathy: Enlargement of a lymph node occurring singly or in multiple nodes anterior to the ear.

Objectives

1.   Be able to describe the characteristics of adenovirus.
2.   Understand how adenovirus causes infection and strategies of prevention.

Discussion

Characteristics of Adenoviruses that Impact Transmission

Adenoviruses are **nonenveloped viruses that contain linear, double-stranded DNA** with a terminal protein attached to both 5' ends of the genome. The **viral capsid** is composed of an **icosadeltahedral** structure that contains a penton base and fiber at each vertex. The fibers contain viral attachment proteins that determine the target cell specificity among viral serotypes. The fiber also serves as a **hemagglutinin.** Over 100 different serotypes have been recognized, more than 49 of which are known to infect humans.

To gain entry into the host cell, the **viral fiber proteins bind to the coxsackie adenovirus receptor on host cell surfaces** and become **internal-**

ized by receptor-mediated endocytosis. The virus then lyses the endosome, and the viral DNA is delivered to the host nucleus by the capsid. Viral DNA replication occurs in the nucleus, and the viral capsid proteins are made in the cytoplasm and then transported to the nucleus for viral assembly. A single viral replication cycle takes approximately 32–36 hours and produces around 10,000 new virions. Figure 24-1 shows the replication cycle. However, errors in assembly and replication are common, resulting in a much lower number of infectious viral particles.

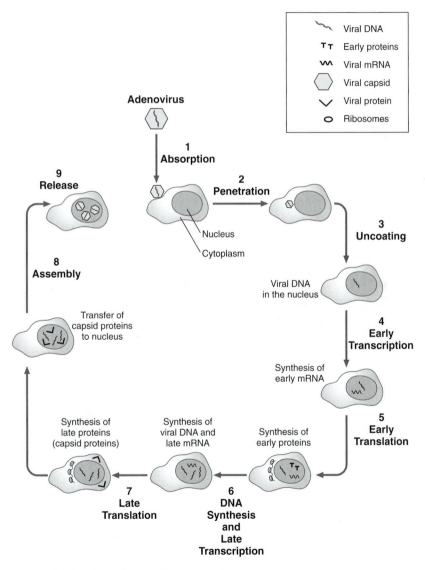

Figure 24-1. Adenovirus replication cycle.

Adenoviruses infect **epithelial cells of the respiratory tract, conjunctiva, and enteric organs.** Infections are **spread from person to person by aerosolized respiratory droplets, close contact, or fecal-oral contact. Fomite** transmission is also common because adenoviruses are nonenveloped, making them more resistant to detergents and desiccation. They can cause **lytic infections** in epithelial cells and tend to cause latent infections in lymphoid tissue. **Persistence in lymphoid tissues** involves integration of viral DNA into the host genome. Reactivation of virus can occur with stress. Viremia may occur and cause spread to distant organs such as the kidney, bladder, liver, and lymphoid tissue. **Viremia is especially common in immunosuppressed patients.**

Diagnosis

Adenoviruses primarily infect **children under 3 years** and appear clinically with a variety of symptoms including **fever, cough, nonstreptococcal exudative pharyngitis, cervical adenitis, conjunctivitis, or gastroenteritis.** Symptoms can last from 3–5 days. More severe respiratory diseases include laryngitis, bronchiolitis, and pneumonia. Reactivated viral disease occurs primarily in immune compromised individuals. Adenoviral follicular **conjunctivitis, or "pink eye,"** outbreaks in children often involve swimming pools as a common source of infection. Gastroenteritis is also a major clinical manifestation of adenoviral infection. Adenoviral types 40, 41, and 42 have been shown to be associated with **gastrointestinal disease** in infants and hospitalized patients.

In addition to clinical presentation of infection, laboratory diagnostic tests, including **cell culture, ELISA** (enzyme-linked immunosorbent assay), **PCR, and DNA-probe analysis** are available and can be used to detect the viral type in clinical samples and tissue culture. However, their primary use is for epidemiological studies, and they are not used widely in clinical practice for diagnostic purposes. Typically, diagnosis is made by clinical presentation and by history.

Treatment and Prevention

Currently, there is no treatment for adenoviral infection. Live oral vaccines have been developed for adenovirus types 4 and 7, which cause acute respiratory tract infections, and have been used primarily in military settings. However, because some adenoviruses are oncogenic, such vaccines have not been made available to the general population. Thus, prevention is the most important aspect involving careful hygiene, handwashing, and isolation of infected individuals.

Comprehension Questions

[24.1] An 11-year-old boy attending summer Boy Scout camp develops symptoms of sore throat, headache, fatigue, and conjunctivitis. He is seen by the camp medical staff and on examination is found to have a slight fever of 39.8°C (103.6°F), but no rash. Within the next 1–2 days, several of the other campers develop similar symptoms, which last for 5–7 days. The larger number of campers with similar symptoms indicates that a common source of infection is causing the outbreak. Which of the following activities is the most likely source of the campers' infection?

    A. Hiking in wooded areas with tall grass
    B. Sharing water canteens with other campers
    C. Sleeping outdoors without protective netting
    D. Swimming in the camp pond
    E. Walking barefoot in the bath house

[24.2] The causative agent in the question above was determined to be an adenoviral infection. Which of the following best describes this viral agent?

    A. Nonenveloped, double-stranded DNA virus with fibers at its vertices
    B. Nonenveloped, double-stranded, circular DNA virus
    C. Enveloped, single-stranded, negative-sense RNA virus
    D. Enveloped, double-stranded, linear DNA virus with glycoprotein spikes
    E. Enveloped, double-stranded, circular DNA virus

[24.3] A 2-year-old child attending daycare develops diarrhea and gastroenteritis as a result of an adenoviral infection. Which of the following adenoviral serotypes would most likely be responsible for this girl's illness?

    A. Type 4
    B. Type 7
    C. Type 19
    D. Type 37
    E. Type 41

Answers

[24.1]   **D.** The campers symptoms are consistent with adenoviral conjunc-
         tivitis, which is commonly spread through contaminated swimming
         pools or ponds; answers A, B, C, and E are incorrect.

[24.2]   **A.** Adenoviruses are nonenveloped, double-stranded DNA viruses with
         fiber structures projecting from their vertices or penton bases; answers
         B, C, D, and E are incorrect: (B) describes polyoma viruses such as
         human papillomavirus; (C) describes viruses such as rhabdoviruses,
         orthomyxoviruses, paramyxoviruses, and the like; (D) describes herpes
         viruses; (E) describes hepatitis B virus.

[24.3]   **E.** Adenoviral types 40, 41, and 42 have been shown to be associated
         with gastrointestinal disease in infants; answers A, B, C, and D are
         incorrect: Adenoviral types 4 and 7, commonly cause upper respira-
         tory infections in military recruits; adenoviral types 19 and 37 have
         been implicated in causing epidemic keratoconjunctivitis.

MICROBIOLOGY PEARLS

  Adenoviruses commonly cause conjunctivitis, in combination with
         pharyngitis, and upper respiratory infections.
  Children under 3 years and immunocompromised adults are at par-
         ticular risk.
  Clinical manifestations are fever, cough, nonstreptococcal exudative
         pharyngitis, cervical adenitis, conjunctivitis, or gastroenteritis.
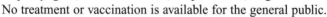 No treatment or vaccination is available for the general public.

REFERENCES

Brooks GF, Butel JS, Morse SA. Jawetz, Melnick, & Adelberg's medical microbiol-
    ogy, 23rd ed. New York: McGraw-Hill, 2004:420–428.
Ryan JR, Ray CG. Sherris medical microbiology, 4th ed. New York: McGraw-Hill,
    2004:507–510.
Shenk TE. Adenoviridae: the viruses and their replication. Fields virology, 4th ed.
    Lippincott Williams & Wilkins, 2001:2111–2135.

You are called to examine a 1-day-old male because the nurse is concerned that he is jaundiced. He was born by spontaneous vaginal delivery to a 19-year-old gravida$_1$ para$_1$ after a full-term, uncomplicated pregnancy. The mother had no illnesses during her pregnancy; she did not use tobacco, alcohol, or drugs; and the only medication that she took was prenatal vitamins. She denied any significant medical history, and there is no family history of genetic syndromes or illnesses among children. The infant is mildly jaundiced but has a notable abnormally small head circumference (microcephaly). His cardiovascular examination is normal. His liver and spleen are enlarged on palpation of the abdomen. Neurologic exam is notable for the lack of a startle response to a loud noise. CT scan of his head reveals intracerebral calcifications. The pediatrician explains to the child's mother that the virus involved is the most commonly transmitted transplacental viral infection in the United States.

◆ **What is the most likely cause of this infant's condition?**

◆ **How did he likely acquire this?**

◆ **What is the test of choice to confirm the diagnosis?**

ANSWERS TO CASE 25: Cytomegalovirus

Summary: A 1-day-old male with microcephaly, jaundice, hepatosplenomegaly, and deafness caused by a viral infection.

◆ **Most likely cause of this infant's condition:** The infant is most likely suffering from a congenital infection with Cytomegalovirus (CMV).

◆ **Likely acquisition of this infection:** Transplacental spread of the virus during a primary CMV infection of the pregnant mother.

◆ **Test of choice to confirm the diagnosis:** The definitive diagnostic test to confirm CMV infection in this patient is to demonstrate the presence of CMV in the infant's urine.

CLINICAL CORRELATION

Human Cytomegalovirus (CMV) is the largest member of the human Herpesviridae family. It is lymphotrophic and commonly produces asymptomatic infections in immune competent hosts. However, it can cause serious primary and recurrent infections in immunosuppressed individuals and neonates. CMV is the most common transplacentally transmitted infection in the United States.

Approach to Suspected CMV Infection

Definitions

Lymphotrophic: Having a specific affinity for lymph cells or their precursors.

Microcephaly: Abnormally smaller sized head, which may be associated with mental retardation.

Hepatosplenomegaly: Enlargement of the liver and spleen.

Subclinical infection: Without the presence of noticeable clinical disease.

Objectives

1. Be aware of the genomic characteristics of Cytomegalovirus.
2. Be able to describe how Cytomegalovirus causes infection, including transplacental infection.

Discussion

Characteristics of CMV that Impact Transmission

CMV belongs to the **Betaherpesvirinae** subunit of the Herpesviridae family and is the **largest known virus to infect humans.** The genome of **linear, double-stranded DNA is housed in an icosadeltahedral capsid.** Between the envelope and the capsid is a layer called the **tegument,** a phosphoprotein-containing matrix that plays a role in initiating replication. CMV, like other herpesviruses, has a lipid envelope that contains glycoproteins that facilitate attachment and entry into host cells. The virus often establishes **latent infection in lymphocytes, leukocytes, and organs like the kidney, heart, and lung.** Cell-mediated immunity is required for the control of CMV infections. Suppression of the immune system by medications or infection, such as **AIDS,** can result in **reactivation of the virus and severe, symptomatic disease.**

CMV has a ubiquitous distribution and approximately **10–15 percent of children are infected before the age of 5.** Most CMV infections in immune competent hosts are asymptomatic, although occasionally a **mononucleosis-like syndrome** can occur. Yet, even in subclinical infections, CMV can be isolated from saliva, cervical secretions, semen, urine, and white blood cells for months to years following infection. Although CMV is found in many host secretions, its major routes of **transmission** are via contact with **blood, oral secretions, sexual contact, organ transplant, or congenital infection.** CMV is the **most common viral cause of congenital disease** and infection, and its spread is thought to occur via **transplacental** transfer. The risk to the fetus is particularly high when the **mother** has a **primary infection during her pregnancy.**

Diagnosis

Although most CMV infections during childhood and in adults are asymptomatic, infants and immunocompromised patients can develop severe clinical symptoms from either primary infection or reactivation. Of the 1 percent of infants infected in utero or during delivery, 90 percent will develop asymptomatic infections, while the other 10 percent will develop symptomatic infections with congenital defects or disorders. **Nearly all of the infants with symptomatic infections are born of mothers with primary infections during their pregnancies.** Congenital CMV can cause a devastating syndrome that includes **microcephaly, intracerebral calcifications, hepatosplenomegaly, thrombocytopenia, chorioretinitis, deafness, mental retardation, jaundice, and rash.** Many of the infants with severe CMV congenital syndrome die within a short time, and those who survive have been shown to have persistent neurologic deficits. Reactivation of a latent infection during pregnancy confers a much lower risk, as the fetus is protected by the maternal immune response.

In addition to assessing the clinical symptoms, more definitive approaches to diagnosing CMV infection include direct detection of **CMV antigen or DNA in tissues or fluids via immunoassays or quantitative PCR.** Diagnosis of CMV infection can be confirmed by identification of the virus in the **infant's urine** during the first week of life. Histologically, CMV infection can also be detected by its ability to produce characteristic **enlarged cytomegaly of infected cells with pronuclear inclusions, or "owl's eyes."**

Treatment and Prevention

CMV infections are primarily treated with **ganciclovir, immune globulin plus ganciclovir, or foscarnet.** Treatment with ganciclovir has been used to prevent CMV disease in AIDS patients and transplant recipients. Use of this agent also reduces the severity of CMV syndromes such as retinitis and gastrointestinal disease. Treatment with both immune globulin and ganciclovir has been used to reduce the high mortality of CMV pneumonia in bone marrow transplant patients.

Unfortunately, congenital and perinatal transmission of CMV cannot be prevented once acquired by the pregnant woman. Thus, hygiene and hand-washing may play a role in prevention. Isolation of infants with CMV infections can prevent spread to other infants. Prevention of transplantation-acquired CMV infection can be obtained by transplanting organs and blood products from seronegative donors into seronegative recipients. In situations where it is not possible to use organ or blood products from seronegative donors, prophylactic treatment of all transplant patients or preemptive therapy of those patients with evidence of active CMV infection should be used. Such therapies include the use of hyperimmune CMV globulin, anti-CMV agents or a combination of both. Additionally, safe sex practices also reduce transmission of new CMV infections. CMV vaccines are currently under development; however, none are currently available.

Comprehension Questions

[25.1] An 18-year-old female presents to her physician with a 1 week history of fever, sore throat, fatigue, and myalgia. Physical examination reveals enlarged tonsils and exudative pharyngitis. Based on her clinical presentation, her physician diagnoses her with infectious mononucleosis. Because there are multiple causes of infectious mononucleosis-like illnesses, which of the following diagnostic assays would rule out CMV as the causative agent of this patient's infection?

A. A negative Gram stain of a throat swab
B. A lack of atypical lymphocytes in the patient's blood
C. A positive histological finding of cytomegaly
D. A positive Monospot test

[25.2] A previously healthy 8-year-old boy develops a classic childhood illness as a result of a primary viral infection. Which of the following agents would most likely produce symptomatic disease in a boy of this age?

A. Cytomegalovirus
B. Epstein-Barr Virus (EBV)
C. Herpes simplex virus 2 (HSV-2)
D. Poliovirus
E. Varicella-zoster virus (VZV)

[25.3] A 32-year old HIV infected male is noted to have acute cytomegalovirus infection causing acute gastrointestinal symptoms. The treating
physician has ordered that antiviral therapy be administered. Which of
the following is most likely to be targeted by the antiviral agent?

A. protease cleavage
B. nuclear transport of virus
C. synthesis of viral DNA
D. transcription of viral proteins
E. viral-cell fusion

Answers

[25.1] **D.** Both CMV and EBV infections can cause infectious mononucleosis
disease; however, only EBV produces heterophile antibodies that
would result in a positive Monospot test; answers A, B, and C, incorrect: A negative Gram stain of the patient's throat culture would rule
out group A *Streptococcus;* atypical lymphocytes are commonly present in EBV infection but not CMV-related infections; and cytomegaly
is typically present in CMV infections.

[25.2] **E.** VZV is a classic childhood disease that produces symptomatic pri-
mary infections; answers A, B, C, and D are incorrect: Most primary
CMV, EBV, and poliovirus infections are asymptomatic, whereas
HSV-2 infections would rarely occur in a child of this age.

[25.3] **C.** Ganciclovir has been used primarily to treat severe CMV infections, and its method of action involves inhibition of DNA synthesis;
answers A, B, D, and E are incorrect methods of antiviral therapy for
CMV infection.

MICROBIOLOGY PEARLS

 CMV is the most common viral cause of congenital infection in the
United States with the mechanism being primarily transplacental
infection.

 CMV establishes latent infection in leukocytes.

❖ CMV can be excreted in saliva, semen, urine, blood, and cervical
secretions for months to years following infection.

 Clinical manifestations include a mononucleosis-like disease in
immune competent individuals; microcephaly, hepatosplenomegaly, deafness, neurological deficits, and jaundice in congenital infections.

❖ CMV cytopathology involves cytomegaly or enlargement of infected
cells with pronuclear inclusions, or "owl's eyes."

REFERENCES

Murray PR, Rosenthal KS, Kobayashi GS, Pfaller MA. Medical microbiology, 4th ed. St. Louis: Mosby, 2002:492–496.

Ryan JR, Ray CG. Sherris medical microbiology, 4th ed. New York: McGraw-Hill, 2004:566–569.

Sia IG, Patel R. New strategies for the prevention and therapy of *Cytomegalovirus* infection and disease in solid-organ transplant recipients. Clin Microbiol Rev 2000;13:83–121.

A 17-year-old female is brought to the office for evaluation of a sore throat and fever. Her symptoms started about 1 week ago and have been worsening. She has been extremely fatigued and has spent most of the last 3 days in bed. She denies any ill contacts. She has no significant medical history, takes no medications, and has no allergies. On examination, she is tired and ill appearing. Her temperature is 38.5°C (101.3°F). Examination of her pharynx shows her tonsils to be markedly enlarged, almost touching in the midline. They are erythematous and covered with white exudates. She has prominent cervical adenopathy, which is mildly tender. A cardiovascular examination is normal, and her abdomen is soft, nontender, and without palpable organomegaly. A rapid streptococcal antigen test in the office is negative. You send a throat culture and decide to start amoxicillin for strep pharyngitis, assuming that the office test was a false negative. Two days later, you get a call from her mother stating that she has had an allergic reaction to the amoxicillin, and she now has a red rash from head to toe.

◆ **What is the most likely diagnosis of this patient?**

◆ **What is the most likely cause of her infection?**

◆ **In what human cells can this virus replicate? In what cells can it cause latent infection?**

ANSWERS TO CASE 26: Epstein-Barr virus

Summary: A 17-year-old female with fever, exudative pharyngitis, and adenopathy develops a prominent macular-papular rash after ampicillin is instituted.

◆ **Most likely diagnosis:** Infectious mononucleosis.

◆ **Most likely etiology:** Epstein-Barr virus (EBV).

◆ **In what human cells can this virus replicate, and in what cells can it cause latent infection?** EBV preferentially replicates in epithelial cells and B cells, and is known to cause latent infections in B cells.

CLINICAL CORRELATION

Epstein-Barr virus (EBV) is a member of the human herpesvirus family, and more specifically a member of the Gammaherpesvirinae subfamily. Humans are the only known natural host for these viruses. EBV infections are most commonly known for causing infectious mononucleosis in adolescents and young adults, and it is often referred to as the "kissing disease." Viral transmission occurs via repeated close intimate contact or through the sharing of items contaminated with saliva, because virus is intermittently shed in the saliva of most seropositive individuals. Secondary attack rates with family and household contacts tend to be low because 90–95 percent of adults have previously been exposed to EBV. Most primary infections are asymptomatic, whereas symptomatic infections are marked with fever, fatigue, pharyngitis, tender lymphadenitis, and possible hepatosplenopathy. Infections with these symptoms can be mistakenly diagnosed as streptococcal pharyngitis, and the resulting inappropriate treatment with amoxicillin can produce an allergic rash.

Approach to Suspected EBV Infection

Definitions

Lymphocytosis: A larger than normal number of T lymphocytes.

Atypical lymphocytes: Enlarged T lymphocytes, also referred to as "Downey cells," with eccentric nuclei and a vacuolated cytoplasm.

Heterophile antibodies: Nonspecific antibodies, including an IgM antibody, that recognizes the Paul-Bunnell antigen on sheep, horse, and bovine erythrocytes.

Objectives

1. Be aware of the genomic and other characteristics of EBV.
2. Be able to describe the clinical disease caused by EBV, mode of transmission, and strategies for treatment.

Discussion

Characteristics of EBV that Impact Transmission

Similar to other members of the **Herpesviridae (Table 26-1), EBV is an enveloped virus** with a **double-stranded linear DNA genome** that is approximately 172 kb in size and encodes more than 70 viral proteins. The DNA core is surrounded by an **icosadeltahedral nucleocapsid, with a protein tegument** located between the capsid and viral envelope, containing viral enzymes and proteins necessary for replication. The outer membrane of EBV contains virally encoded **glycoprotein spikes,** important for host cell attachment to **human B cells and epithelial cells** of the oro- and nasopharynx via the receptor for the C3d component of the complement system. As an **enveloped virus,** EBV is easily disrupted by acids, detergents, and desiccation and, thus, is effectively transmitted via intimate contact and saliva.

There **are two infectious subtypes of EBV, EBV-1 and EBV-2,** which are closely related except for **differences in their nuclear antigens.** The various EBV antigens are expressed in different phases of productive viral replication or in latent infection and can be used in diagnoses. **Early EBV antigens,** such as **early antigens (EAs)** and **nuclear antigens (NAs),** are nonstructural proteins expressed at the onset of lytic viral infection and are followed by the expression of late viral antigens, including the structural components of the viral capsid

Table 26-1
PROPERTIES OF HERPESVIRUSES

VIRUS	TARGET CELL	SITE OF LATENCY	TRANSMISSION
Herpes simplex virus type 1	Epithelial cells of the mucosa	Neurons	Close contact
Herpes simplex virus type 2	Epithelial cells of the mucosa	Neurons	Close contact (sexually transmitted)
Varicella-zoster virus	Epithelial cells of the mucosa	Neurons	Respiratory and close contact
Epstein-Barr virus	B cells and epithelial cells	B cell	Person to person via saliva
Kaposi sarcoma-related virus	Lymphocytes	?	Close contact (sexually transmitted)
Cytomegalovirus	Monocytes, lymphocytes, epithelial cells	Monocytes lymphocytes	Close contact, blood, and tissue transplantation, and congenital

(VCA) and membrane (MA). Latent phase antigens are expressed in latently infected B cells and include Epstein-Barr nuclear antigens (EBNAs), latent proteins (LPs), and latent membrane proteins (LMPs).

EBV was first discovered in association with African **Burkitt lymphoma,** a common malignancy of young children in sub-Saharan Africa. The **highest occurrence of Burkitt lymphoma** appears to occur in regions with **high incidence of malaria,** indicating malaria as a possible disease cofactor. Other EBV-related diseases include **nasopharyngeal carcinoma** and, in immuno-compromised patient populations, B-cell **lymphomas, interstitial lympho-cytic pneumonia,** and **hairy leukoplakia** of the **tongue.**

EBV can cause lytic infections of epithelial cells and latent infection or immortalization of B cells. The lytic infection of epithelial and B cells promotes virus shedding into the saliva of the host, allowing for viral transmission to other hosts and spread within the host. In B cells, EBV promotes cell growth and prevents apoptosis. The proliferating B cells produce an IgM antibody to the Paul-Bunnell antigen, called a **heterophile antibody,** which serves as a diagnostic indicator of infectious mononucleosis. In this stage of infection, antibody is produced against several EBV antigens, and a T-cell response is mounted. This response contributes to the symptoms and signs of mononucleosis, such as lymphadenopathy, splenomegaly, and atypical lymphocytosis. Latent infection of B cells may occur after the resolution of the acute infection, with periodic reactivation and shedding of the virus in the saliva for months, years, or even lifetime. Persons with inadequate T cell immunity may not be able to suppress EBV infection and may progress to lymphoprolifera-tive disease, B-cell lymphomas, or Hodgkin disease. Nasopharyngeal carcinoma, seen primarily in Asian and Aleutian populations, is thought to be associated with EBV infection in conjunction with some other genetic or environmental component.

Diagnosis

EBV-related **infectious mononucleosis** is clinically recognized by **high fever, malaise, lymphadenopathy, pharyngitis, and occasional hepatosplenomegaly.** Young children, who have a less active immune response, tend to have milder or subclinical infections. Symptoms from infection can last for days to weeks and then tend to resolve slowly on their own. Some of the rarer, but serious, complications of EBV infection include laryngeal obstruction, meningitis, encephalitis, hemolytic anemia, thrombocytopenia, and splenic rupture.

Definitive diagnosis of EBV infections involves the finding of lymphocytosis with the presence of **atypical lymphocytes, heterophile-positive antibodies,** and **antibody to EBV antigens.** Atypical lymphocytes appear with the onset of infection, whereas a positive heterophile antibody response can be detected approximately 1 week after the onset of symptoms and remain present for several months. The Monospot test and ELISA (enzyme-linked immunosorbent assay) are widely used for detection of heterophile antibody.

Treatment and Prevention

Currently, there is **no effective treatment** for EBV infection, nor is a viral vaccine available. However, because EBV infections in children tend to be less severe, and the immunity developed is lifelong, it is speculated by some clinicians that early exposure to EBV may be a means of preventing more severe infections and symptomatic disease.

Comprehension Questions

[26.1] Which of the following statements regarding the serologic diagnosis of infectious mononucleosis is correct?

   A. A heterophile antibody is formed that reacts with the membrane protein of EBV.
   B. A heterophile antibody is formed that agglutinates sheep or horse red blood cells.
   C. A heterophile antigen occurs that cross-reacts with atypical lymphocytes.
   D. A heterophile antigen occurs following infection with both EBV and CMV.

[26.2] A transplant patient taking high levels of immunosuppressive drugs becomes infected with EBV and develops a lymphoma. The dosage of immunosuppressive drugs given to the patient is subsequently decreased, and the tumor regresses. Which of the following properties of EBV infection is related to the patient's tumor development?

   A. Immortalization of B cells
   B. Increased white blood cell count
   C. Presence of atypical lymphocytes
   D. Production of heterophile antibodies

[26.3] A 21-year-old man visits the student health center suffering from a sore throat, swollen glands, fatigue, and a temperature of 39.4°C (103°F). Examination of the patient's peripheral blood smear shows 10 percent atypical lymphocytes, an elevated white blood cell count, and a positive heterophile antibody test. The patient asks for antimicrobial therapy. Which of the following statements would best dictate the clinician's response?

   A. Alpha-interferon is helpful in EBV infections but has multiple side effects.
   B. Ribavirin is effective in patients over 60 years.
   C. Attenuated-viral vaccine has been developed but not effective in this case because the infection has already occurred.
   D. There is no effective treatment.

Answers

[26.1]   **B.** A nonspecific heterophile agglutination test (Monospot test) is commercially available and can be used to diagnose EBV infectious mononucleosis within a week to months of infection. Infectious mononucleosis-like infection caused by CMV is heterophile negative.

[26.2]   **A.** Aggressive monoclonal B-cell lymphomas can develop in patients with reduced T-cell function. The immortalization of B cells in the absence of functional T cell immunity can give rise to lymphoproliferative disease such as Hodgkin lymphoma, Burkitt lymphoma, and nasopharyngeal carcinoma.

[26.3]   **D.** Currently, there are no effective treatments or vaccines available for EBV infection. Ribavirin is useful in treating respiratory syncytial virus-related and hepatitis C virus-related infections, while alpha-interferon has been used in treating the following viral infections: condyloma acuminatum, chronic hepatitis B and C, and Kaposi sarcoma.

MICROBIOLOGY PEARLS

❖   EBV-related infectious mononucleosis is heterophile antibody-positive.

❖   Clinical manifestations are fever, malaise, lymphadenopathy, pharyngitis, with presence of lymphocytosis and atypical lymphocytes.

❖   No current treatment or vaccines are available.

REFERENCES

Cohen JL. Epstein-Barr virus infection. N Engl J Med 2000;343:481–492.

Murray PR, Rosenthal KS, Kobayashi GS, Pfaller MA. Medical microbiology, 4th ed. St. Louis: Mosby, 2002:487–492.

Ryan JR, Ray CG. Sherris medical microbiology, 4th ed. New York: McGraw-Hill, 2004:567–573.

A 62-year-old male presents to your office for followup of some abnormal blood test results. You had seen him 2 weeks ago as a new patient for a routine physical examination. You ordered blood tests and found that his liver enzymes were elevated by approximately three times the upper limits of normal. The patient says that to his knowledge he's never had abnormal liver tests before, although he has not been to a doctor in several years. He denies alcohol or drug use and is not taking any medications. He gives no history of jaundice. His past medical history is significant only for hospitalization at the age of 45 for a bleeding stomach ulcer. He required surgery and had transfusion of 4 units of blood. He recovered from this episode without further complication and has had no recurrences. Your complete physical examination 2 weeks ago was normal, and a focused physical examination today shows no signs of jaundice, no hepatosplenomegaly, and no physical exam findings suggestive of portal hypertension. You diagnose an infectious etiology for the laboratory findings (elevated liver enzymes).

◆ **What is the most likely infectious cause of his abnormal liver function tests?**

◆ **How did he most likely acquire this infection?**

ANSWERS TO CASE 27: Hepatitis Viruses

Summary: A 62-year-old man with abnormal liver function tests who had a blood transfusion previously, likely caused by an infectious etiology.

◆ **Most likely infectious etiology:** Hepatitis C virus.

◆ **Most likely route of transmission:** Blood transfusion.

CLINICAL CORRELATION

Hepatitis C virus (HVC) is transmitted parenterally by **blood transfusions or intravenous drug use** and rarely by sexual contact. It is uncommonly diagnosed as a cause of acute hepatitis, often producing subclinical infection, but it is frequently diagnosed later as a cause of chronic hepatitis. The natural history of infection is not completely understood, but 50–85 percent of patients with hepatitis C will develop chronic infection.

On initial infection, approximately 15 percent of persons will develop an acute hepatitis syndrome and recover completely. However, about 80 percent will be asymptomatic yet progress to chronic infection. This chronic infection may progress to cirrhosis, liver failure, or hepatocellular carcinoma. HCV is transmitted from person–to–person, primarily via contact with infected blood or sexual contact. Routine screening of the donated blood supply for HCV was started in 1992. Prior to this, HCV was the primary cause of posttransfusion hepatitis. The high percentage of infections that are asymptomatic contributes to the spread of the virus in the population. Diagnosis is made by the presence of circulating antibody to HCV. HCV-polymerase chain reaction is also used to quantitate the amount of circulating virus present in an infected person. This serves as a measure of disease activity and as a monitor of response to therapy. Recombinant interferon, which induces host antiviral and antiproliferative activity, is the most widely used therapy for HCV.

Approach to Viral Hepatisis

Definitions

Hepatitis: Inflammation of the liver; viral causative agents include hepatitis viruses A, B, C, D, E, and G. The clinical presentation can include fever, nausea or vomiting, jaundice, dark urine, pale feces, and elevated liver enzymes (AST and ALT).

Dane particle: A 42-nm particle that is the hepatitis B virion.

Fulminant hepatitis: Severe acute hepatitis that causes rapid destruction of the liver.

Objectives

1. Know the structure and characteristics of the viruses that cause hepatitis.

2. Know the specific diseases associated with and routes of transmission of the hepatitis viruses.
3. Understand the mechanisms of development of acute and chronic hepatitis infections.

Discussion

Characteristics of Hepatitis Viruses

Because of its rich vascular supply, the liver may be involved in any systemic blood-borne infection, but the most common and clinically significant infections are those with one of five hepatotropic viruses: Hepatitis A, B, C, D, or E. They can produce virtually indistinguishable clinical syndromes. Affected individuals often complain of a prodrome of nonspecific constitutional symptoms including fever, nausea, fatigue, arthralgias, myalgias, headache, and sometimes pharyngitis and coryza. This is followed by the onset of visible jaundice as a result of hyperbilirubinemia, with tenderness and enlargement of the liver, and dark urine caused by bilirubinuria. The clinical course, outcomes, and possible complications then vary depending on the type of virus causing the hepatitis. A comparison of features of these five viruses is shown in Table 27–1.

Hepatitis A

Hepatitis A and **E** are both very contagious and transmitted by **fecal-oral route,** usually by contaminated food or water where sanitation is poor and in daycare by children. **Hepatitis A virus (HAV) is found worldwide,** and is the **most common cause of acute viral hepatitis in the United States. Hepatitis E** is much less common, and it is found in Asia, Africa, and Central America. Both hepatitis A and E infections usually lead to self-limited illnesses and generally resolve within weeks. Almost all patients with hepatitis A recover completely and have no long-term complications.

HAV is a member of the **Picornaviridae family.** It is a nonenveloped, linear, positive-sense, single-stranded RNA virus with only one serotype and seven genotypes. Its average incubation period is about 30 days, and it results in 25,000 symptomatic cases in the United States annually. However, **nearly 95 percent of HAV infections are asymptomatic.** Clinical symptoms vary according to the age of the patient; infections in children are mostly asymptomatic or present with nonspecific symptoms, whereas adults generally have a more severe clinical course. Only 1–4 percent of patients develop fulminant liver failure, and there is 1 percent mortality from HAV infection. It is not **known to cause chronic infection.** The virus is **contagious before symptoms appear.** Serologically, HAV infection can be diagnosed as ALT level rise initially with the appearance of symptoms. Then, **anti-HAV IgM antibodies** are produced and can be detected by enzyme-linked immunoassay. Then 1–3 weeks later, anti-HAV IgG antibodies are made, providing lifelong immunity to the host.

Table 27-1
COMPARISON OF HEPATITIS VIRUS

	VIRUS TYPE	TRANSMISSION	INCUBATION	SEROLOGIC MARKERS	CARRIER STATE	CHRONIC HEPATITIS	PREVENTION
Hepatitis A	RNA	Enteral (fecal-oral)	15–45 days	Anti-HAV igM	No	No	Vaccine, avoid contaminated food and water
Hepatitis B	DNA	Sexual, parenteral	30–180 days (mean 60–90 days)	+HBsAg, anti-HBcIgM (acute)	Yes	Yes	Vaccine, avoid blood and fluids
Hepatitis C	RNA	Parenteral	15–160 days (means 50 days)	Anti-HCV HCV RNA or ELISA	Yes	Yes	No vaccine, avoidance
Hepatitis D	Defective RNA	Parenteral	Same as HBV	Anti-HDV IgM	Yes	Yes	Vaccine for HBV, avoidance
Hepatitis E	RNA	Enteral (fecal-oral)	14–60 days (mean 40 days)	Anti-HEV	No	No	Avoid contaminated food and water

Proper hand washing, avoidance of contaminated food and water, and the administration of a **vaccine** for travelers are all methods for prevention of HAV infection. Alternatively, exposed persons can be treated **with HAV immunoglobulin intramuscularly** within 14 days of exposure. Additional treatment for infected patients is supportive.

Hepatitis B

Hepatitis B virus (HBV) is a member of the Hepadnavirus family and has a **DNA genome,** making it unique among the hepatitis viruses. It is an enveloped virus with a circular and partially double-stranded DNA genome. The HBV virion, known as the **Dane particle,** consists of the viral genome, a DNA polymerase, and P protein. The DNA polymerase also contains reverse transcriptase and ribonuclease H activity, allowing HBV to use an RNA intermediate during replication.

Several viral proteins can be detected during HBV infection and are useful in diagnosis and monitoring of disease. The virion is surrounded by a core protein antigen (HBcAg), and the presence of HBcAg in a patient's serum indicates that the patient has been exposed to HBV. Other HBV antigens include surface antigen (HBsAg) and the "e" antigen (HBeAg). **HBsAg can be detected when live virions** are present in an infection, and HBeAg is a glycoprotein cleavage product of the core which is shed into the serum. The **presence of HBeAg and HBsAg correlate with active HBV infection** and thus, **active disease.** Antibodies to these viral antigens can help to determine whether infection is recent or not. IgM anti-HBc indicates a new infection, whereas IgG anti-HBc indicates past infection. Figure 27-1 shows a hepatitis B serology diagram.

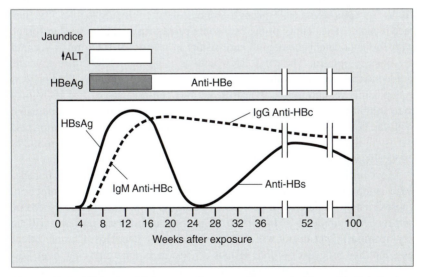

Figure 27-1. Clinical and laboratory features of acute viral hepatitis B infection.

HBV is the **second most common type of viral hepatitis** in the United States, and it is usually **sexually transmitted.** It may also be acquired **parenterally,** such as from intravenous drug use, or during birth, from chronically infected mothers. The outcome then depends on the age at which the infection was acquired. Up to **90 percent of infected newborns develop chronic hepatitis B infection,** which places the affected infant at significant risk of **hepatocellular carcinoma later in adulthood.** For those individuals infected later in life, approximately 95 percent of patients will recover completely without sequelae. Between **5 and 10 percent of patients will develop chronic hepatitis,** which may progress to cirrhosis. Also, a **chronic carrier state** may be seen in which the virus continues to replicate but does not cause hepatic damage in the host.

A **vaccine** consisting of recombinant HBsAg is available and is a scheduled immunization given to all infants and adolescents, as well as to persons with increased risk of exposure (i.e., health care workers and IV drug users). The incidence of HBV infection has decreased with the onset of the HBV vaccine and the screening of pregnant women prior to delivery. Yet, HBV remains in high rates in Southeast Asia and the Mediterranean areas. Nonimmunized persons exposed to HBV can be treated with immunoglobulin within 1 week of exposure. HBV infection can be treated with reverse transcriptase inhibitors or alpha interferon.

Hepatitis C

Hepatitis C virus (HCV) is a member of the **Flaviviridae family.** It is a lipoprotein-enveloped virus with a positive-sense RNA genome. There are hundreds of HCV genotypes as a result of a hypervariable region in the envelope region. The virus is more or less virulent depending on the hypervariable region, thus making it very difficult to produce an effective vaccine against HCV. The virus enters cells through endocytosis after binding to the CD81 surface receptor. The acidity of the endosome causes fusion of the viral envelope with the endosomal membrane and results in release of the viral RNA into the host cytoplasm. The viral RNA acts as messenger RNA, directing the production of the viral polyprotein. The polyprotein anchors to the host cell endoplasmic reticulum and the virus remains cell-associated. The HCV proteins inhibit apoptosis and the action of interferon-a. By remaining associated with the cell and inhibiting apoptosis, HCV can cause chronic infection and persistent liver disease. The incubation period for infection can vary from 2 to 26 weeks, with an average of 6–7 weeks.

Most initial HCV infections are asymptomatic or result in mild nonspecific symptoms such as malaise or abdominal pain. On initial infection, approximately 15 percent of persons will develop an acute hepatitis syndrome and recover completely. **More than 80 percent of infected patients will be asymptomatic, yet many will progress to chronic hepatitis.** Chronic infection can then progress to more serious disease including: cirrhosis, liver failure, or hepatocellular carcinoma. The high percentage of infections that are asymptomatic also contributes to the spread of the virus in the population.

HCV infection is diagnosed by demonstrating the presence of circulating **IgG antibodies** to HCV antigens through enzyme immunoassay. Unfortunately, these antibodies may not be detected until up to 4 months postinfection, making it difficult to diagnose an acute HCV infection. Additionally, such tests cannot distinguish between acute, chronic, or resolved HCV infections. Alternatively, **reverse transcriptase polymerase chain reaction** (RT-PCR) testing can be used to quantitate the amount of circulating HCV RNA in an infected person. This assay serves as both a measure of HCV disease activity and as a monitor of response to therapy.

The most widely used therapy for HCV infection is **recombinant interferon-α**, which helps to induce host antiviral and antiproliferative activity. End-stage chronic HCV hepatitis may require liver transplantation; however, the risk of graft reinfection is 50 percent for HCV. Currently, there is no effective vaccine to prevent HCV infection. However, the establishment of routine screening of donated blood and organs has reduced the spread of HCV via these modes of transfer.

Hepatitis D

Hepatitis D virus (HDV) is a **defective RNA virus** that **requires the presence of the hepatitis B virus** to replicate. Specifically, it lacks genes for envelope proteins, and thus to replicate it requires infection with HBV. It then consists of an envelope, provided by HBV with HBsAg, delta antigen, and RNA. If infection with HDV occurs during a superinfection of preexisting HBV, there is a higher risk of chronic liver infection and chronic HDV infection. This type of superinfection is also more likely to lead to fulminant hepatitis and has a 5–15 percent mortality rate. However, when HDV coinfects a person simultaneously with HBV, it typically presents as severe acute disease with a low risk of developing chronic liver infection or mortality. HDV is spread similarly to HBV, via percutaneously, mucosally, or through sexual contact.

Laboratory diagnosis of HDV is made by ELISA (enzyme-linked immunosorbent assay) detection of HDV antigen or serum IgM antidelta antigen; however, antibodies are present only transiently. To prevent coinfection with HBV, prophylaxis to HBV can be administered. To prevent a HDV superinfection, it is important to educate HBV-positive patients about reducing risk factors for infection. The only treatment available for HDV infection is alpha interferon, which lessens clinical symptoms.

Hepatitis E

Hepatitis E virus (HEV), also called **"enteric non-A, non-B hepatitis,"** is a member of the **Caliciviridae family.** It is nonenveloped, and its genome consists of linear, positive-sense, single-stranded RNA. HEV is similar in many ways to HAV. Both are transmitted by the fecal-oral route, most frequently through contaminated water sources. It is not endemic to the United States and is therefore seen most often in travelers. The average incubation period is 40 days. HEV infection is most often diagnosed by exclusion, because laboratory testing is not available.

Like HAV, it has a **low mortality rate,** except for infection in **pregnancy where a 15–25 percent mortality rate** is noted, and there is **no chronic stage.** Like all of the hepatitis viruses, the clinical severity of infection increases with the age of the patient. The immunological response is also similar to that of HAV. To protect from HEV infection while traveling to endemic areas, travelers are advised not to drink the water (or ice) and not to eat unpeeled fruits or vegetables. There is no vaccine available, and immunoglobulin does not prevent infection with HEV.

Hepatitis Serologies

Clinical presentation does not reliably establish the viral etiology, so serologic studies are used to establish a diagnosis. **Antihepatitis A IgM** establishes an **acute hepatitis A infection.** If Antihepatitis C antibody is present, an acute hepatitis C is diagnosed, but it may be negative for several months. The hepatitis C PCR assay, which becomes positive earlier in the disease course, often aids in the diagnosis. Acute hepatitis B infection is diagnosed by the presence of **hepatitis B surface antigen (HBsAg)** in the clinical context of elevated serum transaminase levels and jaundice. HBsAg later disappears when the antibody (anti-HBs) is produced.

There is often an interval of a few weeks between the disappearance of HBsAg and the appearance of anti-HBsAb, which is referred to as the **"window period."** During this interval, the presence of Antihepatitis B core antigen IgM (anti-HBc IgM), will prove indicate an acute hepatitis B infection. Hepatitis B precore antigen (HBeAg) represents a high level of viral replication. It is almost always present during acute infection, but its persistence after six weeks of illness is a sign of chronic infection and high infectivity. Persistence of HBsAg or HBeAg are markers for chronic hepatitis or a chronic carrier state; elevated or normal serum transaminase levels distinguish between these two entities, respectively.

Comprehension Questions

[27.1] A 33-year-old nurse suffered a needle stick injury. The patient used illicit intravenous drugs. One month later, the nurse develops jaundice. Which of the following findings would implicate hepatitis B as the etiology?

A. Positive antihepatitis B surface antibody
B. Positive antihepatitis B-core antibody
C. Positive hepatitis B surface antigen
D. Positive antihepatitis A antibody

[27.2] A 25-year-old male tests positive for a hepatitis C infection. Which of the following is the most likely method of transmission?

A. Fecal-oral
B. Fomite
C. Intravenous drug (needles)
D. Sexual transmission

[27.3] A 12-year-old teenager is brought into the emergency room with skin "turning yellow" and abdominal discomfort. The liver function tests reveal serum transaminase levels in the 2000 IU/L range. Which of the following is the most accurate statement about probable complications?

A. Significant likelihood of hepatocellular carcinoma
B. Almost no chance of long-term sequelae
C. About a 10 percent chance of a chronic carrier state
D. Long-term complications usually respond to alpha-interferon therapy

[27.4] A 28-year-old woman presents with symptoms of jaundice, right upper quadrant pain, and vomiting. She also has elevated ALT. It is determined that she acquired hepatitis A from a church picnic where several other adults also became infected. What should be done to protect the family members?

A. One dose of HAV immunoglobulin should be administered intramuscularly.
B. No treatment is necessary.
C. A series of three vaccinations should be administered at 0, 1, and 6 months.
D. Alpha interferon should be administered.
E. Household contacts should be quarantined and observed

Answers

[27.1]   **C.** The presence of hepatitis B surface antigen means actively replicating virus, and in the context of the recent needle stick injury, this likely represents a hepatitis B infection. The presence of HBeAg is a marker of active disease and infectivity. For example, pregnant mothers infected with HBV who have the absence of serum HBeAg, there is a greater than 10 percent transmission rate to the fetus, whereas in pregnant mothers with HBeAg in their serum, there is a greater than 90 percent transmission rate to the fetus.

[27.2]   **C.** Intravenous drug use is the primary method of transmission of hepatitis C virus.

[27.3]   **B.** This is most likely hepatitis A infection, which carries a very low chance of long-term sequelae.

[27.4]   **A.** HAV immunoglobulin should be given to household contacts in one IM dose. This must be done within 14 days of exposure to the index patient as prophylaxis against hepatitis A. Answer (C), the series of three vaccinations at time 0, 1, and 6 months, refers to the immunization schedule for hepatitis B, not hepatitis A. This would not be protective for those exposed to HAV. (D) Alpha interferon is used to treat symptomatic patients with HBV and HCV, not prophylaxis of family members of patients with HAV. (E) Quarantining the household contacts of the patient is not the appropriate treatment.

MICROBIOLOGY PEARLS

❖ HCV is an enveloped virus with a positive-sense RNA genome.
❖ HCV transmission occurs primarily via infected blood and sexual contact.
❖ Although most acute infections are asymptomatic, HCV produces high rates of chronic infection and mortality.
❖ Treatment of HCV infection includes recombinant interferon-α.
❖ No vaccine is available for HCV.

REFERENCES

Brooks GF, Butel JS, Morse SA. Jawetz, Melnick, & Adelberg's medical microbiology, 23rd ed. New York: McGraw-Hill, 2004:466–486.
Knipe DM, et al. Fields virology, 4th ed. Lippincott Williams & Wilkins, 2001.
Murray PR, Rosenthal KS, Kobayashi GS, Pfaller MA. Medical microbiology, 4th ed. St. Louis: Mosby, 2002:591–605.
Ryan JR, Ray CG. Sherris medical microbiology, 4th ed. New York: McGraw-Hill, 2004:541–553.

The mother of a 3-year-old girl brings the child in for the evaluation of a "wart" on her thumb. It has been present for 3 or 4 days and seems to cause some pain. The week prior, the child had a "head cold" and "cold sores" around her mouth, all of which have resolved. She has never had warts, and mother says that the child is otherwise healthy. On examination you see a well appearing child who is sitting in her mother's lap and sucking her thumb. Her head and neck exam is normal. On her left thumb, just proximal to the base of the thumbnail, is the lesion about which the mother is concerned. It is a cluster of small vesicles with a faint area of surrounding erythema. The remainder of the child's examination is normal.

◆ **What virus is the most likely cause of this skin lesion?**

◆ **How was it transmitted to this patient's thumb?**

ANSWERS TO CASE 28: Herpes Simplex Viruses

Summary: A 3-year-old girl had "cold sores" previously and now a cluster of small vesicles with a faint area of surrounding erythema on the thumb, consistent with herpetic whitlow.

◆ **Most likely viral cause of this skin lesion:** The most likely cause of the girl's skin lesion is herpes simplex type 1 (HSV-1).

◆ **How was it transmitted to this patient's thumb:** The patient most likely acquired the infection at this secondary site via self-inoculation of the skin by sucking her thumb.

CLINICAL CORRELATION

There are two serotypes of herpes simplex viruses, types 1 and 2 (HSV-1 and HSV-2), which both cause vesicular lesions via infection of mucosal membranes and or compromised epithelial cells. Both HSV-1 and HSV-2 are known to replicate in the basal epithelium of these vesicular lesions and then establish latent and recurring infections within the innervating neurons of these cells.

Approach to Suspected HSV Infection

Definitions

Vesicular lesions: Small, blister-like lesions filled with clear fluid.
Syncytia: Fusion of neighboring cells infected with virus, resulting in multinucleated giant cells.
Gingivostomatitis: Localized inflammation and or ulcerative lesions in the mucous membranes of the oral cavity.
Prodrome: Early symptoms of HSV infection, including itching and tingling of skin 12–24 hours prior to lesion formation.

Discussion

Characteristics of HSV that Impact Transmission

The **herpes simplex viruses (HSV)** are members of the **Alphavirinae subfamily of human herpesviruses.** As with other herpesviruses, they **are large, enveloped viruses** containing **double-stranded DNA** genomes surrounded by an **icosadeltahedral nucleocapsid,** with a protein tegument located between the capsid and viral envelope. The structures of the **HSV-1 and HSV-2 genomes** are similar and share about a **50 percent homology.** They can infect many cell types in humans and in other animals. They tend to cause lytic infections in fibroblast and epithelial cells and latent infections in neurons. HSV enters host cells via fusion at the cell membrane and releases gene transcription proteins, protein kinases, and proteins that are cytotoxic to the host cell. HSV primarily cause clinical symptoms at the site of inoculation of the virus. Although there is some overlap, HSV-1 tends to cause disease above the waist, and HSV-2, which is more commonly transmitted via sexual contact, causes disease below the waist.

The **virus enters through mucosal membranes or breaks in the skin.** It replicates in cells at the infection site and then establishes latent infection of the neuron that innervates the primarily infection site via retrograde transport. HSV avoids antibody-mediated defenses by cell-to-cell spread by the formation of **syncytia. Cell-mediated immunity is necessary for control of HSV infections,** and persons with impaired cellular immunity can get more severe and diffuse disease. The **latent infection of neurons** also helps the virus to avoid host defenses and provides the potential for recurrent disease. **Recurrences** can be triggered by many events, including stress and other illnesses. Recurrent HSV disease is usually less severe than primary disease because of the memory response of the host immune system. HSV-1 tends to be transmitted via contact with saliva or direct contact with skin or mucous membrane lesions. It causes gingivostomatitis, cold sores, and pharyngitis. **Herpetic whitlow,** an infection of the finger with **HSV-1,** results from direct contact with herpes lesions and is most commonly seen in **children who suck their fingers or in healthcare workers** who care for infected patients.

Diagnosis

Clinical signs of HSV-1 and HSV-2 infections include (1) oropharyngeal disease, with symptoms of fever, sore throat, gingivostomatitis, and submandibular lymphadenopathy; (2) keratoconjunctivitis, with recurrent lesions of the eye and eyelid; (3) cutaneous infections, with vesicular lesions of the mouth, fingers, and genital tract (Figure 28-1); and (4) encephalitis. Neonatal infections occur most commonly during vaginal delivery in pregnant mothers experiencing primary or recurrent genital lesions. HSV neonatal infections are nearly always symptomatic and have high mortality rates if not promptly diagnosed and treated. Signs of infection include localized vesicular lesions of the skin, eye or mouth, encephalitis, and/or disseminated disease.

Cytopathologically, HSV can be diagnosed by visualizing **multinucleated giant cells** on direct examination of cells from the base of a vesicular lesion, referred to as a **Tzanck smear.** However, this assay **lacks both sensitivity and specificity,** because it does not distinguish among HSV-1, HSV-2, and varicella-zoster virus (VZV) infections. **Isolation of virus from herpetic lesions,** cerebral spinal fluid, and stool specimens remains the definitive diagnostic approach. HSV-1 and HSV-2 **serotyping** can be performed by several biochemical, nucleic acid, or immunologic methods, with DNA probe analysis being the most widely used in current clinical practice.

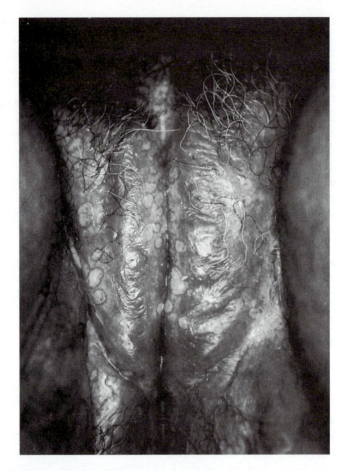

Figure 28-1. First episode primary genital herpes simplex virus infection.

Reproduced, with permission, from Cunningham FG, et al. William's obstetrics, 21st ed. New York: McGraw-Hill, 2001:1495.)

Treatment and Prevention

Several antiviral drugs have been developed to treat HSV infections, including **acyclovir, valacyclovir, and famciclovir.** All of these drugs function as inhibitors of viral DNA synthesis and are capable of shortening the duration of clinical symptoms and suppressing viral reactivation.

   Prevention of HSV infection relies on the avoidance of direct contact with the virus or viral lesions. Asymptomatic shedding of virus can occur in infected persons in saliva, urethral, and cervical sources, and because only about one-fourth of individuals infected with HSV know that they are infected, safe sex practices are highly recommended to avoid spread. The vast majority of HSV infections in newborns can be prevented by cesarean delivery of neonates in women experiencing primary HSV-2 infection or recurrent genital lesions. This practice has significantly decreased the rate of neonatal infection and mortality. Additionally, experimental recombinant HSV-2 vaccines are currently being developed and tested. One prospective trial has shown efficacy in preventing genital herpes infections in HSV-1 and HSV-2 seronegative women.

Comprehension Questions

[28.1] Which of the following cell types are specific to a latent genital infection with HSV-2?

    A. Trigeminal ganglia
    B. Sacral ganglia
    C. Vagal nerve ganglia
    D. Neural sensory ganglia

[28.2] Which of the following viruses, in addition to HSV-1 and HSV-2, produces the cytopathologic findings of multinucleated giant cells?

    A. Adenovirus
    B. *Cytomegalovirus*
    C. Epstein-Barr virus
    D. Human papillomavirus
    E. Varicella-zoster virus

[28.3] Which of the following statements most accurately describes HSV infections?

    A. HSV establishes lytic infection in neural ganglion cells.
    B. Latent HSV infections can be prevented in persons with functional cell-mediated immunity.
    C. Primary and recurrent HSV infections are treated with drugs that inhibit the viral DNA polymerase.
    D. HSV infection is transmitted via direct contact with symptomatic shedding of viral particles in active lesions.
    E. Severe neonatal herpes infections are commonly associated with in utero transmission.

Answers

[28.1]   **B.** Latent infection by HSV-2 has been shown to occur primarily in the sacral ganglia, whereas HSV-1 latency has been demonstrated in trigeminal, superior cervical, and vagal nerve ganglia. Varicella-zoster virus remains latent in neural sensory ganglia.

[28.2]   **E.** A Tzanck smear assay can be used to identify the characteristic cytopathologic effects of multinucleated giant cells in herpetic skin lesions; however, this assay cannot distinguish among HSV-1, HSV-2, and VZV infections.

[28.3]   **C.** Most antiviral therapies for HSV are nucleoside analogues or other inhibitors of the viral DNA polymerase; answers A, B, D, and E are incorrect: HSV establishes lytic infections in fibroblast and epithelial cells and latent infections in neurons; infection with HSV results in lifelong latent infection even in persons with functional cell-mediated immunity; HSV is transmitted most commonly from direct contact with active lesions (however, virus may be shed asymptomatically in saliva and urethral and cervical fluids); although in utero transmission of HSV is possible, it is very uncommon, and most neonatal HSV infections occur via vaginal delivery in mothers with primary genital infections.

MICROBIOLOGY PEARLS

❖   Clinical manifestations include painful vesicular lesions of the mouth, fingers, and genital tract.
❖   Characteristic viral cytopathology includes syncytia, cells with "ballooning" cytoplasm, and Cowdry A type inclusion bodies.
❖   Identification is by viral isolation with HSV-1 and HSV-2 serotyping by nucleic acid restriction mapping or DNA probe analysis.
❖   Effective treatment of primary and recurrent infections is with viral DNA polymerase inhibitors: acyclovir, valacyclovir, and famciclovir.

REFERENCES

Murray PR, Rosenthal KS, Kobayashi GS, Pfaller MA. Medical microbiology, 4th ed. St. Louis: Mosby, 2002:475–484.

Ryan JR, Ray CG. Sherris medical microbiology, 4th ed. New York: McGraw-Hill, 2004:555–562.

Whitley, RJ, Kimberlin, DW, Roizman, B. Herpes simplex viruses. J Clin Infect Dis 1998;26:541–555.

A 28-year-old man presents to the office for evaluation of a rash on his chest. He started with one oval shaped purplish area that he thought was a bruise but has subsequently developed multiple new lesions. The growths don't hurt, itch, or bleed, but he continues to get new ones, and the existing ones are getting larger. He has never had anything like this before, has no history of allergies and denies exposure to any new medications, foods, lotions, or soaps. His past medical and family histories are unremarkable. His review of systems is significant for a 15-lb weight loss in the past 2 months, approximately 6 weeks of diarrhea, and a 3-week history of a sore throat. On examination, he is a thin but generally well appearing male. His vital signs are normal. Examination of his pharynx shows thick white plaques on the posterior pharynx and soft palate. On the skin of his chest are multiple oval shaped purple or brown macules. They are firm on palpation and vary in size from 0.5 to 4 cm in length. Several of them appear to be growing together into larger, confluent plaques. You perform a punch biopsy of one of the lesions. In 5 days you get the pathology report with the diagnosis of Kaposi sarcoma.

◆ **With what virus is this patient likely infected?**

◆ **What specific cell types are most commonly infected with this virus? What cell surface receptor is the binding site of this virus?**

◆ **What serologic testing is most frequently performed to make this diagnosis?**

ANSWERS TO CASE 29: Human Immunodeficiency Virus (HIV)

Summary: A 29-year-old man has weight loss, white plaques on the pharynx, and purple lesions on the abdomen, which on biopsy reveals Kaposi sarcoma.

◆ **Virus with which this patient is most likely infected:** Human immunodeficiency virus (HIV).

◆ **Specific cells infected by and binding site of HIV:** CD4 surface receptor protein on macrophages and T lymphocytes.

◆ **Serologic testing to confirm diagnosis:** HIV enzyme-linked immunosorbent assay (ELISA) and Western-blot analysis, or PCR.

CLINICAL CORRELATION

The human immunodeficiency virus (HIV) is a human retrovirus in the Lentivirinae subfamily. It is a spherical, enveloped RNA virus with a cone-shaped capsid that contains two copies of a positive-strand RNA genome. HIV infects cells of macrophage lineage and helper T cells by binding to the CD4 surface receptor protein on these target cells, resulting in fusion of the viral envelope with the cellular plasma membrane to gain entry. On entry into the host cell cytoplasm, an RNA-dependent DNA polymerase enzyme (reverse transcriptase), which is present in the viral capsid, uses the viral RNA to synthesize viral DNA. The viral DNA is transported to the host nucleus, where it is spliced into the host genome. The integrated viral DNA acts as a host cellular gene and is transcribed by host RNA polymerase II to produce new copies of viral RNA and proteins, which assemble into new HIV virions. HIV initially infects cells of macrophage lineage, but quickly reaches the lymph nodes where CD4 T cells are infected. The immunosuppression caused by HIV is primarily caused by a reduction in the helper and delayed type hypersensitivity responses mediated by CD4 T cells. Infected macrophages probably serve as reservoirs and means of distribution of HIV. HIV avoids the host immune system in several ways. Infection of macrophages and helper T cells inactivates central components of the host immune system. Also, HIV has an intrinsic genetic instability as a result of errors caused by reverse transcriptase which may contribute to an antigenic drift in the virus, resulting in reduced host immune system recognition. Symptomatic disease caused by HIV is proportionate to the loss of CD4 T cells and the resulting immune dysfunction. Acquired Immune Deficiency Syndrome (AIDS) is defined by the presence of HIV, a reduction of CD4 T cells, and the acquisition of characteristic opportunistic infections. Serologic diagnosis of HIV infection is primarily made by ELISA (enzyme-linked immunosorbent assay) testing and, when this is positive, confirmation by Western blot analysis. Current HIV treatment involves using medications, individually or in combinations, which interfere with the actions of reverse transcriptase and block the proteases that activate the virion.

Objectives

1. Know the structure and characteristics of the human immunodeficiency virus.
2. Know the mechanism by which HIV is transmitted, infects target cells, replicates, and causes immune deficiency.
3. Know the diagnosis, treatment, and opportunistic infections associated with AIDS.

Discussion

Characteristics of Human Immunodeficiency Virus (HIV)

Human immunodeficiency virus (HIV) appears to have been derived from primate (chimpanzee, especially) lentiviruses and are the etiologic cause of AIDS. AIDS was described in 1981, and the virus was isolated in 1983. AIDS is one of the most significant public health problems worldwide at the current time.

HIV is a **retrovirus** (reverse transcriptase or RNA-dependent DNA polymerase) in the **lentivirus subgroup.** It is a medium-sized virus (about 100 nm) with two copies of a positive-sense (same as messenger RNA [mRNA]) single-stranded RNA genome. This genome is the most complex of all retroviruses. The **lipid envelope contains glycoproteins** that undergo **antigenic variation,** making vaccine development difficult, if not impossible, at the present time. **Protease enzymes are coded for by the viral genome,** and these are required for the production of infectious viruses. The reverse transcriptase makes a double-stranded DNA copy (provirus) of the viral genomic RNA, which is incorporated into a host chromosome. The proviral DNA later serves as a template for viral mRNA's and new virion genomes. Virions bud from the plasma membrane of the host cell. Heterogeneous populations of viral genomes are found in an infected individual, especially the *env* gene, which codes for envelope glycoproteins. **The gp120 viral receptor** contains binding domains responsible for **viral attachment to the CD4 molecule** (host receptor) and coreceptors and determines cell tropisms (lymphocytes versus macrophages). These glycoproteins cause antibodies to be formed by the host and are only weakly neutralizing to the virus. The **gp41 product** contains a transmembrane domain that **anchors the glycoprotein in the viral envelope** and a **fusion domain** that facilitates viral entry into the target (host) cells. The virus is inactivated by treatment at room temperature for 10 minutes by any of the following: 10% bleach, 50% ethanol, 35% isopropanol, 0.5% paraformaldehyde, or 0.3% hydrogen peroxide. HIV in blood in a needle or syringe, however, requires exposure to undiluted bleach for 30–60 seconds for inactivation. Heating at 56°C for 10 minutes (same as for complement inactivation) will inactivate HIV in 10% serum, but HIV in dried protein-containing mixtures is protected. Lyophilized blood products need to be heated to 68°C for 72 hours to ensure inactivation of contaminating viruses.

Diagnosis

HIV infection can be diagnosed by virus isolation, detection of **antiviral antibodies,** or measurement of **viral nucleic acid or antigens.** HIV may be cultured from lymphocytes in peripheral blood primarily. Virus numbers vary greatly in an individual. The magnitude of plasma viremia is an excellent correlate of the clinical stage of HIV infection compared to the presence of antibodies. The most sensitive viral isolation technique requires cocultivation of the test sample with uninfected mitogen-stimulated peripheral blood mononuclear cells. Virus growth is usually detected in 7–14 days by measuring viral reverse transcriptase activity or virus-specific antigens. Virus isolation of HIV is usually considered a research technique, and most medical center viral diagnostic laboratories will not offer this service.

Antibody detection is the most common way to diagnose HIV infection. Seroconversion in HIV infection is generally found to occur in about 4 weeks. **Most individuals are seropositive within 6–12 weeks after infection,** and essentially all will be antibody positive in 6 months. Commercially available **enzyme-linked immunoassays** (EIA, ELISA) are routinely used as **screening tests.** If done properly, the reported sensitivity and specificity are at least 98 percent. Two separate EIA tests need to be positive for antibodies in the usual screening situation, and a confirmation test (Western blot usually) will be done to rule out EIA false positives. **Western blot tests** (also commercially available) will usually detect antibodies to **viral core protein p24 or envelope glycoproteins gp41, gp120, or gp 160.**

Amplification assays (RT-PCR, DNA PCR. or bDNA tests) are used to detect viral RNA in clinical specimens. These tests may be quantitative when reference standards are used in each test. These molecular-based tests are very sensitive and form the basis for plasma viral load measurements. **HIV RNA levels** are important predictive markers of disease progression and monitors of the effectiveness of antiviral therapies.

Treatment and Prevention

Treatment of HIV infection uses classes of drugs that inhibit the virally-coded **reverse transcriptase** and inhibitors of the **viral protease enzymes.** Unfortunately, current treatments are virostatic, not virucidal. Therapy with combinations of antiretroviral drugs is called **highly active antiretroviral therapy** (HAART). It appears to lower viral replication below the limits of laboratory detection but is not curative. The virus persists in reservoirs of long-lived, latently infected cells. When HAART is discontinued, viral production rebounds. Monotherapy usually results in the rapid emergence of drug-resistant mutants of HIV. HAART therapy has turned HIV infection into a chronic, treatable disease. Unfortunately, large numbers of HIV-infected persons worldwide do not have access to the drugs.

A safe and effective vaccine would be the best hope for controlling HIV infection. Currently, many candidate vaccines are under development and in clinical trials. We have seen that viral vaccines are best when used in a preventative manner. Uninfected individuals are given the vaccine and develop antibodies that prevent infection or disease if the wild-type virus is encountered. HIV vaccine development is difficult because HIV mutates so rapidly. There appears to be so much variation in immune responses in HIV infections that no vaccine has been able to be protective to all individuals in a population. Nothing being currently developed appears to be close to approval in this area, although many organizations are working to produce an effective vaccine. A big hurdle for this, in part, is the lack of an appropriate and cost-effective laboratory animal model for HIV. The SIV-macaque model of simian AIDS is only partially useful for the development of a human HIV vaccine.

Comprehension Questions

[29.1] During a medical check-up for a new insurance policy, a 60-year-old grandmother is found to be positive in the ELISA screening test for antibodies against HIV-1. She has no known risk factors for exposure to the virus. Which of the following is the most appropriate next step?

A. Immediately begin therapy with azidothymidine.
B. Perform the screening test a second time.
C. Request that a blood culture be done by the lab.
D. Tell the patient that she is likely to develop AIDS.
E. Test the patient for *Pneumocystis carinii* infection.

[29.2] In a person with HIV-1 infection, which of the following is the most predictive of the patient's prognosis?

A. CD4+ cell count
B. CD4:CD8 cell ratio
C. Degree of lymphadenopathy
D. Level of HIV-1 RNA in plasma
E. Rate of decline in anti-HIV antibody

[29.3] Highly active antiretroviral therapy against HIV infection includes one or more nucleoside analogue reverse transcriptase inhibitors in combination with representatives of which class of antiretroviral agents?

A. Inhibitors of viral binding
B. Inhibitors of viral protein processing
C. Inhibitors of viral release
D. Inhibitors of viral uncoating
E. Nonnucleoside antiretroviral agents

[29.4] Which of the following is the pathogen responsible for blindness in advanced HIV infections?
A. *Cytomegalovirus*
B. Epstein-Barr virus
C. Fungus
D. Toxoplasma

Answers

[29.1] **B.** Because HIV cannot be safely isolated and grown in the standard medical center diagnostic laboratory, diagnosis of HIV infections relies on detection of antibodies against the virus. The standard screening test is done by ELISA (enzyme-linked immunosorbent assay). ELISA test formats are quite reliable and accurate and can be used for antibody or antigen detection. By definition, however, screening tests are not 100 percent accurate for sensitivity and specificity. HIV infection, especially, is a tragic infection that requires utmost accuracy in laboratory diagnosis results to aid the physician in counseling the involved patient and family. Under the conditions described in Question 29.1, no known risk factors for HIV contact are claimed or identified. For this situation and any other requiring diagnostic laboratory testing for HIV infection, extra effort is taken to ensure accuracy and correct results. Because it is widely accepted that HIV ELISA screening is not 100 percent sensitive and specific (about 98% accurate, however), a second blood sample is collected for retesting by ELISA. If both ELISA results are positive, a second confirming test is done. This is usually a Western blot technique. If the Western blot test is positive, then HIV infection is confirmed and related to the patient.

[29.2] **D.** Amplification assays (RT-PCR, DNA PCR, and b DNA tests) are routinely used to detect viral RNA in clinical specimens. The tests can be quantitative when reference standards are used, and appropriate positive and negative controls must be included in each test. Because these molecular based tests are very sensitive, they form the basis for plasma viral load determinations. It is generally agreed that the amount of HIV in the blood (viral load) is of significant prognostic value. There are continual rounds of viral replication and cell killing in each patient, and the steady-state level of virus in the blood varies with individuals. A single measurement of plasma viral load about 6 months after infection can predict the risk of development of AIDS in men several years later. In women, viral load appears to be less predictive. The plasma viral load appears to be the best predictor of long-term clinical outcome, whereas CD4 lymphocyte counts are the best predictor of short-term risk of developing an opportunistic disease. Plasma viral load measurements are a critical element in assessing the effectiveness of antiretroviral drug therapy.

[29.3]   **B.** A growing number of drugs have been approved for treatment of HIV infections. It must be remembered that all HIV drug treatments are only virostatic and not virucidal at this point in time. Classes of drugs include nucleoside and nonnucleoside inhibitors of the viral reverse transcriptase and inhibitors of the viral protease enzyme. The protease inhibitors are significant because protease activity is absolutely essential for production of infectious virus, and the viral enzyme is distinct from human cell proteases. These inhibitors (approved in 2003) block virus entry into host cells.

[29.4]   **A.** The predominant causes of morbidity and mortality among patients with late-stage HIV infection are opportunistic infections. These are defined as severe infections induced by agents that rarely cause disease in immune-competent individuals. Opportunistic infections usually do not occur until CD4 T cell counts drop from normal (1000 cells per microliter) to less than 200 cells per microliter. The common opportunistic infections in untreated AIDS patients are caused by protozoa, fungi, bacteria, and other viruses. Coinfection with DNA viruses are reported to lead to enhanced expression of HIV in cells in vitro. Herpesvirus infections are common in AIDS patients, and *Cytomegalovirus* (CMV) has been shown to produce a protein that acts as a chemokine receptor and is able to help HIV infect cells. CMV retinitis is the most common severe ocular complications of AIDS.

MICROBIOLOGY PEARLS

 HIV is a retrovirus and requires reverse transcriptase to make a double-stranded DNA copy of the viral genomic RNA.

 Antibody detection is the most common method of diagnosing an infection.

 The treatment of HIV largely depends on targeting viral reverse transcriptase and protease enzymes.

REFERENCES

Brooks GF, Butel JS, Morse SA, Jawetz, Melnick, & Adelberg's medical microbiology, 23rd ed. New York: McGraw-Hill, 2004:605–22.

Knipe DM, Howley PM. Fields virology, 4th ed. Lippincott Williams and Wilkins, 2001:1971–2094.

Murray PR, Rosenthal KS, Kobayashi GS, Pfaller MA. Medical microbiology, 4th ed. St. Louis: Mosby, 2002:574–90.

Ryan JR, Ray CG. Sherris medical microbiology, 4th ed. New York: McGraw-Hill, 2004:601–16.

A 42-year-old woman presents to the office for a routine gynecologic exam. She is feeling well and has no specific complaints at this visit. While reviewing your records, you see that she has not come in for a Pap smear in about 5 years. She admits that she has not come in because she has been feeling fine and didn't think it was really necessary. She has a history of three pregnancies resulting in three full-term vaginal deliveries of healthy children. She was treated at the age of 22 for chlamydia. She has never had an abnormal pap smear. Her social history is notable for a one-pack per day smoking history for the past 25 years. She is divorced from her first husband and is sexually active with a live-in boyfriend for the past 3 years. She has had 7 sexual partners in her lifetime. Her examination today is normal. You perform a Pap smear as part of the examination. The report arrives 10 days later with the diagnosis "high-grade squamous intraepithelial lesion."

◆ **What is the most likely infectious etiology of this lesion?**

◆ **What specific virus types confer a high risk of cervical neoplasia?**

◆ **Where on a cellular level does this organism tend to replicate in benign diseases? In malignancies?**

ANSWERS TO CASE 30: Human Papillomavirus

Summary: A 42-year-old woman has high-grade squamous intraepithelial neoplasia on a Pap smear.

◆ **Most likely infectious etiology of this lesion:** human papillomavirus (HPV)-related infection.

◆ **Specific virus types confer a high risk of cervical neoplasia:** HPV types 16 and 18 are most commonly associated with anogenital neoplasias.

◆ **Location of replication in benign diseases and malignancies:** The site of replication in benign HPV infections occurs in the host neoplasm where the viral DNA remains extrachromosomal. However, in HPV-related malignancies the viral DNA is integrated into the host genome.

CLINICAL CORRELATION

Human papillomavirus (HPV) preferentially infects the squamous epithelium of skin and mucous membranes causing epithelial proliferation and the development of cutaneous warts and genital, oral, and conjunctival papillomas. Although most HPV infections are benign, and most warts or lesions regress spontaneously with time, some HPV viral types have been shown to be linked to cervical and anogenital carcinomas (Table 30-1).

Table 30-1
CLINICAL SYNDROMES AND THEIR ASSOCIATED HPV TYPES

CLINICAL SYNDROME	ASSOCIATED HPV TYPES
Cutaneous warts:	
Plantar wart	1
Common wart	2, 4
Flat wart	3, 10
Benign head & neck tumors:	
Laryngeal papilloma	6, 11
Oral papilloma	6, 11
Conjuncrival papilloma	11
Anogenital warts:	
Condyloma acuminatum	6, 11
Cervical intraepithelial neoplasia	16, 18

Approach to Suspected HPV Infection

Definitions

Koilocytes: Enlarged keratinocytes with shrunken nuclei.

Poikilocytosis: Presence of perinuclear cytoplasmic vacuolization and nuclear enlargement of epithelial cells.

Papillomas: An epithelial neoplasm producing finger-like projections from the epithelial surface.

Condylomas: Epithelial neoplasm and hyperplasia of the skin, resulting in the formation of a large cauliflower-like mass.

Discussion

Characteristics of HPV that Impact Transmission

Human papillomavirus (HPV) is a member of the **papovavirus family.** Over 100 distinct types of HPV have been identified based on DNA sequence studies. It has **circular, double-stranded DNA genome** contained within a small, nonenveloped capsid. HPV has a predilection for infecting the squamous epithelium of skin and mucous membranes. HPV is transmitted from **person to person by direct contact, sexual intercourse,** or via **delivery through an infected birth canal.** As a nonenveloped virus, HPV is more environmentally resistant to acids, detergents, and desiccation, which allows for transmission via contaminated fomites.

HPV gains entry through breaks in the skin and **replicates in the basal cell layer** of the epithelium. HPV DNA is replicated, and the viral particles are assembled in the nucleus of epithelial cells with late viral gene expression occurring in the upper layers of differentiated keratinocytes. In **benign lesions,** such as **common skin warts,** the viral DNA **remains extrachromosomal in the nucleus of the infected epithelial cell.** However, more commonly in **carcinomas or high-grade intraepithelial lesions** viral DNA becomes **integrated into the host genome.** The viral genome encodes transforming genes, which have been shown to cause the inactivation of proteins that inhibit cellular growth, making infected cells more susceptible to mutation or other factors that may lead to the development of dysplasia and cancer.

HPV DNA, primarily **types 16 and 18,** has been shown to be present in more than 95 percent of cervical carcinoma specimens. Because of their high occurrence in cervical cancers, these HPV types are considered to be high-risk, whereas **HPV types 6 and 11 are considered low-risk** and many other HPV types are considered benign. Yet, because many HPV-related infections (even those with types 16 and 18) are benign with lesions that can regress spontaneously, the utility of characterizing specific HPV types in clinical specimens remains to be determined.

Diagnosis

HPV infection presents clinically with the growth of a variety of cutaneous warts and papillomas. Warts result from HPV replication stimulating **excessive growth** of the **epidermal layers above the basal layer** (Figure 30-1). Different types of warts (flat, plantar, or common), genital condylomas, and laryngeal papillomas can develop depending on the infecting viral type and the site of infection. Laryngeal papillomas can occur in infants born to mothers with active HPV genital lesions. While rare, these papillomas often require repeated surgical removal. Anogenital warts occur on the squamous epithelium of the external genitalia and anorectum and are most commonly caused by HPV types 6 or 11, however, these lesions rarely undergo malignant transformation. HPV types 16 and 18 are responsible for most cases of cervical intraepithelial neoplasia and cancer. Cervical cancer usually develops after a progression of cellular changes from cellular atypia to low-grade intraepithelial lesion, high-grade intraepithelial lesion and subsequently to carcinoma. Although the mechanisms of host defenses against HPV are not well understood, the immune system, especially cellular immunity, are important in the control of HPV infections. HPV diseases occur more frequently and tend to be more severe in immunocompromised hosts.

Treatment and Prevention

Although many HPV infections are benign with the resulting warts or lesions regressing spontaneously with time, because of the strong association of HPV with cervical carcinomas and transmission via vaginal delivery, physical treat-

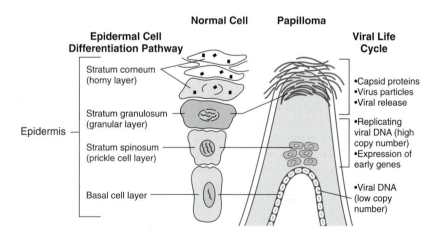

Figure 30-1. Schematic representation of a papilloma wart. HPV is incorporated in the basal layer and affects the maturing cells (left) and results in the skin wart or papilloma (right).

ment and removal of lesions is often performed. **Physical treatment** of warts and other lesions involves local cellular destruction by means of cryotherapy, acid application or electrocautery. Alternatively, **immune stimulant therapy** is used to promote immunologic clearance of the abnormal cells using either the injection of interferon or topical applications of imiquimod. Cervical cancer usually develops after a progression of cellular changes from cellular atypia to low-grade intraepithelial lesion, high-grade intraepithelial lesion, and subsequently to carcinoma. The introduction of routine screening of women for cervical cancer with Papanicolaou (Pap) smears has resulted in finding more abnormalities in earlier, more treatable stages, and a marked reduction in the death rate from cervical cancer. Most deaths from cervical cancer now occur in women who have not had adequate Pap smear screening. Research on HPV-vaccine development is ongoing. A prospective study of an HPV-16 virus-like particle vaccine has indicated the potential for prevention of persistent infection with the HPV type 16. Infection with HPV can be prevented by avoiding direct contact with infected skin lesions. Sexual transmission of HPV can be prevented by safe sex practices.

Comprehension Questions

[30.1] Which of the following types of cancers is HPV most commonly associated with?

    A. Anogenital

    B. Breast

    C. Lung

    D. Oral

    E. Prostate

[30.2] HPV-related cervical intraepithelial neoplasia can be diagnosed by the presence of which of the following histologic features?

    A. Central, basophilic intranuclear cellular inclusions

    B. Cowdry type A intranuclear cellular inclusions

    C. Enlarged multinucleated cells

    D. Cytoplasmic vacuolization and nuclear enlargement of cells

    E. Numerous atypical lymphocytes

[30.3] Which of the following viral families is known to be causally associated with tumor formation in healthy appearing human adults?

    A. Flaviviruses

    B. Papovaviruses

    C. Paramyxoviruses

    D. Polyoma viruses

Answers

[30.1]   **A.** of the types of cancers listed, HPV is most commonly associated
with anogenital carcinomas, which includes cervical carcinomas.

[30.2]   **D.** HPV produces characteristic cytoplasmic vacuolization and
nuclear enlargement of squamous epithelial cells, referred to as koilo-
cytosis; answers A, B, C, and E are incorrect: Both Cowdry type A
intranuclear inclusions and enlarged multinucleated cells can be seen
with herpes simplex virus (HSV) and varicella-zoster virus (VZV)
infections; central, basophilic intranuclear inclusion bodies are seen
in CMV infections, whereas the presence of atypical lymphocytes is
seen specifically in Epstein-Barr virus (EBV) infections.

[30.3]   **B.** HPV is a member of the Papovavirus family and is causally associated with cervical cancer in otherwise healthy individuals; answers
A, C, D, and E are incorrect: Hepatitis C virus is a member of the
Flaviviruses family and causes chronic hepatitis and in severe cases
is a factor in liver cancer development; Paramyxoviruses include
agents such as respiratory syncytial virus and measles virus and are
not associated with carcinomas; human polyoma viruses include BK
and JC viruses, which have been associated with immunocompromised patients, and their role in formation of human tumors is still
under investigation.

MICROBIOLOGY PEARLS

❖ HPV has a tropism for squamous epithelium of skin and mucous
membranes.

❖ 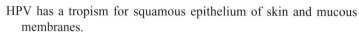 HPV types 16 and 18 are most commonly associated with cervical
carcinomas.

❖ 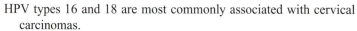 Treatment of HPV-related lesions include immunologic agents,
cryotherapy, acid application, and electrocautery.

REFERENCES

Bosch FX, et al. The causal relationship between human papillomavirus and cervical cancer. J Clin Pathol 2002;55:244.
Murray PR, Rosenthal KS, Kobayashi GS, Pfaller MA. Medical microbiology,
4th ed. St. Louis: Mosby, 2002:458–465.
Ryan JR, Ray CG. Sherris medical microbiology, 4th ed. New York: McGraw-Hill,
2004:617–620.

A 4-year-old girl is brought in by her mother for the evaluation of multiple skin growths on her neck and upper chest. They have been present for a month or two. They are not pruritic or painful. The mother thinks that they are "pimples" because she squeezed a couple of them and some white material was expressed. She has been treating the lesions with an over-the-counter acne preparation, but it hasn't helped. The child has no significant medical history, takes no medications, and has no allergies. On examination you see multiple discrete, isolated 1–2 mm papules on her upper chest and lower neck. They are flesh colored, have a central umbilication, and feel firm on palpation. The remainder of her examination is normal. You suspect Molluscum contagiosum.

◆ **How did the girl most likely acquire this infection?**

◆ **What would you see microscopically on a stained slide of material expressed from the core of one of these lesions that would confirm your diagnosis?**

ANSWERS TO CASE 31: Molluscum contagiosum

Summary: A 4-year-old girl with multiple discrete 1–2 mm papules on her upper chest and lower neck that are flesh colored, have a central umbilication, consistent with Molluscum contagiosum.

◆ **Most likely mechanism of acquisition of infection:** Direct contact with the virus or via contact with contaminated fomites.

◆ **Microscopic findings of expressed material confirming diagnosis:** Microscopic observation of the core material would show eosinophilic cytoplasmic inclusions, also known as molluscum bodies.

CLINICAL CORRELATION

Molluscum contagiosum is a poxvirus that causes benign cutaneous disease worldwide. It is transmitted via direct contact with infected cells or with objects contaminated with virus particles. It causes small wart-like growth on infected skin, and occurs more frequently in children than adults.

Approach to Suspected Infection

Definitions

Molluscum bodies: Eosinophilic cytoplasmic inclusions seen in epidermal cells infected with Molluscum contagiosum.
Umbilicated lesions: Lesions with cup-shaped crater and a white core.
Papules: Lesions that are raised and well circumscribed.

Objectives

1. Be aware of the characteristics of the poxvirus.
2. Be able to describe the mechanism of infection and strategies for prevention and treatment.

Discussion

Characteristics of Molluscum contagiosum that Impact Transmission

Poxviruses are among the **largest, most complex viruses known.** They have a linear, **double-stranded DNA genome** that is fused at both ends. The virion binds to a cell surface receptor and enters the target cell by fusion of the outer envelope with the cell membrane. Replication of poxviruses occurs entirely in the host cytoplasm, making them unique among DNA viruses and requiring them to provide all enzymes necessary for viral replication. For example, poxviruses encode proteins for mRNA synthesis, DNA synthesis, nucleotide scavenging, and immune escape mechanisms. Viral DNA replication and virion assembly occurs in **cytoplasmic inclusions** called **Guarnieri's inclusions.** The newly assembled virions are released on cell lysis.

Because the worldwide eradication of smallpox has been documented, **Molluscum contagiosum is the only poxvirus specific for humans.** Viral inoculation occurs through small skin abrasions, either from direct contact with infectious particles or via contaminated fomites. The **incubation period** for Molluscum contagiosum infection is approximately **2 weeks to 6 months.** Some documented forms of viral spread include direct contact with lesions during **wrestling matches, in swimming pools,** sharing of **towels,** and **sexual contact.** Molluscum contagiosum infection is more common in children than in adults, and in adults it is most often transmitted by sexual contact. Immunocompromised persons who are infected with Molluscum contagiosum may develop hundreds of lesions. Patients who are at greatest risk for this presentation are those with late-stage AIDS, with a CD4 count < 200 cells/microliter.

Diagnosis

Molluscum contagiosum clinically causes discrete, flesh-colored papules with a central umbilication. These nodular lesions most commonly form in groups of 5–25 occurring on the trunk, genitalia, and extremities. They are also known to cause **"kissing lesions"** via direct contact of a lesion with an uninfected area of skin on the same host; such as a lesion on the lateral chest may cause a "kissing lesion" on the inner arm. The semisolid core of these lesions can be expressed and examined **microscopically** for the presence of **large, eosinophilic inclusions, known as molluscum bodies.**

Treatment and Prevention

The lesions of Molluscum contagiosum generally develop within 2–3 months of contact and usually resolve within 1–2 years. Cell-mediated and humoral immunity both appear to be important for disease resolution. When indicated, the lesions can be removed by **curettage, electrocautery, or liquid nitrogen** applications.

Comprehension Questions

[31.1] The incidence of Molluscum contagiosum as a sexually transmitted disease is increasing in young adults and results in the formation of small wartlike lesions in the genital region. Which of the following viruses might also be suspected in such a case of sexually acquired lesions?

    A. Cytomegalovirus
    B. Varicella-zoster virus
    C. Human papillomavirus
    D. Human immunodeficiency virus

[31.2] Which of the following statements best describes the viral characteristics of Molluscum contagiosum?

    A. A large and complex virus containing single-stranded linear RNA
    B. A double-stranded DNA virus encoding a DNA-dependent RNA polymerase
    C. A double-stranded linear DNA virus that integrates into the chromosome
    D. A single-stranded DNA virus that replicates in the host cytoplasm
    E. A double-stranded circular DNA virus

[31.3] A sexually active 17-year-old man presents to the local free clinic to check some small papules that appeared on his penis. The papules are small and white and contain a central depression in their center. There is no penile discharge, nor is there pain on urination. To what group is the organism most likely associated with?

    A. Poxviridae
    B. Papovaviridae
    C. Adenoviridae
    D. Parvoviridae
    E. Arenaviridae

Answers

[31.1]   **C.** Human papillomavirus; answers A, B, and D are incorrect; Cytomegalovirus is known as a sexually transmitted disease but does not characteristically form lesions in or around the genitalia; varicella-zoster virus does form vesicular lesions but appears clinically as a vesicular rash of the head, trunk, or extremities in a dermatomal pattern, not as a genital infection; human immunodeficiency virus is also known to be transmitted via sexual contact, yet it manifests clinically primarily through suppression of the host immune response, not through the formation of genital lesions.

[31.2] **B.** Molluscum contagiosum is a poxvirus and therefore is a double-stranded DNA virus encoding a DNA-dependent RNA polymerase; answers A, C, D, and E are incorrect: (A) describes the characteristics of rabies virus; (C) more appropriately describes herpes simplex viruses; (D) poxviruses do replicate in the host cytoplasm, and Molluscum contagiosum is a double-stranded DNA virus; (E) more appropriately describes human papillomaviruses.

[31.3] **A.** The disease in question is Molluscum contagiosum, which belongs to the Poxviridae and is characterized by small white papules with a central umbilication usually found in the genital region; answers B, C, D, and E are incorrect: (B) Papovaviridae include human papillomavirus and BK, JC polyomavirus, and although HPV causes genital warts, they do not have the central umbilication present in Molluscum contagiosum; (C) Adenoviridae include a variety of viral serotypes which cause respiratory, ocular, and gastrointestinal diseases; (D) Parvoviridae include erythema infectiosum characterized by the slapped cheek appearance; (E) Arenaviridae include lymphocytic choriomeningitis and Lassa virus, which are not described in the question stem.

MICROBIOLOGY PEARLS

❖ Molluscum contagiosum is a poxvirus transmitted via direct contact with infected cells, sharing of towels, or via sexual contact.
❖ Clinical manifestations are small flesh colored umbilicated lesions occurring on the trunk, extremities, or genitalia.
❖ Lesions will resolve spontaneously over time, or can be removed via scraping or treatment with liquid nitrogen.

REFERENCES

Brooks GF, Butel JS, Morse SA. Jawetz, Melnick, & Adelberg's medical microbiology, 23rd ed. New York: McGraw-Hill, 2004:463–464.

Murray PR, Rosenthal KS, Kobayashi GS, Pfaller MA. Medical microbiology, 4th ed. St. Louis: Mosby, 2002:499–504.

Ryan JR, Ray CG. Sherris medical microbiology, 4th ed. New York: McGraw-Hill, 2004:528–529.

A 6-year-old boy is brought to your office for evaluation of fever, ear pain, and swollen cheeks. His mother reports that he's had 3 or 4 days of low-grade fever and seemed tired. Yesterday he developed the sudden onset of ear pain and swelling of the cheeks along with a higher fever. He is an only child, and neither of the parents has been ill recently. He has had no significant medical illnesses in his life, but his parents decided not to give him the measles, mumps, rubella (MMR) vaccine because they read that it could cause autism. On examination, his temperature is 38.6°C (101.5°F), and his pulse is 105 beats per minute. He has swollen parotid glands bilaterally to the point that his earlobes are pushed up, and the angle of his mandible is indistinct. His tympanic membranes appear normal. Opening his mouth causes pain, but the posterior pharynx appears normal. You do note some erythema and swelling of Stensen duct. He has bilateral cervical adenopathy.

◆ **What is the cause of this child's illness?**

◆ **What factor has reduced the incidence of this disease by over 99 percent in the United States?**

ANSWERS TO CASE 32: Mumps

Summary: A 6-year-old boy with has tender inflammation of the parotid glands (parotitis) and fever.

◆ **Most likely cause of this child's disease:** Mumps virus.

◆ **Factor decreasing disease incidence by over 99 percent in the United States:** Routine vaccination with live, attenuated mumps virus.

CLINICAL CORRELATION

The mumps virus is primarily a childhood disease that causes acute, painful swelling of the parotids and other glands. It is a highly communicable disease that has one known serotype and infects only humans. Mumps is endemic around the world, with approximately 90 percent of children being infected by the age of 15. It is now an uncommon illness in countries such as the United States, where a live attenuated vaccine is widely used. The MMR vaccine, a combination vaccine of measles, mumps, and rubella, has resulted in a greater than 99 percent reduction in the incidence of mumps. Almost all cases of mumps now seen are in the unvaccinated or in persons with depressed cellular immunity.

Approach to Suspected Mumps Virus Infection

Definitions

Parotitis: Inflammation of the parotids; large salivary glands located on each side of the face below and in front of the ear.

Hemagglutinin-neuraminidase protein: A viral capsid glycoprotein involved with viral attachment, fusion, and enzymatic hydrolysis of various proteins; also produces nonspecific agglutination of red blood cells used for diagnostic assay.

Orchitis: Inflammation of the testes.

Oophoritis: Inflammation of one or both ovaries.

Objectives

1. Be able to describe the characteristics of the mumps virus.
2. Be able to describe the strategies for prevention and treatment of the infection.

Discussion

Characteristics of the Mumps Virus that Impact Transmission

The mumps virus is a member of the genus **Rubulavirus** of the family **Paramyxoviridae.** It is an **enveloped, spherical virus with a single-stranded, negative-sense RNA genome.** The viral envelope contains two glycoproteins: a **hemagglutinin-neuraminidase protein** involved in attachment and a **membrane fusion protein.** The mumps virus is transmitted to epithelial cells of the mouth or nose via direct contact with contaminated respiratory droplets or saliva or via fomites. The virus then fuses with the host cell membrane via the specific viral attachment and surface fusion proteins, which results in binding to sialic acid on the target cell membrane. Transcription, replication, protein synthesis, and assembly occur in the cytoplasm of the host cell. Newly formed virions acquire their outer envelope by budding through the host cell membrane and are released to infect other host cells. After initial infection and replication in the nasal or upper respiratory tract, viral infection spreads to the salivary glands. Virus infects the **parotids or other salivary glands** either by ascending infection into the gland through Stensen duct or by viremia. Viral particles are also transmitted to distant organs, such as the kidneys, testes, ovaries, and central nervous system (CNS) through viremic spread.

The symptoms of mumps are often the result of the inflammatory response of the host immune system. Many mumps infections are subclinical, and this, along with the fact that infected persons are contagious even 1–2 weeks prior to developing symptoms, promotes person-to-person spread of the disease. The cell-mediated immune system is responsible for defense against this infection and acquired immunity is lifelong. Passive immunity is transferred from mothers to newborns, and thus, mumps is rarely seen in infants less than 6 months old.

Diagnosis

Cases of mumps are now relatively uncommon, but can be diagnosed primarily by clinical presentation along with a patient history that lacks mumps virus immunization. Clinical symptoms include acute onset of **fever and malaise, followed with painful bilateral or unilateral swelling of the parotid or other salivary glands.** 10–20 percent of cases may progress to more severe infections with CNS involvement, resulting in aseptic meningitis or meningoencephalitis. In adolescent children and adults, additional complications may occur including: orchitis, oophoritis, and pancreatitis. These more severe symptoms are more rare and occur primarily in immunocompromised hosts.

Laboratory diagnosis is not typically required; however, rapid confirmation of mumps infection can be obtained through direct **viral antigen detection** via immunofluorescence analysis. Appropriate clinical samples for analysis include saliva, CSF, and urine. Additionally, clinical specimens can be cultured in cells for observation of cytopathic effects such as cell rounding and syncytia formation. Alternately, serology can be used to detect a fourfold rise in mumps-specific IgM or IgG antibody in clinical samples.

Treatment and Prevention

There is no specific antiviral therapy for mumps. However, immunization with the live attenuated mumps virus vaccine provides effective protection against infection.

Comprehension Questions

[32.1] A 6-year-old child presents to their pediatrician with symptoms of fever, fatigue, and swollen glands. Which of the following patient information would confirm a diagnosis of infection with the mumps virus?

   A. A history of exposure to mumps
   B. Clinical evidence of orchitis
   C. Detection of mumps-specific IgM antibody
   D. Resolution of fever followed by signs of encephalitis

[32.2] Which of the following statement regarding infection with the mumps virus is correct?

   A. After initial replication, viremic spread can occur to various organs.
   B. Diagnosis is made solely on symptoms, as virus cannot be cultured.
   C. Passive immunization is the only means of preventing infection.
   D. Reinfection is possible, because of the presence of two viral serotypes.
   E. Virus is transmitted via the fecal-oral route.

[32.3] Which of the following organs would most commonly exhibit signs of mumps infection?

   A. CNS
   B. Ovaries
   C. Pancreas
   D. Parotids
   E. Testes

Answers

[32.1]   **C.** The detection of mumps-specific IgM antibody indicates active
         mumps virus infection; answers A, B, D, and E; are incorrect; (A)
         exposure to mumps does not necessarily cause infection, particularly
         if the child has been immunized; (B) symptoms of orchitis because of
         mumps infection occurs only in adolescent males; (D) encephalitis is
         a more rare complication of mumps infection and is not specific to
         the mumps virus.

[32.2]   **A.** After initial replication in the upper respiratory tract and salivary
         glands, viral particles are also transmitted to distant organs such as
         the kidneys, testes, ovaries, and CNS through viremic spread; answers
         B, C, D and E are incorrect.

[32.3]   **D.** Swollen parotid glands are a common symptom during infection
         with the mumps virus; answers A, B, C, and E are possible compli-
         cations of infection with the mumps virus, but are less commonly
         occurring.

MICROBIOLOGY PEARLS

 Nearly all cases of mumps are seen in unvaccinated children or per-
     sons with depressed cellular immunity.

 Clinical manifestations: acute fever and painful swelling of the
     parotids and other glands.

❖ Immunization with a live attenuated mumps virus vaccine has resulted
     in nearly 100 percent reduction in the incidence of infection.

REFERENCES

Brooks GF, Butel JS, Morse SA. Jawetz, Melnick, & Adelberg's medical microbiol-
    ogy, 23rd ed. New York: McGraw-Hill, 2004:560–562.
Ryan JR, Ray CG. Sherris medical microbiology, 4th ed. New York: McGraw-Hill,
    2004:513.

An 8-year-old boy is brought in to the office with a 3-day history of fever and a rash. He has also had a mild sore throat and felt somewhat fatigued. His mother is concerned that he could have "scarlet fever." The rash started on his face and then spread to his arms and legs. He has only been given acetaminophen for the fever. He takes no other medications, has no known allergies, has no significant medical history, and has had no contact with anyone known to be ill. On examination, his temperature is 37.7°C (99.8°F), and his other vital signs are normal. His cheeks are notably red, almost as if they had been slapped. His pharynx is normal appearing, and the remainder of his head and neck exam is normal. On his extremities there is a fine, erythematous, maculopapular rash but no vesicles or petechiae. A rapid group A streptococcal antigen test done in the office is negative.

◆ **What virus is the likely cause of this illness?**

◆ **In which human cells does this virus cause lytic infections?**

ANSWERS TO CASE 33: Parvoviruses

Summary: An 8-year-old boy with fever and "slapped cheek" appearance has erythema infectiosum or fifth disease.

◆ **Most likely viral cause of this illness:** Infection with parvovirus B19.

◆ **Human cells in which the virus causes lytic infections:** Mitotically active erythroid precursor cells.

CLINICAL CORRELATION

Parvovirus B19 is the only parvovirus known to cause disease in humans. Infection occurs typically in school-age children resulting in a mild febrile upper respiratory illness followed by an exanthematous rash on the face or "slapped cheek" appearance which later spreads to the extremities. It is classically described as fifth disease because it was the fifth childhood exanthem to be described after varicella, rubella, roseola, and measles. Adults are less commonly infected, and primarily present with polyarthritis of the hands, knees, and ankles, occurring with or without rash. Chronic infection occurs in immunodeficient patients with more serious consequences, such as severe anemia and aplastic crisis. Additionally, infection occurring in pregnant seronegative mothers can lead to serious infection and fetal death.

Approach to Suspected Parvoviral Infection

Definitions

Exanthem: An eruptive disease or eruptive fever appearing on the skin.
Enanthem: An eruptive disease appearing on mucous membranes.
Petechiae: Tiny reddish or purplish spots containing blood and appearing on the skin or mucous membranes.
Hydrops fetalis: Serious edema of the fetus which can result in congestive heart failure.
Erythroid progenitor cells: Precursors to erythrocytes.

Objectives

1. Be able to describe the characteristics of the virus.
2. Be able to describe the strategies for prevention and treatment of the infection.

Discussion

Characteristics of Parvovirus that Impact Transmission

Parvoviruses are small, **nonenveloped viruses with a linear, single-stranded DNA** genome. They are the **smallest of the DNA animal viruses,** and their virions contain either a positive- or negative-sense copy of the viral genome.

Parvovirus B19 belongs to the **Parvoviridae family** and is the only parvovirus known to cause human disease. It is spread from **person–to person by respiratory and oral secretions,** replicating first in the nasopharynx, then spreading by viremia to the bone marrow. It binds to the **erythrocyte blood group P antigen on erythroid precursor cells** and is internalized through coated pits. After internalization, the viral DNA is uncoated and transported to the nucleus, where a complementary DNA strand is created by the host DNA polymerase. Inverted repeat sequences on the 5' and 3' ends of the viral DNA are used as primers to initiate DNA replication. The resultant double-stranded viral DNA is then further replicated and transcribed via host cell machinery, and newly formed virions are assembled in the nucleus. Additionally, other factors only available in the S phase of mitosis are required for parvoviral replication. The newly assembled infectious particles are then released by lysis of the host nuclear and cytoplasmic membranes, resulting in cell death. The major site for parvoviral replication is in adult bone marrow and fetal liver cells. Because replication in these cells results in cell lysis and death, there is a **disruption of red cell production and resultant anemia** that occurs with viral infection.

Clinical symptoms caused by parvovirus B19 are related to the immune system response to the infection. The most common clinical illness associated with parvovirus B19 is **erythema infectiosum, or fifth disease.** It is commonly seen in children and usually causes a biphasic infection with mild upper respiratory symptoms, low-grade or no fever, and a rash. The initial stage lasts for approximately 1 week and involves the infection and killing of erythroid cells followed by viremic spread. This stage is the infectious stage and produces flu-like symptoms with mild fever and upper-respiratory symptoms. The second stage of infection is immune-mediated, with the formation of host antibody-virus immune complexes, a reduction in viremia, and the emergence of a lacy skin rash. The rash usually starts on the face and is classically described as causing a **"slapped cheek"** appearance. A maculopapular rash will then frequently develop on the extremities. Adults may get a rash, but more often develop arthralgias or frank arthritis. The production of rash, arthralgias, and arthritis are all results of circulating antibody-virus immune complexes. These symptoms are usually self-limited; however, persistent infections can occur in immune-compromised hosts who fail to produce virus-neutralizing antibodies, because host antibody-mediated immunity is necessary for defense against the infection and prevention of reinfections.

More rare but potentially life-threatening complications of parvovirus B19 infection can occur. **Aplastic crisis** can occur in hosts with a chronic hemolytic anemia, such as **sickle cell disease** or other acquired hemolytic anemias. In this setting, the combination of viral replication in red cell precursors along with the reduced circulatory life span of existing red cells may result in a profound anemia. Additionally, parvoviral B19 infection in immunodeficient patients can result in persistent infections with chronic bone marrow suppression and anemia. There is also an increased risk of fetal loss because of anemia caused by **transplacental infection of the fetus** when a seronegative mother becomes infected during pregnancy. Fetal parvoviral infection can result in hydrops fetalis, severe anemia, and often, fetal death before the third trimester. The fetus of a seropositive mother is protected from infection by maternal circulating antibodies.

Diagnosis

Definitive diagnosis of parvovirus B19 infection relies on the detection of **viral DNA** via **PCR or DNA hybridization** assays using patient serum, blood or tissue samples. Additionally, **serologic detection of viral IgM or IgG antibodies** via ELISA (enzyme-linked immunosorbent assay) can be used for diagnoses.

Treatment and Prevention

At present, there is **no specific treatment** for parvovirus B19 infections. Infection control measures are used in hospitals to avoid parvoviral spread, such as rigorous hand washing and isolation of infected patients. Although vaccines are available for dogs and cats, there is currently no parvoviral B19 vaccine available for humans.

Comprehension Questions

[33.1] Which of the following statements is most accurate regarding infection with parvovirus B19?

    A. Parvovirus B19 replicates in the host cell nucleus utilizing a virally encoded DNA polymerase to create a double-stranded DNA intermediate.

    B. Parvovirus B19 causes severe anemia because it preferentially infects erythrocyte precursors

    C. Parvovirus B19 can be diagnosed by detection of viral RNA using PCR or hybridization assays.

    D. Parvovirus B19 can cause hydrops fetalis via transplacental infection of a fetus in a seropositive mother.

    E. Parvovirus B19 is transmitted primarily by fecal-oral transmission and is highly prevalent in infants and young children.

[33.2] A normally healthy 7-year-old girl is sent home from school with a suspected case of fifth disease as a result of her presenting with the initial symptoms of the infection. After being at home for a few days, her symptoms change indicating her transition into the second phase of the illness. Which of the following symptoms is the girl most likely experiencing during the second phase of parvoviral infection?

    A. Aplastic crisis

    B. Diarrhea

    C. High fever

    D. Skin rash

    E. Swollen glands

[33.3] Which of the following conditions would put an individual at increased risk for serious chronic illness following an infection with parvovirus B19?

A. Immunization with a live measles vaccine
B. Having sickle cell disease
C. Caring for a pet with canine parvoviral infection
D. Coinfection with influenza A virus
E. Not being immunized for poliovirus

Answers

[33.1]   **B.** Parvovirus B19 binds preferentially to the erythrocyte blood group P antigen on erythroid precursor cells; answers A, B, C, and E are incorrect: (A) after entry the single-stranded viral DNA genome is transported to the cell nucleus where the host DNA polymerase synthesizes the complimentary DNA strand; (C) Parvovirus B19 infection can be diagnosed by direct detection of viral DNA not RNA; (D) the fetus of a seropositive mother is protected from infection by maternal circulating antibodies; (E) Parvovirus B19 is transmitted primarily by respiratory secretions and is prevalent in school-age children.

[33.2]   **D.** The second stage of parvoviral B19 infection is immune-mediated, and results in formation of a lacy skin rash occurring first on the face and then moves to the extremities; answers A, B, C, and E are incorrect: (A) aplastic crisis occurs in hosts with sickle cell disease or other acquired hemolytic anemias, not in normally healthy individuals; (B) parvoviral infection does not cause gastrointestinal symptoms; (C) mild fever, not high fever, is a symptom that occurs in the initial stage of fifth disease; (E) parvoviral infection does not result in swollen glands.

[33.3]   **B.** More serious complications of parvoviral B19 infection, such as aplastic crisis, can occur in hosts with sickle cell disease or other chronic hemolytic anemias; answers A, C, D, and E are incorrect as they are not associated with serious complications of parvovirus B19 infection.

MICROBIOLOGY PEARLS

❖ Parvovirus B19 is the smallest human DNA virus and replicates in mitotically active erythroid progenitor cells.

❖ Clinical manifestations in children: mild fever followed by rash with "slapped cheek" appearance; fetal infections: hydrops fetalis and death.

❖ Clinical manifestations in adults: polyarthritis of hands, knees, and ankles with or without rash; chronic infection may result in chronic anemia or aplastic crisis.

❖ No specific treatment or vaccination.

REFERENCES

Brooks GF, Butel JS, Morse SA. Jawetz, Melnick, & Adelberg's medical microbiology, 23rd ed. New York: McGraw-Hill, 2004:414–419.

Heegaard ED, Hornsleth A. Parvovirus: the expanding spectrum of disease. Acta Paediatr 1995;84:109–117.

Ryan JR, Ray CG. Sherris medical microbiology, 4th ed. New York: McGraw-Hill, 2004:522–523.

A 62-year-old man presents to the emergency room after suddenly losing the use of his right leg. He reports that he had a few days of headache, fever, and sore throat, which was treated with oral antibiotics and resolved about 4 days ago. He was feeling fine until this morning, when he could not lift his right leg to get out of bed. All of his other limbs are functioning normally, and he has normal sensation in them. He has a medical history significant for lung cancer for which he is receiving chemotherapy, with his most recent cycle having been completed a few days prior to the onset of his febrile illness. He denies having any recent falls, injuries, current headache, or neurologic symptoms other than in the right leg. He has not traveled outside of the United States. His only current medication is amoxicillin/clavulanic acid, which was prescribed for his recent febrile illness. He lives with his son, daughter-in-law, and two young grandchildren. The children are healthy, and each had their routine well-child checkups and vaccinations about a month ago, including an oral vaccine. On examination, he is anxious appearing but has normal vital signs and has unremarkable head and neck, cardiovascular, pulmonary, and abdominal examinations. He has flaccid paralysis with normal sensation of the right leg, with normal movement and strength in all other extremities and a normal cranial nerve examination. A head CT scan and lumbar magnetic resonance imaging (MRI) are also normal.

◆ **What is the most likely infectious cause of this man's flaccid paralysis?**

◆ **Assuming that he was infected at home, what is the most likely source of his infection?**

ANSWERS TO CASE 34: Poliovirus

Summary: A 62-year-old man with flaccid paralysis of the right leg. He lives with his grandchildren, who were recently given an oral vaccine.

◆ **Most likely infectious cause of this man's flaccid paralysis:** Poliomyelitis, caused by poliovirus.

◆ **Most likely source of his infection:** fecal-oral transmission of viral particles shed from one of his grandchildren recently vaccinated with live attenuated poliovirus vaccine.

CLINICAL CORRELATION

Poliovirus is an exclusive human pathogen, which causes an acute infectious disease that can result in flaccid paralysis from the destruction of motor neurons in the spinal cord. Although most childhood infections tend to be subclinical, the risk of more serious paralytic disease increases with age. Infections are spread through fecal-oral transfer and poor sanitation and crowded conditions help to promote viral spread. Both attenuated live and inactivated oral viral vaccines have been available for over 40 years, and most industrialized countries have been free from wild poliovirus infections since the late 1990s or early 2000s. Use of the killed-virus vaccine for childhood immunizations is currently recommended in the United States because of safety issues with the live-attenuated vaccine, including possible transfer of live virus to close contacts. Efforts are being continued to globally eradicate poliovirus from residual areas such as Africa and India.

Approach to Suspected Infection

Definitions

Poliomyelitis: Inflammation and destruction of the gray matter of the spinal cord, which can result in paralysis.

Attenuated live poliovirus vaccine or oral polio vaccine (OPV): A viral vaccine consisting of a less virulent form of poliovirus, obtained through multiple passages of three types of poliovirus through tissue culture cells.

Inactivated poliomyelitis vaccine (IPV): A viral vaccine consisting of a large dose of viral antigen that will elicit a protective antibody response without risk of spreading the infection.

Objectives

1. Be able to describe the characteristics of the virus.
2. Be able to describe the strategies for prevention and treatment of the infection.

Discussion

Characteristics of Poliovirus that Impact Transmission

Poliovirus is a member of the **Enterovirus genus of the Picornaviridae family.** It is a **small, nonenveloped virus with a single-stranded, positive-sense RNA genome** that resembles cellular mRNA. It is contained within an icosahedral capsid composed of four polypeptides (VP1-VP4) that are necessary for maintaining virion structure, attachment to specific host cell receptors, and entry into cells. The viral genome contains a small protein at the 5' end, termed VPg, and is polyadenylated at the 3' end. The genome is transcribed into a single polyprotein that is proteolytically cleaved to produce all of the virally encoded proteins. One of these proteins is a viral protease, which specifically degrades the 5' cap proteins from cellular mRNAs and thus preferentially inhibits translation of host mRNA. The 5' viral VPg protein promotes cap-independent association of the poliovirus genome with host cell ribosomes and allows translation of viral proteins to occur. Polioviruses are **cytolytic** and cause direct damage to infected cells.

As with other *Enteroviruses,* poliovirus is transmitted primarily by the **fecal-oral route.** Viral particles enter through the mouth and primary replication is thought to occur in the oropharynx, tonsils, and lymph nodes or in the intestinal epithelium and adjacent lymphoid tissue. The virus is resistant to a wide range of pH levels, allowing it to survive the acidity of the stomach. Depending on the host immune response and the ability of the virus to spread, infection with poliovirus can result in one of four different types of infection: asymptomatic illness, abortive poliomyelitis, nonparalytic poliomyelitis, or paralytic poliomyelitis. After initial viral replication, an immune competent host will make specific antibodies to the virus, and if the infection is limited to this stage the infection remains asymptomatic. Host antibodies provide the major immune response to poliovirus infections. However, if infection is not contained by the host antibody response, there may be a "minor" viremic spread to cells containing a specific receptor recognized by the capsid VP proteins. The specificity of poliovirus infection via these receptors restricts the tropism for poliovirus to cells such as the **anterior horn cells of the spinal cord, dorsal root ganglia, motor neurons, skeletal muscle cells, and lymphoid cells.**

After binding to the receptor, the RNA genome is inserted into the host cytoplasm through a channel created in the cell membrane. Viral transcription and replication occur in the cytoplasm, and new virions are released by cell lysis. Replication in these cells can then lead to a "major" viremia that, when controlled by host antibody response, produces the "minor" illness of abortive poliomyelitis. Abortive poliomyelitis causes nonspecific symptoms that include fever, sore throat, and headache. In a small percentage of infected people, the virus may continue to spread to involve the central nervous system (CNS) or the meninges. This can occur either as a result of viremic dissemination or ascending infection through peripheral nerves into the CNS. This can then result in nonparalytic poliomyelitis, aseptic meningitis, or, when anterior horn cells of the spinal cord or motor cortex are involved, paralytic poliomyelitis. Paralytic poliomyelitis is the least common complication of poliovirus infection and appears less than a week following initial symptoms of abortive poliomyelitis. Paralytic disease is caused by cytolytic damage caused by the virus, not by the immune response.

Diagnosis

In addition to the presentation of the above clinical findings, a suspected poliovirus infection can be diagnosed by the **recovery and culture of the virus from clinical samples.** The best clinical specimens include throat swabs if collected shortly after the onset of infection or rectal swabs and stool specimens collected up to 30 days post onset. Cells inoculated with poliovirus will show cytopathic effects of viral infection in less than a week of culture. Even when there is CNS and meningeal involvement, poliovirus is rarely recovered from CNS fluid. RT-PCR can also be used to detect RNA sequences in tissues and body fluids, increasing the sensitivity and speed of diagnosis.

Treatment and Prevention

Universal vaccination has eliminated wild-type polio from the western hemisphere and has greatly reduced the incidence of the disease worldwide. Two vaccine types exist—a **live, attenuated virus vaccine given orally** and an **inactivated vaccine given by injection.** The live, attenuated virus vaccine has the advantages of creating a secretory antibody in the gastrointestinal (GI) tract and is easily administered. However, viral shedding in the stool of the vaccinated person does occur and has been a source of polio infections during the era of widespread vaccination. In very rare cases, the polio vaccine caused disease either in the vaccinated individual or a close, usually immunocompromised, contact. Because of this, the current recommendation in the United States is to give only the inactivated vaccine, which induces humoral antibodies, but does not carry the risk of vaccine-induced disease. A primary series of four inoculations is recommended within a 1–2 year period, with periodic boosters administered as necessary later in life. However, the inactivated vaccine does not induce local intestinal immunity, allowing poliovirus to still replicate in the GI tract.

Comprehension Questions

[34.1] Which of the following statements best describes an advantage of the oral polio vaccine when compared to the inactivated poliomyelitis vaccine?

    A. It can be administered to immunocompromised patients.

    B. It is not associated with vaccine-related cases of poliomyelitis.

    C. It induces local intestinal immunity.

    D. It is easily administered as a series of multiple injections.

    E. It can be given to young children with other scheduled immunizations.

[34.2] The primary pathologic effect of polioviral infection is a result of which of the following:

A. Destruction of infected cells
B. Paralysis of muscle cells
C. Immune complex formation
D. Aseptic meningitis
E. Persistent viremia

[34.3] The majority of nonimmunized patients infected with poliovirus would be expected to experience:

A. Flu-like illness
B. Aseptic meningitis
C. Muscle spasms and pain
D. Flaccid paralysis of one or more extremities
E. Asymptomatic infection

Answers

[34.1] **C.** The oral polio vaccine or "live" vaccine produces not only IgM and IgG antibodies in the blood but also secretory IgA antibodies in the intestine, resulting in intestinal immunity; the inactivated poliomyelitis vaccine produces humoral immunity, but not localized intestinal immunity. Answers A, B, D, and E are incorrect: (A) only the inactivated poliomyelitis vaccine is administered to immunocompromised patients; (B) the oral polio vaccine has been associated with transfer of live poliovirus to close contacts of immunized patients, and therefore, use of the inactivated poliomyelitis vaccine is currently recommended in the United States for childhood immunizations; (D) it is easily administered in multiple oral doses, not injections; (E) both the oral polio vaccine and the inactivated poliomyelitis vaccine can be given to young children with other scheduled immunizations.

[34.2] **A.** polioviruses are cytolytic and cause direct damage to infected cells; answers B, C, D, and E are incorrect: (B) paralysis results in less than 2 percent of patients infected with poliovirus and is a direct result of the destruction of infected neurons in the spinal cord and brain; (C) paralytic disease is caused by cytolytic damage because of the virus, not by the immune response; (D) aseptic meningitis is a result of poliovirus infection which occurs in less than 1–2 percent of patients infected, and is a result of the destruction of infected cells; (E) if not contained by the host antibody response, polioviral infection may result in "minor" and "major" viremic spread within the patient, however, the primary pathologic effect of poliovirus is still the cell lysis of infected cells.

[34.3]   **E.** Greater than 90 percent of infections with poliovirus result in asymptomatic infections; answers A, B, C, and D are incorrect; all are potential outcomes of polioviral infections that remain uncontrolled by a host immune response, but are much less common outcomes of poliovirus infection.

MICROBIOLOGY PEARLS

❖ Poliovirus is a small, nonenveloped virus with a single-stranded, positive-sense RNA genome.

❖ More than 90 percent of poliovirus infections are asymptomatic.

❖ Clinical manifestations: "minor" illness of abortive poliomyelitis includes fever, sore throat, and headache; "major" illness of non-paralytic poliomyelitis or paralytic poliomyelitis also includes back pain, muscle spasm, aseptic meningitis, and spinal paralysis of one or more limbs.

❖ Vaccines available: attenuated live poliovirus vaccine or oral polio vaccine (OPV) and inactivated poliomyelitis vaccine (IPV).

REFERENCES

Brooks GF, Butel JS, Morse SA. Jawetz, Melnick, & Adelberg's medical microbiology, 23rd ed. New York: McGraw-Hill, 2004:491–492.

Ryan JR, Ray CG. Sherris medical microbiology, 4th ed. New York: McGraw-Hill, 2004:532–537.

A 3-year-old male infant is brought to the emergency room in the middle of January with fever, vomiting, and diarrhea for the past day. He has not been able to keep anything down by mouth and has had profuse, very watery stools. He attends day care, and several of his classmates have been out sick recently as well. No adult members of the household have been ill. He has no significant past medical history. On examination, his temperature is 37.9°C (100.2°F), and he has tachycardia. His mucous membranes are dry, and eyes appear somewhat sunken. His abdomen has active bowel sounds and is nontender. His stool is watery and pale. The stool tests negative for blood and fecal leukocytes.

◆ **What is the most likely cause of this child's illness?**

◆ **How is this virus activated to form an infectious particle?**

ANSWERS TO CASE 35: Rotavirus

Summary: A 3-year-old boy who attends day care develops gastroenteritis in the winter.

◆ **Most likely cause of this child's illness:** Rotavirus.

◆ **How is this virus activated to form an infectious particle:** Activation of Rotavirus occurs when the outer capsid layer is lysed by gastrointestinal (GI) proteases to create an infectious subviral particle (ISVP).

CLINICAL CORRELATION

Rotaviruses are ubiquitous worldwide and are estimated to cause more than 50 percent of gastroenteritis cases occurring in children less 2–3 years of age, resulting in approximately 4 billion annual cases. Infections typically occur in the cooler months and result in abrupt onset of vomiting followed with frequent watery diarrhea. Illness is typically self-limiting; however, severe infection can result in immunocompromised or malnourished children and may be fatal. Outbreaks are common in daycare, preschool, and hospital settings. Adults may also become infected but usually have few if any symptoms.

Approach to Suspected Rotavirus Infection

Definitions

Tachycardia: An increased heart rate.
Reassortment: The formation of new virions with hybrid genomes assembled in cells with mixed viral infections, which occurs among viruses containing segmented genomes (i.e. influenza viruses and reoviruses), resulting in high genetic variation.
Intussusception: Blockage of the intestines as a result of the bowel telescoping into itself.

Objectives

1. Be able to describe the characteristics of the virus.
2. Be able to describe the strategies for prevention and treatment of the infection.

Discussion

Characteristics of Rotavirus that Impact Transmission

Rotavirus is one of the **four genera of the family Reoviridae** and is a common cause of childhood gastroenteritis around the world. The virus consists of a **double-layered protein capsid** that contains a genome made of **11 segments**

of double-stranded RNA. The double capsid **looks like a wheel with short spokes** connecting the outer capsid to the inner capsid and core, thus the name **Rotavirus.** As a nonenveloped virus, it retains its infectivity in a wide range of pH and temperatures and is resistant to many common detergents as well. **Rotavirus** is spread through fecal-oral contact, and because of its stability, fomite transmission can also occur. The virus would be inactivated by the pH of a normal, empty stomach but can survive in a buffered stomach or in the gastric environment following a meal. The outer capsid of the virus is partially digested by GI proteolytic enzymes, creating an infectious subviral particle (ISVP). A surface protein of the virus, VP4, is also cleaved by GI proteases, allowing it to bind to the surface of intestinal epithelial cells and allow the ISVP to enter by direct penetration. The RNA genome remains in the viral core and is transcribed into mRNA by a viral polymerase. The mRNA is then transported out of the core to the cell cytoplasm, where it is translated and assembled into new virions. The newly created viral particles are released by cell lysis.

Rotaviruses have been classified into at least **three different major subgroups** and nine different serotypes based on antigenic epitopes of the inner capsid protein VP6. There are primarily four serotypes that are important in causing human disease. Because of the segmented nature of the genome, Rotaviruses are capable of producing virions with high genetic variation as a result of the reassortment of genome sequences in mixed infections. This high genetic variability results in increased numbers of serotypes for this viral group and allows for reinfection of persons previously exposed to one rotaviral serotype. Reinfections are common, yet successive infections appear to cause less severe symptoms.

The mechanism by which rotaviral infection causes diarrhea is not entirely understood. Rotaviral particles infect the cells of the small intestinal villi and multiply in the cytoplasm of enterocytes. Damaged cells are sloughed off, releasing large numbers of viral particles into the stool. Virus can be excreted for days to weeks after infection. The infection prevents absorption of water, sodium, and glucose, resulting in a loss of water and electrolytes. A virally encoded nonstructural protein also acts as an enterotoxin, similar to those of *Escherichia coli* and *Vibrio cholerae.* Typical symptoms of rotaviral infection include fever, vomiting, abdominal pain, and watery diarrhea without blood or mucus. The net result is a profuse watery diarrhea that can cause dehydration without appropriate fluid and electrolyte replacement. Symptoms may last for approximately 1 week, with viral excretion lasting weeks longer. Severe and prolonged illness can occur in immunodeficient and malnourished children and without supportive therapy infection can be fatal. Infection with rotavirus stimulates a humoral response; however, protection against reinfection is temporary and incomplete. The presence of high levels of rotavirus IgA in the lumen of the intestine confers relative protection.

Diagnosis

Because the symptoms of rotaviral infection resemble those of other viral diarrhea producing agents, the definitive diagnoses of rotaviral infection requires the **detection of viral antigens in stool samples.** Enzyme immunoassay and latex agglutination are two easy, rapid assays used to confirm rotaviral infection. Additionally, PCR can be used for genotyping viral nucleic acid in stool specimens. Viral culture is both difficult and unreliable and therefore is not used for diagnoses.

Treatment and Prevention

Treatment of rotaviral infection is **supportive,** including the replacement of fluids and electrolytes to restore physiologic balance and prevent dehydration. Both oral and intravenous rehydration therapy are effective, and which one is used depends on the severity of dehydration. Because Rotaviruses can retain infectivity over a wide range of pH and temperatures and are resistant to many common detergents, strict hand washing and use of gloves is necessary to limit nosocomial spread.

An **attenuated recombinant Rotavirus vaccine** was developed and used in children for several years. However, its **approval was withdrawn,** and its use stopped because of concerns with the development of **intussusception** among vaccine users. Another difficulty with the production of such a vaccine is that a single vaccine may not protect against all Rotavirus serotypes.

Comprehension Questions

[35.1] You isolate a virus from the stool of a 1-year-old infant with signs of fever, vomiting, and diarrhea. Laboratory results show that the viral genome is composed of multiple segments of double-stranded RNA, which leads you to suspect that rotavirus is the causative agent of infection. Which of the following statements is true regarding rotavirus replication?

A. The viral genome integrates into the host chromosome.
B. The virus uses the host RNA polymerase for replication of its genome.
C. The segmented genome contributes to the antigenic variation of the virus.
D. The viral agent has a single antigenic type.
E. The newly assembled viral particles are released via budding through the host cell membrane.

[35.2] Similar to Rotavirus, which of the following viral agents is also a nonenveloped RNA virus known to cause gastroenteritis diarrhea in young children?

A. Calicivirus
B. Paramyxovirus
C. Parainfluenza virus
D. Coxsackie virus
E. None of the above

Answers

[35.1]   **C.** The segmented genome of Rotaviruses, allows for the assembly of new virions with mixed genomes in cells multiply infected as a result of reassortment; answers A, B, D, and E are incorrect: (A) the rotaviral genome consists of double-stranded RNA and replicates in the cytoplasm and thus does not integrate into the host chromosome; (B) as an RNA virus that replicates in the cytoplasm, the rotoviral genome is replicated by a viral RNA polymerase; (D) the high genetic variability of rotaviruses because of reassortment results in multiple viral serotypes, at least nine different serotypes have currently been classified in human illness; (E) newly assembled nonenveloped rotaviral particles are released by cell lysis.

[35.2]   **A.** Like Rotaviruses, Caliciviruses are nonenveloped RNA viruses that cause watery diarrhea, especially in children; answers B, C, D, and E are incorrect: (B) paramyxoviruses are enveloped RNA viruses that cause childhood respiratory and exanthemous infections; (C) parainfluenza viruses are enveloped RNA viruses which cause respiratory infections such as croup, bronchiolitis, and pneumonia in children; (D) Coxsackie viruses are nonenveloped RNA viruses that cause nonspecific respiratory tract infections, febrile rashes, and meningitis.

MICROBIOLOGY PEARLS

❖ Rotaviruses are ubiquitous, causing greater than 50 percent of gastroenteritis cases in children under 2–3 years.
❖ Rotaviruses are composed of a double-layered protein capsid and a segmented double-stranded RNA genome, allowing the new virions to have high genetic variation as a result of reassortment.
❖ Clinical manifestations: abrupt onset of fever, vomiting, abdominal pain, and watery diarrhea without blood or mucus.
❖ Only supportive treatment of infection including fluid and electrolyte replacement; no vaccine is currently available.

REFERENCES

Brooks GF, Butel JS, Morse SA. Jawetz, Melnick, & Adelberg's medical microbiology, 23rd ed. New York: McGraw-Hill, 2004:505–508.

Centers for Disease Control and Prevention. Intussusception among recipients of rotavirus vaccine—United States, 1998–1999. Morb Mortal Wkly Rep 1999;48:577–581.

Ryan JR, Ray CG. Sherris medical microbiology, 4th ed. New York: McGraw-Hill, 2004:577–581.

A 10-month-old female is brought to the pediatric emergency room in late December with a cough and fever. She started getting sick with a mild cough and runny nose about 3 days prior, but has progressively worsened. She is now coughing frequently and has vomited after coughing. She has no history of asthma or other respiratory illness. She was born after an uncomplicated, full-term pregnancy and has no significant medical history. She attends daycare 3 days a week. On examination, her temperature is 38.3°C (100.9°F), pulse is 110 beats per minute, respiratory rate is 30 breaths per minute, and her oxygen saturation is low at 91 percent by pulse oximetry. Her head and neck examination shows her to have a right otitis media but is otherwise normal. Her cardiac exam is notable only for tachycardia. Her pulmonary examination shows her to be in moderate respiratory distress. She has prominent nasal flaring and subcostal retractions on inspiration. She has loud expiratory wheezes in all lung fields. The remainder of her examination is normal. A chest x-ray shows hyperaeration but no infiltrates.

◆ **What is the likely infectious cause of her respiratory illness?**

◆ **Following resolution of this illness, her mother asks whether she is protected from getting this disease again. How do you respond?**

ANSWERS TO CASE 36: Respiratory syncytial virus

Summary: A 10-month-old female presents with bronchiolitis. A chest x-ray shows hyperaeration but no infiltrates.

◆ **Likely infectious cause of her respiratory illness:** Respiratory syncytial virus (RSV).

◆ **Is she protected from getting this disease again:** The immunity developed with an RSV infection is incomplete, and reinfections are common. However, the severity of disease with repeat infections appears to be reduced, especially in older children and adults.

CLINICAL CORRELATION

RSV is a ubiquitous and highly contagious viral infection and is the single most common cause of fatal respiratory tract infections in infants under 12 months of age. It accounts for approximately 25 percent of pediatric hospitalizations of this age group, resulting in severe respiratory illnesses such as bronchiolitis, pneumonia, and respiratory failure. It is also highly prevalent in childcare settings, with 70–95 percent of children attending daycare being infected by 3–4 years of age. Less severe illness occurs in older children and adults and may present as a common cold.

Approach to Suspected Infection

Definitions

Bronchiolitis: Inflammation of the bronchioles or thin-walled branches of the lungs.

Right otitis media: Inflammation of the right middle ear marked with pain, fever, dizziness, and abnormal hearing.

Objectives

1. Be able to describe the characteristics of the virus.
2. Be able to describe the strategies for prevention and treatment of the infection.

Discussion

Characteristics of RSV that Impact Transmission

RSV belongs to the Pneumovirus genus of the family Paramyxoviridae. It is a common cause of upper and lower respiratory tract infections in all age groups, but tends to cause more severe, lower respiratory disease in **infants and young children.** RSV is an **enveloped virus with a single-stranded, negative-**

sense RNA genome. It is transmitted by the inhalation of aerosolized respiratory droplets. It can survive on nonporous surfaces, such as countertops, for 3–30 hours but is inactivated by many detergents and does not tolerate changes in temperature or pH well. RSV infections primarily remain localized in the respiratory tract. The virus infects target respiratory epithelial cells by fusion of its envelope with the host cytoplasmic membrane via the action of two viral envelope glycoproteins. However, unlike the related influenza and parainfluenza viruses, RSV envelope glycoproteins do not possess hemagglutinin or neuraminidase activities. RNA transcription, protein synthesis, replication, and assembly all occur in the cytoplasm and newly formed virions are released by budding from the host cell. RSV is also capable of promoting cell-cell fusion, resulting in multinucleated giant cells known as syncytia, an ability for which it derives its name.

RSV is initially transmitted to the nasopharynx through contact with **infected secretions and fomites,** resulting in localized infections of respiratory epithelium. Although viremia is rare, progressive infections can extend to the middle and lower airways. Disease caused by RSV is primarily the result of the host immune system mediating damage to infected respiratory epithelial cells. In adults and older children, mild upper respiratory tract symptoms such as a runny nose or mild cough usually develop with clinical symptoms lasting for 1–2 weeks. In **infants or younger children,** more serious illness such as **bronchiolitis** can occur. This occurs when there is inflammation and plugging of the bronchi and bronchioles with mucous and necrotic tissue from immune-mediated cellular damage. The smaller airways of infants and young children are especially susceptible and may result in cough, tachypnea, respiratory distress, wheezing, and hypoxia.

Mortality is high in infants with underlying disease or reduced immune function, and causes of death often include respiratory failure, cor pulmonale (right-sided heart failure), or bacterial superinfection. The immune response to RSV is not entirely understood, but both humoral and cell-mediated systems appear to play a role. The immunity developed with an infection does not appear to be complete. Repeat infections with RSV are common, but symptoms tend to be less severe with subsequent infections. Although outbreaks of RSV infection can occur in **elderly patients** resulting in severe illness, particularly in those residing in long-term care facilities.

Diagnosis

In addition to the presenting clinical symptoms, RSV can be diagnosed more definitively through **viral isolation and antigen detection.** Direct identification of RSV antigens is performed via immunofluorescence analysis on exfoliated epithelial cells or with ELISA (enzyme-linked immunosorbent assay) testing on nasal secretions. Large amounts of viral particles are present in **nasal washings,** particularly from infected children, making it a good clinical specimen for viral isolation. Because of the labile nature of RSV, clinical samples should be inoculated immediately into cell cultures. The presence of RSV can be recognized by the formation of giant cells or syncytia formation in inoculated cultures in 1–2 weeks.

Treatment and Prevention

Treatment of RSV infections relies mainly on **supportive care including oxygenation, ventilatory support, IV fluids, and nebulized cold steam.** These modalities are used in an effort to remove or reduce mucus secretions in the airways and allow for adequate oxygen exchange. The antiviral agent ribavirin has been approved for use via aerosolization in high-risk infants exposed to RSV and in severe lower respiratory tract illnesses caused by RSV infection. Additionally, close observation of severe cases is critical. Currently there is no vaccine approved for RSV.

Additionally, preventative measures are particularly important in hospital and specifically neonatal intensive care units, because **RSV is highly contagious.** Prevention of nosocomial spread requires strict enforcement of the following precautions: hand washing; isolation of RSV infected infants; and changing of gloves, gowns, and masks between patients.

Comprehension Questions

[36.1] Which of the following paramyxoviruses lacks an envelope viral attachment protein with hemagglutinin activity?

    A. Parainfluenza virus

    B. Mumps virus

    C. Measles virus

    D. Respiratory syncytial virus

[36.2] An 8-month-old infant is brought to the emergency room with a suspected RSV infection. Which of the following clinical illnesses would you be most concerned about this child having as a result of infection with this virus?

    A. Bronchiolitis

    B. Encephalitis

    C. Meningitis

    D. Pancreatitis

    E. Pharyngitis

[36.3] Which of the following statements most accurately describes the chemical and physiologic properties of RSV?

A. RSV is a nonenveloped virus with a single-stranded, negative-sense RNA genome.

B. Newly formed RSV viral particles are released via cell lysis by budding from the host cell.

C. RSV infects erythroid precursor cells via fusion of its viral envelope glycoproteins with the host cytoplasmic membrane.

D. Transcription of the RSV genome occurs in the nucleus of the host cell, while protein synthesis, replication, and assembly occur in the cytoplasm.

E. RSV is sensitive to detergents and is inactivated by changes in temperature and pH.

Answers

[36.1]   **D.** Respiratory syncytial virus, differs from other paramyxoviruses in that it does not have a hemagglutinin protein in its viral envelope; answers A, B, and C all have viral envelope proteins with hemagglutinin activity.

[36.2]   **A.** Bronchiolitis is a common clinical manifestation of RSV infection in infants, which results from inflammation and plugging of the bronchi and bronchioles with mucous and necrotic tissue; answers B, C, D, and E are incorrect as they are not symptoms specific to infection with RSV.

[36.3]   **E.** RSV is an enveloped virus and is inactivated by many detergents as well as changes in temperature and pH.; answers A, B, C, and D are incorrect: (A) RSV is an enveloped virus with a single-stranded, negative-sense RNA genome; (B) RSV virions are released by budding from the host cell membrane, not by cell lysis; (C) RSV infects respiratory epithelial cells, not erythroid precursor cells, via fusion with the host membrane; (D) RSV is an RNA virus, and transcription, protein synthesis, replication, and assembly of new virions occurs in the cytoplasm of the host cell.

MICROBIOLOGY PEARLS

❖ RSV is highly contagious and is the primary cause of respiratory tract infections in infants under 1 year of age.

❖ Clinical manifestations: respiratory symptoms including rhinitis, pneumonia, and blockage of airways leading to respiratory distress.

❖ No vaccine is available for RSV.

❖ Treatment with ribavirin in severe cases or in high risk infants exposed to the virus.

REFERENCES

Brooks GF, Butel JS, Morse SA. Jawetz, Melnick, & Adelberg's medical microbiology, 23rd ed. New York: McGraw-Hill, 2004:558–560.

Ryan JR, Ray CG. Sherris medical microbiology, 4th ed. New York: McGraw-Hill, 2004:503–506.

You are asked to consider being vaccinated with smallpox vaccine to serve as a first-responder in the event of a biological warfare attack. After considering the risks and benefits, you consent. You are given the vaccine by the standard technique—a small, bifurcated needle is used to create multiple punctures in the skin overlying your deltoid. The area is covered, and you are instructed not to touch the actual site. In two days, a small papule and erythema appear at the vaccine site. A few days later, multiple vesicles are noted. These progress to form larger pustules. In about two weeks, the whole vaccine site has formed a scab and this subsequently falls off in another week. When complete recovery has occurred, you have a scar left at the vaccine site.

◆ **What is the actual virus used as the smallpox vaccine?**

◆ **Why must variola carry or encode its own enzymes for DNA and mRNA synthesis?**

ANSWERS TO CASE 37: Smallpox

Summary: A physician has received the smallpox vaccine.

◆ **Actual virus used as the smallpox vaccine:** Vaccinia, which is a form of the cowpox virus.

◆ **Reason variola carries or encodes its own enzymes for DNA and mRNA synthesis:** Variola virus must produce its own enzymes for DNA and mRNA synthesis because viral replication occurs entirely in host cell cytoplasm, and therefore it cannot use the enzymes located in the host nucleus.

CLINICAL CORRELATION

Variola, the virus that causes smallpox, is a member of the poxvirus family. Smallpox is a highly contagious and severe disease that once caused high mortality in human populations. It was discovered in 1798 by Edward Jenner that the closely related but less virulent cowpox virus could confer resistance to smallpox. This discovery, along with the fact that humans were the only reservoir for variola, eventually lead to an effective global vaccination program, using the vaccinia virus as the live viral vaccine. Vaccinia shares antigenic determinants with variola but primarily causes clinical disease in nonhuman animals. Rare, but potentially severe, adverse events such as postvaccinial encephalitis, progressive vaccinia necrosum, or fetal vaccinia can occur after vaccination, primarily in persons with suppressed immunity, severe allergies, eczema, or pregnant women. Additionally, smallpox vaccination is also contraindicated for persons in close contact with individuals with the conditions listed.

Because of worldwide vaccination and disease control efforts, the last case of indigenously acquired smallpox was seen in Somalia in 1977. The World Health Organization declared that smallpox was eradicated in 1980. Routine smallpox vaccination was discontinued after 1980, as the risk of vaccination was thought to outweigh the risk of acquiring smallpox. Concerns about the risk of smallpox being used as a bioterror weapon have led to the reinstitution of vaccination programs, primarily among military, public health, and safety workers.

Approach to Suspected Infection

Definitions

Bifurcated needle: A specialized needle that forks into two prongs at its distal end; the prongs use capillary action to administer a specific amount of smallpox vaccine via multiple inoculations at the same site.

Maculopapular: The clinical presentation combination of both macules (rash) with papules (lesions).

Guarnieri's inclusion bodies: Electron-dense intracytoplasmic acidophilic inclusions within infected cells which serve as assembly sites for new smallpox virions.

Objectives

1. Be able to describe the characteristics of the virus.
2. Be able to describe the strategies for prevention and treatment of the infection.

Discussion

Characteristics of Smallpox that Impact Transmission

Variola is a member of the poxvirus family, and a member of the genera Orthopoxviridae. There are several diseases caused by orthopoxviruses: variola, vaccinia, cowpox, and monkeypox. **Variola** is the causative agent of smallpox, a virulent human virus that causes high mortality, while cowpox and monkeypox are zoonotic viruses causing accidental cutaneous infections in humans. **Vaccinia** is a form of the **cowpox** virus and has been used effectively as a live viral vaccine against smallpox disease. **Poxviruses are the largest and most complex viruses known.** Poxviruses are **enveloped and contain a linear, double-stranded DNA genome,** which is fused at both ends. They are the only DNA viruses, which replicate entirely in the host cell cytoplasm. Because of this, poxviruses must carry and/or encode all of the proteins required for mRNA and DNA synthesis.

Transmission of the smallpox virus occurs via **inhalation of infected respiratory droplets,** exposure to infectious skin lesions, or through contact with contaminated fomites. Once inhaled, initial replication of the virus occurs in the respiratory tract, where the virus binds to a target cell surface receptor and the envelope fuses with the cell membrane. The core of the virus is then released into the cellular cytoplasm where DNA replication and transcription takes place. New virions are assembled in cytoplasmic inclusions, referred to as **Guarnieri's inclusion bodies.** Unlike other enveloped viruses, poxviruses assemble their own viral membranes around these viral inclusions instead of acquiring them from host membranes. The new viral particles are then released either by cell lysis or budding. After initial infection of the respiratory tract occurs, the virus spreads through lymphatic channels causing primary viremia and infection of reticuloendothelial cells. Viral replication in these cells causes a secondary viremia and results in clinical manifestations of the skin and internal organs. Variola virus exists as at least two strains—**variola major and variola minor. Variola major** is associated with **high mortality rates** (20–50%), whereas **variola minor** is associated with a **mortality rate of less than 1 percent.**

Diagnosis

Clinical smallpox has an incubation period of approximately 2 weeks, followed by an **abrupt onset of malaise, fever, chills and myalgia.** A few days post-onset, a characteristic **maculopapular rash begins** to develop and progresses in a centrifugal pattern over the head and extremities. During approximately a 2-week period, the rash progresses to a **single crop of maculopapular lesions to firm vesicles, then to pustules** that scab and slowly heal. The high mortality associated with this smallpox results from either the overwhelming primary viral infection or from potential secondary bacterial superinfection.

Treatment and Prevention

As previously discussed, successful **global vaccination** efforts have eliminated naturally acquired cases of smallpox worldwide, with routine smallpox vaccinations ending in 1980 in the United States. However, new concerns of biological weapons development has led to the testing of old vaccine stocks and the development of new stocks for use primarily among military, public health, and safety workers. Chemotherapeutic agents such as **methisazone or cidofovir** may have some efficacy as prophylaxis against smallpox infection; however, currently there are no treatments available for use in established smallpox disease.

Comprehension Questions

[37.1] Which of the following statements describes a characteristic that enabled the worldwide eradication of smallpox in 1980?

    A. The inactivated smallpox vaccine is easily prepared and safe.

    B. Smallpox has no known reservoir outside of humans.

    C. Mass vaccination of the world was possible as a result of easy administration of the vaccine in the field.

    D. Subclinical smallpox infections were also inhibited through worldwide mass vaccinations.

    E. All stocks of smallpox virus were destroyed worldwide in 1979.

[37.2] Due to the potential of a bioterrorist threat, emergency healthcare responders in New York City are being considered for smallpox vaccination. Which of the following would be a candidate for vaccination?

    A. Household contact is breast-feeding

    B. Mild asthma

    C. Is pregnant

    D. Has eczema

    E. Household contact is HIV-positive

[37.3] A college student is reading about the Middle Ages and notices that many people during that era contracted a deadly disease with similar symptoms including acute fever, chills, and myalgia followed by a characteristic rash with small blister-like lesions. Those that did not die from the illness were left with disfiguring scars. The inciting agent has a double-stranded linear DNA genome that replicates in the cytoplasm. Which of the following agents is the most likely culprit?

A. Varicella virus
B. Herpes Simplex virus
C. Rubeola virus
D. Papilloma virus
E. Variola virus

Answers

[37.1] **B.** Smallpox has no known reservoir outside of humans, which was one of the factors which enabled its eradication; answers A, C, D, and E are all incorrect: the vaccination for smallpox consists of a live vaccinia virus and does not contain smallpox virus; mass vaccination of the world was not performed or required because there are no known nonhuman reservoirs of smallpox and subclinical infections do not occur. Thus, large numbers of vaccinations occurring in many populations, such as in the United States, along with strict epidemiologic reporting of smallpox cases worldwide allowed for immunization of those exposed and the elimination of smallpox disease. Not all stocks of smallpox virus were destroyed, and there are still two locations where smallpox virus strains are held: one in Atlanta, and one in Moscow.

[37.2] **B.** Smallpox is a live attenuated vaccine and is contraindicated for individuals or those who are household contacts who are immunocompromised or who may be susceptible to the adverse effects of the vaccine. Those with eczema and similar skin conditions, infection with HIV, transplant patients, those on high dose corticosteroids, those patients who are pregnant or who are breast feeding are a partial listing of patients for whom the vaccine is contraindicated.

[37.3] **E.** Smallpox (variola virus) killed many people during the Middle Ages. The clinical presentation was that of fever, malaise, and myalgia followed by pus-filled or vesicular rash, which often left disfiguring scars.

MICROBIOLOGY PEARLS

❖ Variola is a poxvirus and etiologic agent of smallpox.
❖ Vaccinia is a form of the cowpox virus and has been used effectively as a live viral vaccine against smallpox disease.
❖ Clinical manifestations of smallpox: a severe rash followed by a single crop of maculopapular lesions that transition into vesicles and pustules, and then slowly crust and heal. The lesions are at the same stage.
❖ Contraindications for vaccinia vaccination: suppressed immunity, severe allergies, eczema, pregnancy, or close contact with such persons.

REFERENCES

Brooks GF, Butel JS, Morse SA. Jawetz, Melnick, & Adelberg's medical microbiology, 23rd ed. New York: McGraw-Hill, 2004:561–566.

Cono J, Casey CG, Bell DM: Smallpox vaccination and adverse reactions. Guidance for clinicians. MMWR Recomm Rep 2003;52(RR-4):1.

Ryan JR, Ray CG. Sherris medical microbiology, 4th ed. New York: McGraw-Hill, 2004:525–527.

A 65-year-old man comes to your office for the evaluation of lower back pain. For the past 3 days, he has had a sharp, burning pain in his left lower back, which would radiate to his flank and, sometimes, all the way around to his abdomen. The pain comes and goes, feels like an "electric shock," is unrelated to activity, and can be severe. He has had no injury to his back and has no history of back problems in the past. He denies fever, urinary symptoms, or gastrointestinal symptoms. His examination today, including careful back and abdominal examination, is normal. You prescribe a nonsteroidal antiinflammatory for the pain. The next day, he returns to your office stating that he has had an allergic reaction to the medication because he's developed a rash. The rash is in the area where he had the pain for which he was seen the day before. On examination now, he has an eruption consisting of patches of erythema with clusters of vesicles extending in a dermatomal distribution from his left lower back to the midline of his abdomen.

◆ **What is the cause of this rash?**

◆ **What is the mechanism for the dermatomal distribution of the rash?**

ANSWERS TO CASE 38: Varicella zoster

Summary: A 65-year-old man has a painful, dermatomal rash.

◆ **Cause of this rash:** The most likely cause of this man's rash is reactivation of varicella-zoster virus, causing the appearance of shingles.

◆ **Mechanism for the dermatomal distribution of the rash:** The dermatomal distribution of this rash is caused by reactivation of a latent varicella infection of a dorsal root ganglion with viral spread along the pathway of the nerve distribution.

CLINICAL CORRELATION

Varicella-zoster virus (VZV) is the causative agent of both chickenpox and shingles. Primary infection with chickenpox occurs mostly in children, with 90 percent of the population acquiring antibodies to VZV by age 10. After primary infection, the virus becomes latent in the dorsal root ganglia, where it may be reactivated later in life. Reactivation of VZV infection results in the unilateral eruption of a painful rash known as herpes zoster or shingles.

Approach to Suspected VZV Infection

Definitions

Dermatome: An area of skin served by one sensory spinal nerve.
Neuropathic pain: Pain disseminating from the peripheral nervous system.

Objectives

1. Be able to describe the characteristics of the virus.
2. Be able to describe the strategies for prevention and treatment of the infection.

Discussion

Characteristics of VZV that Impact Transmission

Varicella-zoster virus (VZV) is a member of the **Alphaherpesvirinae** subfamily of the **herpesviruses,** which also include HSV-1 and HSV-2. Similar to other herpesviruses, VZV is a **large, enveloped virus with a double-stranded DNA genome.** Only enveloped virions are infectious and the envelope is sensitive to drying and many detergents, necessitating its spread from **person to person via respiratory droplets or direct contact with skin lesions.** Initial VZV infection and replication occur in the epithelium of the **respiratory tract.** The virus binds to specific receptors, and the viral envelope fuses with the cell membrane. The capsid delivers the genome to the host cell nucleus where transcription and replication occur.

VZV can cause both lytic and latent infections. In lytic infections, new virions are assembled in the host nucleus, acquire an envelope from the nuclear or Golgi membrane, and are released by exocytosis or lysis of the host cell. In latent infections, the viral genome is not replicated, and only certain viral genes are transcribed. Latent infection of dorsal root or cranial nerve ganglia can occur during the initial infection. The virus spreads by viremia or lymphatic dissemination to the reticuloendothelial system. A secondary viremia then occurs, which disseminates VZV to the skin and other organs. VZV can also form syncytia and spread directly from cell to cell.

Diagnosis

Viremic spread to the skin results in classic varicella infection or chickenpox. Typically, **crops of vesicles and pustules form on erythematous bases,** starting on the head and trunk and progressing centripetally to the extremities. The appearance of these lesions is often described as **"dewdrops on a rose petal."** Both humoral and cell-mediated immunity contribute to control of the infection. VZV is a common childhood disease, and infection usually confers lifelong immunity against future disseminated disease. However, reactivation of latent VZV infections of **nerve root ganglia** may result and is classically described as herpes zoster or shingles. The causes of the reactivation are not entirely known, but it tends to be more common in older persons as cellular immunity decreases, in immunosuppressed individuals or in otherwise immunecompetent individuals during times of emotional stress. The **reactivated virus replicates and is released along the dermatomal distribution of the nerve,** causing the characteristic **unilateral vesicular eruption of shingles.** The rash is frequently preceded by pain along the course of a sensory nerve days to weeks prior to the onset of rash. Neuropathic pain may continue to persist for weeks or months after the rash clears, indicating damage to the nerve root. Secondary bacterial infections may also complicate reactivation. Reactivations of VZV tend to be infrequent and sporadic.

Similar to HSV-1 and HSV-2, VZV can be diagnosed by examining a **Tzanck smear** of cells scraped from vesicular lesions for the presence of **multinucleated giant cells.** However, **direct fluorescent-antibody staining** of vesicular lesion scrapings remains the most rapid, sensitive, and specific assay for diagnosing VZV infections.

Treatment and Prevention

Several **viral DNA polymerase inhibitors** are available for treating VZV infections including: **acyclovir, famciclovir, and valacyclovir.** Treatment with these drugs has shown to be effective in reducing fever and skin lesions if treatment is begun within 3 days of onset of infection, prior to the eruption of lesions. These drugs have also shown some efficacy in reducing viral dissemination in immunocompromised patients.

Prevention of infection spread involves respiratory and contact isolation of infected patients. **Passive immunization of high-titer Varicilla Zoster immune globulin (VZIG)** can be administered to immunocompromised patients if given within 3 days of exposure. This treatment is effective only for inhibiting primary infection in high-risk patients. More recently, a **live vaccine** has been used in the United States since 1995 to prevent primary childhood infections. A single dose has been shown to be 80 percent effective in children 1–13 years of age, and two doses has been shown to be 70 percent effective in adults.

Comprehension Questions

[38.1] A Tzanck smear is obtained from a scraping of a patient's skin lesion, and analysis of the smear shows the presence of multinucleated giant cells. Which of the following viruses are known to cause this type cytopathic effect in infected cells?

A. Cytomegalovirus
B. Epstein-Barr virus
C. Human papillomavirus
D. Human herpesvirus 8
E. Varicella virus

[38.2] A 3-year-old girl presented to her pediatrician's office with fever, swollen lymph nodes, and a vesicular rash on her chest and upper arms. The vesicles were at various stages of development: some were newly forming, while some were crusted over. Which of the following infectious agents is the most likely cause of this girl's rash?

A. Smallpox
B. Parvovirus B19
C. Epstein-Barr virus
D. Measles virus
E. Varicella-zoster virus

[38.3] Based on information provided in the previous question, which of the following clinical specimens should be collected to confirm diagnosis of VZV infection?

A. Saliva
B. Blood
C. Vesicle fluid
D. Cerebral spinal fluid
E. Urine

Answers

[38.1]   **E.** HSV-1, HSV-2, and VZV are all known to produce multinucleated giant cells resulting in a positive Tzanck smear, whereas CMV, EBV, HPV, and human herpesvirus 8 do not.

[38.2]   **E.** VZV produces a vesicular rash commonly seen in children, and different "crops" of vesicles generally appear on the head and trunk then moving outward; answers A, B, C, and D are incorrect, smallpox infection produces a vesicular rash with all lesions being at the same stage of development, whereas parvovirus B19, EBV, and the measles virus does produce a rash, but not consisting of vesicular lesions.

[38.3]   **C.** VZV-specific antigens or viral DNA can be detected in vesicle fluid leading to a definitive diagnosis of VZV infection; answers A, B, D, and E are incorrect: CMV can be detected in saliva, blood, and urine; VZV is not commonly detected in CSF specimens.

 ## MICROBIOLOGY PEARLS

 Primary lytic infection: chickenpox or varicella; recurrent latent infection: shingles or zoster.

 Clinical manifestations: unilateral eruption of a painful rash in a single dermatome.

 Prevention: a live vaccine, respiratory and contact isolation of infected persons.

Treatment: viral DNA polymerase inhibitors such as acyclovir, famciclovir, and valacyclovir.

REFERENCES

Fields BN, et al. Herpesviridae. Fields virology, 3rd ed. Lippincott-Raven, 1996:2525–2541.

Murray PR, Rosenthal KS, Kobayashi GS, Pfaller MA. Medical microbiology, 4th ed. St. Louis: Mosby, 2002:475–487.

Ryan JR, Ray CG. Sherris medical microbiology, 4th ed. New York: McGraw-Hill, 2004:562–566.

A 42-year-old woman with chronic asthma presents for evaluation of a cough. She has had severe asthma for most of her life and currently uses both inhaled and oral corticosteroids, oral leukotriene modifiers, and inhaled albuterol to manage her symptoms. While in the process of tapering down her dose of oral steroids, she developed a cough productive of brown mucous and, occasionally, blood. She has had a low-grade fever as well. Her asthma control has been significantly worsened since she developed the cough. On examination, she has a temperature of 37.7°C (99.9°F) and a respiratory rate of 22 breaths per minute, and her saturation of oxygen is slightly low (96% on room air). She is coughing frequently. Her head and neck exam is unremarkable. Her pulmonary examination is notable for diffuse expiratory wheezing. A chest x-ray shows a lobular infiltrate that is reminiscent of a cluster of grapes. A complete blood count (CBC) shows a mildly elevated white blood cell count with a markedly elevated eosinophil count. A microscopic examination of her sputum is also notable for the presence of numerous eosinophils.

◆ **What organism is most likely causing her cough?**

◆ **What is the characteristic morphology of this organism seen on microscopic examination?**

ANSWERS TO CASE 39: *Aspergillus*

Summary: A 42-year-old asthmatic woman has allergic bronchopulmonary aspergillosis.

◆ **Most likely etiologic agent:** *Aspergillus fumigatus*

◆ **Characteristic morphology of this organism seen on microscopic examination:** septate hyphae with 45° angle branching.

CLINICAL CORRELATION

Aspergillus is a ubiquitous fungal organism that is capable of causing disease in both healthy and immunocompromised hosts. Infection occurs following either inhalation of the organism into the respiratory tract or introduction through the skin via a wound or surgery. *A. fumigatus* causes about 90 percent of invasive disease in humans, with *A. flavus* causing about 10 percent. Other *Aspergillus* species can cause disease but are less common. *Aspergillus* primarily infects the lungs and may cause a hypersensitivity reaction, chronic necrotizing pneumonia, aspergillomas ("fungal balls"), or systemic infection. *Aspergillus* can also cause keratitis and sinusitis. The hypersensitivity reaction, known as allergic bronchopulmonary aspergillosis (ABPA), is seen primarily in chronic asthmatics and persons with cystic fibrosis (CF). About 25 percent of asthmatics and about half of patients with CF are allergic to *Aspergillus,* although the percentages that develop symptomatic disease are much lower. ABPA causes a cough productive of brown mucous plugs and, often, blood. Examination of the mucous will reveal eosinophils and the characteristic fungus. The symptoms initially tend to be mild but become more severe as the patient ages. Repeated episodes may cause bronchiectasis and chronic fibrotic pulmonary disease.

Systemic disease most often occurs in patients who are severely immunocompromised such as subsequent to bone marrow transplantation

Approach to the Suspected *Aspergillus* Patient

Definitions

Allergic bronchopulmonary aspergillosis (ABPA): A hypersensitivity response to inhaled Aspergillus in patients with underlying asthma or lung disease.

Aspergilloma: A fungal ball most commonly in the sinus or within an old tuberculous cavity.

Bronchiectasis: Chronic inflammation of the bronchi with dilatation and loss of elasticity of the walls.

Objectives

1. Know the morphology, environmental sources, and pathogenic properties of *Aspergillus* species.
2. Know the clinical syndromes and diseases associated with *Aspergillus* infections.

Discussion

Characteristics of *Aspergillus* Species

Aspergillus **species** is found in every country in the world, and its **primary habitat is decomposing vegetation.** It is an **opportunistic pathogen** of animals and humans that causes a spectrum of disease ranging from **allergic bronchopulmonary disease** to **disseminated disease** in severely immunosuppressed patients. There are more than 40 species of *Aspergillus*, not all of which cause disease in humans. Therefore species identification is helpful in determining the clinical significance of an isolate. *Aspergillus fumigatus* is responsible for the majority of serious infections as a result of these organisms; however, *A. terreus* and *A. flavus* can be associated with disease in patients on cancer chemotherapy.

A **virulence factor** common to most *Aspergillus* species is **mycotoxin production.** One of the toxins, **gliotoxin,** can affect phagocytosis by macrophages as well as induce apoptosis.

Several factors contribute to the ability of *A. fumigatus* to cause infection. *A. fumigatus* grows more readily at normal human body temperature than other *Aspergillus* species. It has a very small spore size, which allows the spores to penetrate deep into the lung. It also is the most rapidly growing of all *Aspergillus* species.

Diagnosis

Diagnosis of allergic aspergillosis is usually made clinically, although these patients may have **positive respiratory cultures** for *Aspergillus*. Patients typically have a long-standing **history of asthma** with a history of **infiltrates on chest x-ray.** Other diagnostic criteria include presence of **specific antibody to** *Aspergillus* as well as elevated levels of IgE in the serum and **peripheral blood eosinophils.** The lack of systemic symptoms helps differentiate ABPA from *Aspergillus* pneumonia or disseminated disease. Diagnosis of disseminated disease is by culture of the organism from a normally sterile site and/or demonstration of hyphae invading blood vessels in a tissue biopsy. Disseminated disease can also be presumptively diagnosed by presence of antibody or galactomannan antigen in the patient's serum.

Fungal hyphae can be seen on **direct smear using KOH or calcofluor white,** which is a more sensitive fluorescent stain. *Aspergillus hyphae* can be identified by their **frequent septae, and branching at regular intervals at a**

45° angle (Figure 39-1); however, these characteristics are not specific or diagnostic for *Aspergillus*. Definitive diagnosis would be made by microscopic observation of the fungus after culture of the organism. *Aspergillus* species can be **cultured from sputum or bronchoalveolar lavages** of infected patients. The fungus grows rapidly on most laboratory media including blood agar, although a more selective media such as Sabouraud agar is commonly used to culture fungus. Growth is enhanced by incubation at room temperature versus 35°C. Visualization of the characteristic structure with a conidiophore, a vesicle to which the phialides are attached would confirm the diagnosis of *Aspergillus*. Although speciation can be preliminarily made by the color of the front and reverse of the colony on Sabouraud dextrose agar and their microscopic features, *A. fumigatus* is differentiated from the others by growth at a temperature at or above 50°C.

Treatment and Prevention

Treatment of ABPA is usually not warranted; however because this is a hypersensitivity reaction, systemic **corticosteroids** are effective treatment, whereas inhaled corticosteroids are not. Therapy for **invasive aspergillosis** is with **amphotericin B, itraconazole, or voriconazole.** Antifungal agents may be used for prophylaxis of patients who are severely immunocompromised to prevent disseminated disease, particularly bone marrow transplant patients. These patients should also be protected from exposure to the organism by use of air filters.

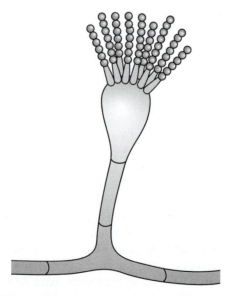

Figure 39-1. *Aspergillus fumigatus.* Frequent septa with branching pattern is characteristic.

Comprehension Questions

[39.1] A biopsy of an infected lung from a 76-year-old woman who suffered a third-degree burn 2 months ago revealed uniform hyphae with regularly spaced septation and a parallel arrangement. No yeast cells were observed. Which of the following is the most probable diagnosis?

A. Actinomycosis
B. Aspergillosis
C. Blastomycosis
D. Cryptococcosis
E. Zygomycosis

[39.2] Which of the following is the probable source of infection in aspergillosis in the patient [39.1]?

A. Contact with an infected animal
B. Implantation
C. Ingestion
D. Inhalation
E. Water used in preparing lemonade

[39.3] An examination of sputum for a suspected case of fungal infection may reveal hyphae in which of the following?

A. Aspergillosis
B. Cryptococcosis
C. Histoplasmosis
D. Paracoccidioidomycosis
E. Sporotrichosis

Answers

[39.1 and
39.2] **B.** Aspergillosis is a spectrum of diseases that may be caused by a number of *Aspergillus* species. These species are widespread in nature. *Aspergillus* species grow rapidly in vivo and in vitro and bear long conidiophores with terminal vesicles on which phialides produce chains of conidia. In healthy individuals, alveolar macrophages are able to phagocytize and destroy the conidia. Macrophages from immunocompromised patients have a diminished ability to do this. In the lung, conidia swell and germinate to produce hyphae that have a tendency to invade preexisting cavities (abnormal pulmonary space as a result of tuberculosis, sarcoidosis, or emphysema). Sputum and lung tissue specimens produce colonies which are hyaline, septate and uniform in width. Blastomyces and Cryptococcus from yeast cells, while Zygomycoses species have hyphae that are sparsely septate. Actinomyces may be considered a branching bacterium.

[39.3]   **A.** Cryptococcosis, histoplasmosis, paracoccidioidomycosis and
sporotrichosis are all caused by dimorphic fungi. At 37°C, the yeast
form predominates. Aspergillosis, on the other hand, is caused by an
organism that produces only hyphae (no-yeast component).

MICROBIOLOGY PEARLS

 Aspergillus is commonly found in the environment and cause a spectrum of disease ranging from allergic bronchopulmonary disease to disseminated disease.

 Microscopically *aspergillus* has septated, hyphae that branch at 45° angles and a vesicle with condida in either a single row (uniserate) or a double row (biserate).

 Although steroids are used to treat allergic disease, disseminated disease is difficult to treat and has a high mortality rate in severely immunosuppressed patients such as following bone marrow transplant.

REFERENCES

Denning DW. Aspergillus species. In: Mandell GL, Bennett JE, Dolin R, eds. Principles and practice of infectious diseases, 5th ed. Philadelphia: Churchill Livingstone, 2000:2674–85.

Murray PR, Rosenthal KS, Kobayashi GS, Pfaller MA. Opportunistic mycoses In: Murray PR, Rosenthal KS, Kobayashi GS, Pfaller MA. Medical microbiology, 4th ed. St. Louis: Mosby, 2002:664–72.

A 52-year-old man presents to the office for the evaluation of a cough and fever. He has had these symptoms for about a week. He has also noted a sharp chest pain that is worse when he coughs or takes a deep breath. He has had some associated fatigue, headaches, achy joints, and sweatiness at night. He has been using an over-the-counter flu medication, which helps to reduce the cough, but he wanted to be checked because his symptoms are lingering. He has no history of pulmonary diseases and has never smoked cigarettes. He has had no exposure to ill contacts. His only recent travel was a weeklong golf vacation to Phoenix, which he took 3 weeks ago. On examination, he is comfortable appearing and in no respiratory distress. His temperature is 37.7°C (99.9°F), and his vital signs are otherwise normal. His pulmonary examination is notable for some faint expiratory wheezing and crackles in the left upper lung field. The remainder of his physical examination is unremarkable. A chest x-ray shows hilar adenopathy. A CBC shows a normal total white blood cell count but with a high percentage of circulating eosinophils. Microscopic examination of a fresh sputum sample treated with KOH reveals numerous spherules.

◆   **What organism is the likely cause of this patient's symptoms?**

◆   **For this organism, how do spherules form and what is their role in propagating infection?**

ANSWERS TO CASE 40: *Blastomycosis, Coccidiodomycosis,* and *Histoplasmosis*

Summary: A 52-year-old man who recently traveled to Phoenix complains of a cough, fatigue, and night sweats. A chest x-ray shows hilar adenopathy. The sputum reveals numerous spherules.

◆ **Organism most likely to cause his symptoms:** *Coccidioides immitis.*

◆ **How do spherules form and what is their role in propagating infection:** Inhaled arthroconidia lose their hydrophobic outer wall and remodel into spherical cells, or spherules. Nuclear division and cell multiplication occur and multiple septae develop within the circular cell, dividing it into endospore-containing compartments. The external wall of the spherule thins as growth occurs and then ruptures, releasing multiple spores and propagating the infection.

CLINICAL CORRELATION

C. immitis is a dimorphic fungus endemic in the western hemisphere. It is typically found in semiarid climates within the north and south 40° latitudes. Common endemic regions in the United States include the San Joaquin Valley, southern Arizona, and southwestern Texas. Transmission occurs by inhalation of the arthroconidia from the soil. The arthroconidia are taken into the bronchioles, where they form a spherule. When symptoms do occur, they usually start 1–3 weeks after exposure and typically include cough, fever, and fatigue. Chest pain, dyspnea, arthralgias, and skin rashes may occur as well. Most infections are self-limited, but it can take several weeks to months for symptomatic resolution. A small percentage of infections result in progressive pulmonary disease or chronic pulmonary complications, and an even smaller percentage may result in dissemination outside of the lung the most common site being the skin. Other areas of dissemination include the bones, joints, and the central nervous system (CNS). Most patients who develop disseminated disease have an underlying risk factor of severe immunosuppression, including those infected with HIV.

Approach to the Suspected *Coccidoides* Patient

Definitions

Dyspnea: Shortness of breath or difficulty breathing.

Dimorphic fungi: Fungi that grow as a mold at room temperature and in the environment and as yeast at 35°C or in the body.

Arthroconidia: Barrel-shaped structures that are the mold and infectious form of *C. immitis.*

Objectives

1. Know the morphology, growth, and reproductive characteristics of *C. immitis.*
2. Know the sources of infection, modes of transmission, and clinical diseases associated with *C. immitis* infection.

Discussion

Characteristics of *Coccidioides* Species

Coccidioides is one of several **systemic and dimorphic fungi.** *Histoplasma capsulatum*, *Blastomyces* dermatitidis, and *Paracoccidioides* braziliensis are the others. *Cryptococcus neoformans* is also a **systemic** fungus but is **not dimorphic.** *Sporothrix schenckii* is dimorphic but not usually systemic. These fungi are commonly found in the environment in differing parts of the world and are transmitted by the aerosol route. In the majority of cases, fungi are inhaled into the lungs, and disease is unrecognized because patients remain asymptomatic.

C. immitis **grows in the soil as mycelia by apical extension.** Maturation results in the development of arthroconidia, which have a hydrophobic outer layer and can remain viable for a long period of time. They form fragile attachments to adjacent cells that are easily broken. Physical trauma, even a mild wind, can break these attachments and result in airborne dissemination of arthroconidia. If inhaled, the arthroconidia can deposit in the lung, where they lose their hydrophobic outer wall. The cell remodels into a spherical form known as a spherule. Within the spherule, cells multiply and septae form that divide the spherule into multiple compartments. These compartments contain endospores that are released as the spherule grows and eventually ruptures. The endospores are capable of generating new spherules or reverting to mycelial growth if removed from the site of an infection.

Spherule growth and rupture result in a host inflammatory response that includes the action of neutrophils and eosinophils. T lymphocytes also play an important role in the control of *C. immitis* infection. Most infections with this organism are asymptomatic or cause mild, nonspecific upper respiratory symptoms that are not diagnosed.

Diagnosis

Initial preliminary diagnosis is made by consistent clinical symptoms in a patient with recent travel to a *Coccidioides* endemic area of the country. **Definitive diagnosis is made by direct observation of spherules** with subsequent culture of the organism in a specimen, usually of respiratory origin. Direct examination can be made using either KOH or calcofluor white stains. *Coccidioides* **immitis is a dimorphic fungus** that forms spherules in the patient

(35°C) and arthroconidia in the environment (room temperature). The **arthroconidia are the infectious form** and can be transmitted in the laboratory if proper biosafety precautions are not adhered to. *C. immitis* grows rapidly (within 1 week) on routine laboratory media. Colonies appear as a white fluffy mold, whose appearance is indistinguishable from the other dimorphic fungi, including *Histoplasma capsulatum* and *Blastomyces dermatitidis*. *C. immitis* can be specifically identified by immunodiffusion of extracted *C. immitis* antigen and commercially prepared antibody or by DNA probes specific for *C. immitis* RNA.

In cases in which culture is not possible, or negative, serology or skin testing may be helpful for diagnosis. The disadvantage of both is that a positive conversion may last for life and make diagnosis of a current infection difficult.

Treatment and Prevention

Treatment is not usually provided to patients with uncomplicated respiratory disease without risk factors for dissemination. Patients with complicated disease are treated with either an **azole or amphotericin B.**

Comprehension Questions

[40.1] A 35-year-old man is HIV antibody-positive and has a CD4 count of 50 cells/mm^3 (normal: 500–1000 cells/mm^3). He has had a fever of 38.3°C (101°F) for a few weeks and "feels tired all the time." He has no other symptoms, and findings on physical examination are normal. Complete blood count (CBC), urinalysis, and chest x-ray are normal. A bone marrow biopsy reveals granulomas, and a culture grows an organism that is a budding yeast at 37°C, but produces hyphae and tuberculated chlamydospores at 25°C. Of the following, which is the most likely cause?

A. *Aspergillus fumigatus*
B. *Coccidioides immitis*
C. *Cryptococcus neoformans*
D. *Histoplasma capsulatum*
E. *Mucor* species

[40.2] A 4-year-old girl who lives in Bakersfield, CA, has had a low-grade fever. Skin tests performed for the first time give the following results:

Tuberculin (PPD)	Positive (10 mm induration)
Coccidioidin test	Positive (15 mm induration)
Dick test	Positive (with erythema)
Dick control test (heated toxin)	Negative (no erythema)
Schick test	Negative (no erythema)
Schick control test (heated toxin)	Negative (no erythema)

The test results suggest that the patient:

A. Has been exposed to *Coccidioides immitis.*
B. Has been immunized against *Coccidioides immitis.*
C. Has had scarlet fever.
D. Has IgG antibody to *Mycobacterium tuberculosis.*
E. Lacks immunity to *Corynebacterium diphtheriae.*

[40.3] A 50-year-old immunocompromised woman is diagnosed as having meningitis. A latex agglutination test on the spinal fluid for capsular polysaccharide antigen is positive. Of the following organisms, which one is the most likely cause?

A. *Aspergillus fumigatus*
B. *Cryptococcus neoformans*
C. *Histoplasma capsulatum*
D. *Nocardia asteroides*
E. *Toxoplasma gondii*

[40.4] Which of the following is the most common portal of entry in *Blastomyces dermatitidis* infection?

A. Genitourinary tract
B. Lymphatic system
C. Mouth
D. Respiratory tract
E. Skin

Answers

[40.1] **D.** An HIV-positive individual may have normal immune capacity as measured by laboratory parameters, but still be more at risk for opportunistic organisms. Respiratory infections may be caused by fungi, bacteria, or viruses. As a result, laboratory results may be crucial in determining the exact organism causing an infection. In this case, the bone marrow biopsy revealed a budding yeast form at 37°C, but hyphae and tuberculated chlamydospores at room temperature (25°C). In disseminated histoplasmosis, bone marrow cultures are often positive. Tuberculate macroconidia are characteristic for *H. capsulatum's* mycelial form.

[40.2] **A.** The Dick and Schick tests are related to streptococcal infections, specifically scarlet fever. The young girl has been exposed to a *Mycobacterium,* most likely *M. tuberculosis,* but the positive reaction observed is based on a cellular immune reaction, not one mediated by antibodies. The location is a region where *coccidioides* is endemic and should be one of the suspected pathogens to be considered. No vaccine is available for *C. immitis.* Therefore, a positive coccidioidin test indicates that the young girl has been exposed to the agent and has developed a cellular immune reaction in response.

[40.3]   **B.** *Cryptococcus neoformans* is a yeast characterized by a thick poly-saccharide capsule. It occurs worldwide in nature and in very large numbers in pigeon feces. Cryptococcus infection is usually associated with immunosuppression. Tests for capsular antigen can be performed on cerebrospinal fluid and serum. The latex agglutination test for cryptococcal antigen is positive in 90 percent of patients with cryptococcal meningitis. With effective treatment (amphotericin B and possibly flucytosine), the antigen titer usually drops except for AIDS patients.

[40.4]   **D.** *Blastomyces dermatitidis* grows as a mold culture, producing septate hyphae and conidia. In a host, it converts to a large, singly budding yeast cell. It is endemic in North America. Human infection is initiated in the lungs. Diagnosis may be difficult because no skin or serologic tests exist. Chronic pneumonia is a common presentation. Sputum, pus, exudates, urine, and lung biopsy material can be examined microscopically, looking for thick walled yeast cells with broadly attached buds. It may also be cultured.

MICROBIOLOGY PEARLS

❖   *Coccidioides immitis* is a dimorphic, systemic fungus, commonly found in the soil of arid areas.

❖   Most patients exposed to the arthroconidia of *C. immitis* develop an asymptomatic or respiratory infection. Disseminated disease occurs rarely in severely immunosuppressed patients.

❖   Person-to-person transmission of *C. immitis* is not known to occur.

REFERENCES

Galgiani J. Coccidioides immitis. In: Mandell GL, Bennett JE, Dolin R, eds. Principles and practice of infectious diseases, 5th ed. Philadelphia: Churchill Livingstone, 2000:2746–57.

Murray PR, Rosenthal KS, Kobayashi GS, Pfaller MA. Systemic mycoses In: Murray PR, Rosenthal KS, Kobayashi GS, Pfaller MA. Medical microbiology, 4th ed. St. Louis: Mosby, 2002:651–63.

A 28-year-old woman presents to the office complaining of 2-days of itchy vaginal discharge. One week ago you saw and treated her for a urinary tract infection (UTI) with sulfamethoxazole and trimethoprim (SMX-TMP). She completed her medication as ordered and developed the vaginal discharge shortly thereafter. She denies abdominal pain, and her dysuria has resolved. She is not currently taking any medications. On examination, she is comfortable appearing and has normal vital signs. Her general physical examination is normal. A pelvic examination reveals a thick, curd-like, white discharge in her vagina that is adherent to the vaginal sidewalls. There is no cervical discharge or cervical motion tenderness, and bimanual examination of the uterus and adnexa is normal.

◆ **What is the most likely cause of these symptoms?**

◆ **What are the most likely reservoirs of this organism in this patient?**

ANSWERS TO CASE 41: *Candida*

Summary: A 28-year-old woman who recently took antibiotics now presents with a vaginal discharge consistent with candidiasis.

◆ **Most likely etiologic organism:** *Candida albicans.*

◆ **Most likely reservoirs of infection:** Gastrointestinal (GI) and vaginal colonization.

CLINICAL CORRELATION

Most *Candida* infections come from the host's endogenous flora. Both humoral and cell-mediated immune functions play a role in defense against *Candida* infections. Those with impaired or suppressed immunity are predisposed to more severe or diffuse disease. Neutropenic persons, such as those on chemotherapy or posttransplant patients, are at risk for severe disease, which disseminates in the blood stream. In contrast, AIDS patients often develop oral, pharyngeal, or esophageal candidiasis but rarely disseminated disease. Intact skin also plays a key role in preventing cutaneous infections, because breaks in the skin of even healthy hosts may result in *Candida* skin infections. The use of antibiotics is probably the most significant predisposing factor for the development of *Candida* infections. Antibiotics that suppress the growth of the normal host bacterial flora can allow *Candida* to proliferate. This is a frequent contributing cause of the development of vaginal candidiasis in women and *Candida* diaper dermatitis in infants.

    Candida is the cause of a wide range of infections from oral lesions (thrush) to disseminated disease including endocarditis and meningitis. *Candida albicans* is the most common cause of vaginitis. Predisposing factors include diabetes, previous antimicrobial use, pregnancy, and use of oral contraceptives. Although the pathogenesis and the virulence mechanisms of *Candida* infection is unclear, the presence of pseudohyphae seems to indicate active disease versus colonization. Pseudohyphae are able to adhere to epithelial cells, then the blastoconidia.

Approach to the Suspected *Candida* Patient

Definitions

Neutropenia: A decrease in the number of neutrophils circulating in the blood to less than 2.0×10^9/L, with significant neutropenia being less than 0.5×10^9/L.

Thrush: Form of oral candidiasis in which a membrane forms in the oral cavity consisting of *Candida,* desquamated cells and white blood cells and debris. The appearance is of a creamy white, curd-like exudative plaque on the tongue and in the mouth.

Objectives

1. Know the morphology, reservoirs, and reproduction of *Candida* species.
2. Know the clinical syndromes, risk factors, and routes of transmission of diseases associated with *Candida* infection.

Discussion

Characteristics of *Candida*

Candida are **yeasts** that **exist as both sexual and asexual forms, reproduce by budding** and form **blastospores,** which are small, thin-walled ovoid cells. Blastospores, **pseudohyphae** may be seen on examination of clinical specimens. There are over 150 species of *Candida,* nine of which appear to cause disease in humans. *C. albicans* is the most common cause of human candidiasis. It can be found in soil and on inanimate objects and foods. It is also found in the normal flora of the human GI tract, vagina, and skin.

Diagnosis

Diagnosis of vaginitis is made by a combination of physical examination and testing the vaginal exudate. Ruling out other causes of vaginitis may be aided by determining the pH of the exudates as well as stain and culture of the material. **Yeast cells are larger than bacteria** and can be visualized easily by direct wet preparation of the exudates with KOH. *Candida* will grow with 24–48 hours on most routine laboratory media; however, Sabouraud dextrose agar can be used to inhibit the normal flora bacteria in cultures for mucosal candidiasis. *Candida* colonies are smooth and creamy, although some species may be dry and can be identified as yeast by a wet preparation. *Candida* species produce round or oval blastoconidia, and some species also produce **pseudohyphae** (chains of elongated blastoconidia), as in Figure 41–1. Preliminary differentiation of *Candida albicans* from the other *Candida* species can be made by observation of the presence of a germ tube. *Candida albicans* will make a germ tube after several hours incubation in the presence of serum. *Candida albicans* can also be differentiated from other yeast based on their microscopic morphology on corn meal agar. *C. albicans* produce chlamydospores, large rounded structures in the middle of the pseudohyphae. Yeast that are germ tube–negative can be further identified by assimilation of different substrates. Several commercial kits are available that identify *Candida* to the species level.

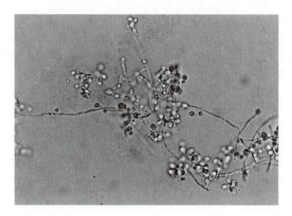

Figure 41-1. *Candida albicans.* Pseudohyphae noted on microscopy.

Reproduced, with permission, Brooks G, Butel J, Morse S. Jawetz, Melnick, & Adelberg's medical microbiology, 23rd ed. New York: McGraw-Hill, 2004:646.

Treatment and Prevention

Therapy for *Candida* vaginitis is usually topical **antifungal agent such as nystatin** or **clotrimazole.** It is not uncommon for patients to remain or be recurrently colonized with vaginal yeast after appropriate therapy. This may or may not lead to a symptomatic recurrence. **Oral or intravenous therapy with either an azole antifungal such as fluconazole, amphotericin B,** or the new agent, **caspofungin,** are used for treatment of disseminated infections with *Candida.* The agent of choice is dependent on the species of *Candida* isolated and the susceptibility of the isolate to the antifungal. Prophylaxis for *Candida* infections is not routinely recommended because of the selection of strains of *Candida* that are resistant to antifungal agents. The only population in which some benefit has been seen with prophylaxis is in bone marrow transplant patients. Partly as a result of the increased use of fluconazole, the incidence of *Candida* species not *albicans,* or the species more likely to be fluconazole resistant have also increased.

Comprehension Questions

[41.1] *Candida albicans* can be differentiated from other *Candida* species on cornmeal agar by its unique ability to form which of the following?

A. Arthrospores
B. Aseptate hyphae
C. Chlamydospores
D. Germ tubes
E. Tuberculate macroconidia

[41.2] A young man in his mid-20s presented with mucosal lesions in his mouth. Based on his CD4 cell count and other signs during the past few months, he was diagnosed as having AIDS. Which of the following is the most likely etiology of the oral lesions?

A. *Aspergillus*
B. *Candida*
C. *Cryptococcus*
D. *Mucor*
E. *Rhizopus*

[41.3] Which of the following morphologic structures is not associated with *Candida albicans?*

A. Chlamydospore
B. Hyphae
C. Pseudohyphae
D. Sporangium
E. Yeast

[41.4] Which of the following is the main reason that individuals taking tetracycline often develop candidiasis?

A. *Candida albicans* is capable of degrading the antibiotic.
B. The action of the antibiotic is neutralized by the protein of *C. albicans.*
C. The antibiotic damages the host mucous membrane.
D. The antibiotic is nutritionally favorable for the growth of *C. albicans.*
E. The normal bacterial flora is drastically altered by tetracycline.

Answers

[41.1]   **C.** Although multiple *Candida* species may cause disease in humans, *C. albicans* is the most frequent species identified. Chlamydospores (chlamydoconidia) are round, thick-walled spores formed directly from the differentiation of hyphae in which there is a concentration of protoplasm and nutrient material. They may be intercalary (within the hyphae) or terminal (end of hyphae). Germ tubes appear as hyphal-like extensions of yeast cells, usually without a constriction at the point of origin from the cell. Approximately 75 percent of the yeasts recovered from clinical specimens are *C. albicans,* and the germ-tube test can usually provide identification within 3 hours. The morphologic features of yeasts on cornmeal agar containing Tween 80 allow for the differentiation of *C. albicans* from five other *Candida* species.

[41.2]   **B.** The risk factors for cutaneous and mucosal candidiasis include AIDS, pregnancy, diabetes, young or old age, birth control pills, and trauma. Oral thrush can occur on the tongue, lips, gums, or palate. It may be patchy to confluent, and it forms whitish lesions composed of epithelial cells, yeasts, and pseudohyphae. Oral thrush commonly occurs in AIDS patients. Although the other genera listed may be opportunistic, only *Candida* routinely presents with mucosal lesions.

[41.3]   **D.** A sporangium is a sac enclosing spores, seen in certain fungi, but not *Candida* species. Spores produced within a sporangium, usually located at the tip of a long hyphal stalk are released by rupture of the sporangial wall. All other options (chlamydospore, hyphae, pseudohyphae, and yeasts) are routinely observed in *Candida albicans* cultures, depending on conditions of growth.

[41.4]   **E.** Patients with compromised host defenses are susceptible to ubiquitous fungi to which healthy people are exposed but usually resistant. *Candida* and related yeasts are part of the normal microbial flora, but are kept at low numbers by faster-growing normal flora bacteria. If broad-spectrum antimicrobials are used, much of the usual flora bacteria may be eliminated. No longer held in check, the opportunist yeast may become more predominant and opportunistic. Discontinuation of use of the broad-spectrum antibiotic is an important first step in patient management, allowing for reestablishment of the normal or usual flora and control of the yeast species.

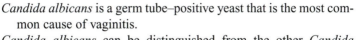

MICROBIOLOGY PEARLS

 Candida albicans is a germ tube–positive yeast that is the most common cause of vaginitis.

 Candida albicans can be distinguished from the other *Candida* species by formation of a germ tube after incubation in serum.

 The incidence of *Candida* species other than albicans has increased because of the increased use of azoles and their propensity to develop resistance to those antifungal agents.

REFERENCES

Edwards JE. Candida species. In: Mandell GL, Bennett JE, Dolin R, eds. Principles and practice of infectious diseases, 5th ed. Philadelphia: Churchill Livingstone, 2000:2656–74.

Murray PR, Rosenthal KS, Kobayashi GS, Pfaller MA. Opportunistic mycoses In: Murray PR, Rosenthal KS, Kobayashi GS, Pfaller MA. Medical microbiology, 4th ed. St. Louis: Mosby, 2002:664–72.

A 32-year-old man with known AIDS is brought to the emergency room with headache and fever for the past 3 days. According to family members who are with him, he has been confused, forgetful, and irritable for a few weeks prior to the onset of these symptoms. They state that he has advanced AIDS with a low CD4 count and has had bouts of pneumocystis pneumonia, candidal esophagitis, and Kaposi sarcoma. He is on multiple medications, although they don't know whether he is actually taking them. On examination, he is cachetic and frail appearing. He is confused and only oriented to his name. His temperature is 37.8°C (100°F), and his other vital signs are normal. Examination of his cranial nerves is normal. He has minimal nuchal rigidity. Cardiovascular, pulmonary, and abdominal examinations are normal. He is hyperreflexic. A head CT scan is normal. A report of the microscopic examination of his cerebrospinal fluid obtained by lumbar puncture comes back from the lab and states that there were numerous white blood cells, predominantly lymphocytes, and no organisms identified on Gram stain but a positive India ink test.

◆ **What organism is the likely cause of this illness?**

◆ **What characteristic of this organism is primarily responsible for its virulence?**

ANSWERS TO CASE 42: *Cryptococcus neoformans*

Summary: A 38-year-old male with advanced AIDS presents with meningitis. The India ink test is positive.

◆ **Most likely etiology for this man's meningitis:** *Cryptococcus neoformans.*

◆ **Characteristic of this organism is primarily responsible for its virulence:** *Cryptococcus neoformans* is known characteristically to produce a mucopolysaccharide capsule. This is a key feature of this organism's virulence, because it is antiphagocytic and also interferes with leukocyte migration to sites of infection.

CLINICAL CORRELATION

Cryptococcus neoformans is an encapsulated monomorphic fungi that commonly causes chronic meningitis in immune-suppressed individuals and occasionally in immune-competent persons. The lungs are the primary site of infection, although the organism appears to have specific affinity for the brain and meninges on systemic spread. *C. neoformans* is the leading cause of fungal meningitis and is an important cause of mortality in AIDS patients.

Approach to Suspected *Cryptococcus neoformans* Infection

Definitions

Meningitis: Inflammation of the meninges.
Nuchal rigidity: Stiffness of the neck associated with meningitis.
Cachetic: Weight loss or wasting because of disease or illness.

Objectives

1. Be aware of the characteristics, disease presentation, and methods of diagnosis of this organism.
2. Be able to describe the treatment and prevention of infection.

Discussion

Characteristics of *Cryptococcus neoformans* that Impact Transmission

C. neoformans is an **encapsulated yeast, 4–6 mm in diameter,** which is distributed globally. The most common serotypes are found in high concentrations in **pigeon and other bird droppings,** although they do not appear to cause disease in these hosts. The most common route of transmission to humans is via aerosolization of the organism followed by inhalation into the lungs. Direct animal-to-person transmission has not been shown. Unlike other systemic fungi, *C. neoformans* is **monomorphic,** not dimorphic, and **grows as budding yeast cells** at both 25°C in culture and at 37°C in tissues. When grown in culture, *C. neoformans* produces white- or tan-colored mucoid colonies in 2–3 days on a variety of common fungal media. Microscopically, the organism appears as spherical budding yeast, surrounded by a thick capsule. *C. neoformans* differs from the other nonpathogenic cryptococcal strains by its ability to produce phenol oxidase and growth at 37°C.

The **capsule** is an **important virulence factor** of *Cryptococcus,* and it consists of long, unbranched polysaccharide polymers. Capsule production is normally repressed in environmental settings and is stimulated by physiological conditions in the body. The **capsule is antiphagocytic,** because of its large size and structure and has also been shown to interfere with antigen presentation and the development of T-cell-mediated immune responses at sites of infection. This suppression of an immune response can allow for multiplication of the organism and promotion of its spread outside the respiratory tract. Once outside the lung, the organism appears to have an affinity for the central nervous system (CNS), possibly because of its ability to bind C3 and the low levels of complement found in the CNS.

Diagnosis

Inhalation of these aerosolized yeast cells leads to a primary pulmonary infection. The infection may be asymptomatic or may result in a flu-like respiratory illness or pneumonia. Commonly, cryptococcal pulmonary infection is identified only as an incidental finding on a chest x-ray being performed for other reasons. Often the infection and resulting lesions appear suspicious for a malignancy, only to be diagnosed properly after surgical removal. The most commonly diagnosed cryptococcal disease is meningitis, which results from hematogenous spread of the organism from the lung to the **meninges.** It occurs most commonly in persons with **AIDS** or those who are **immunosuppressed** for other reasons, but it can occasionally occur in persons without underlying conditions. Outside the lungs, *C. neoformans* appears to have a preference for the cerebrospinal fluid (CSF), but disseminated disease can also cause infections of the skin, eye, and bone. Cryptococcal meningitis may be insidious in its onset, slowly causing mental status changes, irritability, or confusion that occurs over weeks to months, or it can occur acutely, with immediate changes in mentation and meningeal symptoms. Clinical disease may present with intermittent headache, irritability, dizziness, and difficulty with complex cerebral functions and may even be mistaken as psychoses. Seizures, cranial nerve signs, and papilledema may appear in late clinical course.

A diagnosis of *C. neoformans* infection is made primarily by clinical presentation and examination of CSF for increased pressure, increased number of white cells, and low glucose levels. Serum and CSF specimens should also be tested for polysaccharide capsular antigen by latex agglutination or enzyme immunoassay. Another classic test for *C. neoformans* is the India ink test, which is an easy and rapid test that is positive in approximately 50 percent of patients with cryptococcal disease. **A drop of India ink** is placed on a glass slide and mixed with a loopful of CSF sediment or a small amount of isolated yeast cells. A cover slip is added and the slide is examined microscopically for encapsulated yeast cells that exclude the ink particles.

Treatment and Prevention

C. neoformans infections can be treated with antifungal agents such as **amphotericin B or fluconazole.** Amphotericin B is a broad-spectrum chemo-therapeutic agent and is the most effective drug for severe systemic mycoses. However, it is an extremely nephrotoxic agent to which all patients have adverse reactions such as fever, chills, dyspnea, hypotension, and nausea. Fluconazole is less toxic than amphotericin B and produces fewer side effects; however, resistance to fluconazole has been shown to occur. AIDS patients with cryptococcosis are required to continue lifelong suppressive therapy with fluconazole to prevent relapse of fungal infection.

Comprehension Questions

[42.1] A 32-year-old man who lives in downtown Philadelphia presents to his physician with a 4-day history of terrible headache, fever, and stiff neck. He has always been in good health and attributes this to his healthy eating habits and his daily running through the city parks near his apartment. The physician suspects the man may have cryptococcal meningitis and collects CSF for examination. Which of the following results would you most likely expect from this patient's CSF studies?

A. Elevated CSF pressure with increased white cell counts
B. Elevated polymorphonuclear cells with high protein levels
C. Elevated lymphocytes with normal glucose levels
D. Normal CSF pressure with a positive Gram stain reaction
E. Normal CSF pressure with negative Gram stain reaction

[42.2] Which of the following laboratory tests would best definitely diagnose cryptococcal infection in the above patient?

A. Quelling reaction capsular swelling
B. Latex agglutination test for polysaccharide capsular antigen
C. Ouchterlony test for fungal infection
D. India ink test for the presence of capsulated yeast
E. Gram stain reaction

[42.3] A 35-year-old man with AIDS presents to the local clinic with complaints of nausea, vomiting, confusion, fever and staggering gait. A lumbar puncture is performed, and an organism with a halo is noted with India ink preparation. What drug would be most beneficial?

A. Ketoconazole and amphotericin B
B. Flucytosine and amphotericin B
C. Nystatin and ketoconazole
D. Nystatin and miconazole
E. Griseofulvin

[42.4] A 34-year-old white homeless man in New York city is brought in by the police to the emergency room because he was found wandering the streets confused with a staggering gait. On physical exam he is noted to have acne like lesions over a large part of his body accompanied with skin ulcers. He is febrile and has some cranial nerve deficits. A short time later the man becomes short of breath, which was determined to be caused by severe cerebral edema compressing the medulla. Which of the following is the most likely causative agent?

A. *Histoplasma capsulatum*
B. *Coccidioides immitis*
C. *Exophiala werneckii*
D. *Sporothrix schenckii*
E. *Cryptococcus neoformans*

Answers

[42.1] **A.** meningitis caused by *C. neoformans* infection typically results in increased CSF pressure with an increased number of white cells and low glucose levels; answers B, C, D, and E are incorrect: both (B) and (D) appropriately describe meningitis caused by a bacterial agent such as *Neisseria meningitides;* (C) appropriately describes meningitis caused by a viral agent such as herpes simplex virus; (E) describes normal CSF findings

[42.2] **B.** answers A, C, D, and E are incorrect: (A) is a test useful for diagnosing *Streptococcus pneumoniae* and uses capsule-specific antibody to cause capsule swelling; (C) is an immunodiffusion test useful in diagnosing *Histoplasma* and *Blastomyces* fungal infections; (D) does provide rapid diagnosis of *Cryptococcus neoformans;* however, this assay is positive in only 50 percent of cryptococcal cases; (E) the Gram stain is more useful in diagnosing bacterial infections, because it would show the presence of yeast cells, but the capsule would not be visible.

[42.3]   **B.** The organism present is *C. neoformans,* the usual treatment for
cryptococcosis is amphotericin B and flucytosine. The other drugs
listed are not indicated for cryptococcosis. Ketoconazole is usually
used for chronic mucocutaneous candidiasis. Nystatin is used for candidiasis, and griseofulvin is indicated for dermatophytes of the hair,
skin, and nails. Miconazole is used for topical fungal infections, oral
thrush and vaginitis.

[42.4]   **E.** The symptoms described including acne-like lesions, skin ulcers,
fever, confusion, staggering gait and cranial nerve deficits are a
classic example of *Cryptococcus neoformans* infection. In some
patients the cerebral edema progresses to a fatal stage compressing
the medulla reducing respiratory efforts. The other yeast listed do not
cause cerebral edema. *E. werneckii* causes tinea nigra characterized
by dark patches on the hands and soles of the feet. *S. schenckii* is usually associated with a prick from a rose thorn. *C. immitis* is associated
with the desert southwest. *H. capsulatum* is usually associated with
the Mississippi river valley and lesions that calcify.

MICROBIOLOGY PEARLS

 Cryptococcus neoformans is transmitted via aerosolized pigeon or
   bird droppings.

 Clinical manifestations: headache, altered mental state, nuchal rigidity, often associated with AIDS.

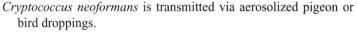 Identification: clinical symptoms, examination of CSF for increased
   pressure and number of white cells with low glucose levels, and
   a positive India ink test.

 Current treatment: amphotericin B or fluconazole.

REFERENCES

Brooks GF, Butel JS, Morse SA. Jawetz, Melnick, & Adelberg's medical microbiology, 23rd ed. New York: McGraw-Hill, 2004:647–649.
Murray PR, Rosenthal KS, Kobayashi GS, Pfaller MA. Medical microbiology,
   4th ed. St. Louis: Mosby, 2002:651–655.
Ryan JR, Ray CG. Sherris medical microbiology, 4th ed. New York: McGraw-Hill,
   2004:647–649.

A 29-year-old woman comes into the clinic for evaluation of a cough. Her symptoms started a few weeks ago and have progressively worsened. The cough is not productive. She has had intermittent, low-grade fevers and feels short of breath. She has tried some over-the-counter cough medications, which don't seem to help. She smokes about a half-pack of cigarettes a day. She denies any history of pulmonary diseases. On examination, her temperature is 37.5°C (99.5°F), pulse is 100 beats per minute, respiratory rate is 26 breaths per minute, and oxygen saturation is 89 percent on room air. Her blood pressure is normal, but when applying the blood pressure cuff, you notice numerous scars in her antecubital region consistent with "needle tracks." In general, she is a thin woman who appears to be in moderate respiratory distress and is coughing frequently. Her head and neck examination is normal. Her lung examination is notable for decreased breath sounds and rhonchi in all fields. Her cardiovascular and abdominal examinations are normal. A chest x-ray shows a bilateral interstitial infiltrate with a "ground-glass" appearance. She confides that she is HIV positive.

◆ **What organism is the likely cause of her symptoms?**

◆ **Describe the sexual phase of reproduction of this organism.**

ANSWERS TO CASE 43: *Pneumocystis carinii*

Summary: A 29-year-old woman IV drug user who is HIV positive has an interstitial pneumonia.

◆ **Most likely etiologic agent:** *Pneumocystis carinii.*

◆ **Sexual phase reproduction of *P. carinii:*** Haploid trophic forms conjugate to form diploid zygotes that become sporocysts; sporocysts undergo meiosis and mitosis to form the spore case that contains eight haploid spores. The spores are released by rupture of the spore case wall.

CLINICAL CORRELATION

Pneumocystis is an opportunistic organism found primarily in the lungs of humans and other animals. The reservoir of the organism in the environment is at this point unknown. Transmission of the organism is from person–to person by respiratory droplet inhalation into the lungs. It is unclear whether disease results from the reactivation of a latent infection or acquisition of a new infection. The cellular immune system is primarily responsible for host defenses, with alveolar macrophages and CD4 cells playing a particularly important role. In HIV patients, the risk of developing symptomatic disease from *Pneumocystis* is highly correlated to the number of circulating CD4 cells, with the highest risk in those persons with CD 4 counts below $200/mm^3$. The use of corticosteroids or other immunosuppressive drugs, treatment for malignancies, or severe malnutrition are risk factors for disease in non-HIV infected people. Classic *Pneumocystis* pulmonary infection is an interstitial pneumonia with plasma cell infiltrates. Typical symptoms are nonproductive cough, fever, dyspnea, and hypoxia. Chest x-rays commonly show a bilateral interstitial infiltrate extending from the hilum with a "ground-glass" appearance. In severely immunosuppressed patients *Pneumocystis* can disseminate most commonly to the thyroid, liver, bone marrow, lymph nodes, or spleen.

Approach to the Suspected *Pneumocystis* Patient

Definitions

Hypoxia: Reduction of oxygen supply to the tissues despite adequate blood perfusion.

Dyspnea: Shortness of breath leading to labored breathing.

Objectives

1. Know the life cycle, morphology, and reproduction of *Pneumocystis*.
2. Know the epidemiology, modes of transmission, and clinical syndromes associated with *Pneumocystis* infection.

Discussion

Characteristics of *Pneumocystis*

Pneumocystis was **originally characterized as a trypanosome;** however, advanced molecular biological techniques have shown it to be closely related to fungi. It is unusual among fungi because it **lacks ergosterol in its cell membranes** and is insensitive to many antifungal drugs. Its life cycle has **both sexual and asexual components.** The trophic form of *Pneumocystis* is small and often seen in clusters. It multiplies asexually by binary fission and sexually by conjugation of haploid trophic forms to diploid cells that become sporocysts. These uninuclear cells undergo miosis then mitosis to form a spore case, which contains eight haploid spores. The spores are released by rupture of the cell wall, although the cyst wall remains and can be identified as empty structures.

    Pneumocystis is thought to be ubiquitous in the environment, and most adults have been exposed to the organism during childhood and develop an asymptomatic infection. *Pneumocystis* is found in many mammalian species and is not thought to cross species lines. *Pneumocystis* that infects humans was recently renamed *P. jirovecii.*

Diagnosis

The **diagnosis** is confirmed by the **presence of the organisms in sputum or bronchial samples** obtained by bronchoalveolar lavage or other techniques, such as sputum induced by respiratory therapy. *Pneumocystis* can be identified microscopically by using numerous stains, such as **methenamine silver, Giemsa, chemofluorescent agents such as calcofluor white, or specific** immunofluorescent monoclonal antibodies. The monoclonal antibody fluorescent stain increases the sensitivity and specificity of the test. The diagnostic stage seen is usually the cyst form. The organism cannot be grown in culture.

Treatment and Prevention

Treatment for *Pneumocystis* is usually with **sulfamethoxazole and trimethoprim (SMX-TMP);** however, in allergic patients there are other options such as **dapsone** or **pentamidine.** Prophylaxis with SMX-TMP is recommended for severely immunosuppressed patients including HIV patients with a **CD4 count of less than 200 cells/mm³.**

Comprehension Questions

[43.1] *Pneumocystis carinii* is now considered a fungus. Which of the following statements accurately describes this organism?

    A. In immunocompromised patients the organism invades blood vessels causing thrombosis and infarction.

    B. It grows best in a culture medium containing tissue fluid.

    C. It is now classified as a fungus because it grows into septate hyphae in Sabouraud agar.

    D. It is sensitive to antifungal agents such as amphotericin B.

    E. Methenamine silver stain is used to visualize the organism in the clinical specimen.

[43.2] Which of the following statements best describes the laboratory diagnosis of *Pneumocystis carinii?*

    A. India ink stain of bronchoalveolar lavage material

    B. KOH stain of lung biopsy tissue

    C. Growth of the organism on Sabouraud agar

    D. Methenamine silver stain of induced sputum

[43.3] *Pneumocystis carinii* produces disease under what conditions listed below?

    A. In individuals with CD4 lymphocyte counts above 400/uL

    B. In the presence of immunosuppression

    C. Infection in early childhood

    D. Prophylaxis with SMX-TMP

Answers

[43.1]   **E.** *Pneumocystis carinii* is often reported as the organism responsible for the described case. Evidence points to *P. carinii* being primarily found in rats, whereas *P. jirovecii* is the human species. These species are not grown in the laboratory and do not respond to traditional antifungal chemotherapy. Being found primarily in the lungs, respiratory infections occur in immunocompromised individuals, and dissemination is rare. Specimens of bronchoalveolar lavage, lung biopsy, or induced sputum are stained (Giemsa or methenamine silver, e.g.) and examined for cysts or trophozoites.

[43.2]   **D.** Because *Pneumocystis* species are not able to be grown in the laboratory, staining procedures constitute the primary diagnostics techniques used. See the answer to Question 43.1 for further discussion.

[43.3]   **B.** *Pneumocystis carinii* and *P. jirovecii* are present in the lungs of many animals, including humans. This organism rarely causes disease except in immunocompromised hosts. No other natural reservoir has ever been demonstrated, and the mode of infection is unclear. Transmission by aerosols may be possible.

MICROBIOLOGY PEARLS

❖   *Pneumocystis* that infects humans was recently renamed from *P. carinii* to *P. jirovecii.*
❖   *Pneumo*cystis has a predilection for the lungs of humans and animals.
❖   Diagnosis of *Pneumocystis* is made by induced sputum or bronchoscopy with microscopic visualization of the cyst forms with either Papanicolaou, Giemsa, silver stain, or monoclonal antibodies.

REFERENCES

Murray PR, Rosenthal KS, Kobayashi GS, Pfaller MA. Opportunistic mycoses. In: Murray PR, Rosenthal KS, Kobayashi GS, Pfaller MA. Medical microbiology, 4th ed. St. Louis: Mosby, 2002:664–72.

Thomas CF, Limper AH. Pneumocystis pneumonia. NEJM 2004;350:2487–98.

Walter PD. Pneumocystis carinii. In: Mandell GL, Bennett JE, Dolin R, eds. Principles and practice of infectious diseases, 5th ed. Philadelphia: Churchill Livingstone, 2000:2781–95.

❖ CASE 44

A 44-year-old woman presents to the office for evaluation of skin growths on her right arm. She reports that a few weeks ago she developed some small, red bumps on her right palm, which seemed to come together into a larger nodule. This then ulcerated, but it never was painful. She has been putting topical antibiotic on this area, and it seemed to be improving. However, in the past week she has noticed new growths extending up her forearm that appear just like the original lesion. She denies having skin lesions anywhere else, denies systemic symptoms such as fever, and has no history of anything like this before. She has no significant medical history and takes no medications. She is employed as a florist and floral arranger. On examination she is comfortable appearing and has normal vital signs. On her right palm you see a circular, 1 cm diameter, ulcerated area with a surrounding red, raised border. There are two identical appearing, but smaller, lesions on the forearm. Microscopic examination of a biopsy taken from one of the lesions reveals numerous white blood cells and cigar-shaped yeast forms.

◆ **What is the most likely infectious cause of these lesions?**

◆ **What is the most likely route by which this infection was transmitted?**

ANSWERS TO CASE 44: *Sporothrix schenckii*

Summary: A 44-year-old florist has painless, ulcerated lesions on her right hand and arm.

◆ **Most likely infectious etiology:** *Sporothrix schenckii.*

◆ **Most likely route by which this infection was transmitted:** Most likely mechanism of infection is inoculation into the skin via a puncture of the hand with an infected plant (most likely a rose thorn).

CLINICAL CORRELATION

Cutaneous sporotrichosis results from the inoculation of the organism into the skin via a puncture or other minor trauma. Most cases occur in persons with occupational or avocational exposure to infected material, such as in gardening or farming. The most common exposures are to rose thorns and sphagnum moss. The initial lesions are usually in areas that are prone to trauma, such as the extremities. They are often erythematous papules or nodules, which then ulcerate. Secondary lesions develop along the lines of lymphatic drainage. The lesions are usually painless, can wax and wane, and systemic symptoms are rare. Extracutaneous infections with *S. schenckii* have occurred, most commonly involving the joints, particularly hand, elbow, ankle, or knees. Cases of pulmonary sporotrichosis as well as meningitis have been described. Invasive and disseminated disease may occur in the severely immunosuppressed, particularly patients with advanced HIV disease.

Approach to the Suspected Sporotrichosis Patient

Definitions

Dematiaceous fungi: Fungi with dark colored (brown or black) conidia and/or hyphae.
Lymphadenitis: Inflammation of the lymph node(s).

Objectives

1. Know the morphologic characteristics of the yeast and mycelial forms of *Sporothrix schenckii.*
2. Know the common sources, routes of transmission, and clinical syndromes associated with *Sporothrix schenckii* infections.

Discussion

Characteristics of *Sporothrix schenckii*

S. schenckii is a **dimorphic fungus** that is most often isolated from **soil, plants, or plant products.** When cultured at 37°C or *in vivo,* it exists as a **cigar-shaped yeast.** At lower temperatures, it exists as a white, fuzzy mold that on further incubation develops a brown pigment. The hyphal form has numerous conidia, which develop in a rosette pattern at the ends of conidiophores. The fungus is found in the soil and on vegetation in all parts of the world, but most commonly in the tropical regions of North and South America. Transmission from animals to man has also been rarely described.

Diagnosis

Skin lesions associated with sporotrichosis can resemble those of other infectious and noninfectious entities, such as other fungal infections, *Mycobacterium* infections, or collagen vascular diseases. Diagnosis can be made by culture of biopsy material or demonstration of the **characteristic cigar-shaped yeast forms** on microscopic examination of a biopsy specimen. Multiple attempts at biopsy and culture may be required to recover the organism.

    S. schenckii grows well within several days to several weeks on routine fungal media such as Sabouraud dextrose agar. Colonies initially are small and white to cream color that eventually turn brown to black. Laboratory confirmation of *S. schenckii* can be established by demonstration of characteristic mold structures after culture at room temperature. The **rosette formation of the conidia** on the conidiophore is characteristic, but not diagnostic. Conversion from the hyphal form to the yeast form on subculture of a specimen at 37°C can aid in the specific identification of the fungus.

Treatment and Prevention

Cutaneous sporotrichosis is usually **treated orally with either a saturated solution of potassium iodide** or an **antifungal agent such as itraconazole.** Extracutaneous or disseminated disease is difficult to treat, but usually treated with **itraconazole.** Patients with concomitant HIV and sporotrichosis are usually treated prophylactically for the rest of their life with oral itraconazole.

Comprehension Questions

[44.1] Which of the following fungi is most likely to cause cutaneous disease?

  A. *Aspergillus fumigatus*
  B. *Candida albicans*
  C. *Cryptococcus neoformans*
  D. *Histoplasma capsulatum*
  E. *Sporothrix schenckii*

[44.2] A woman who pricked her finger while pruning some rose bushes develops a local pustule that progressed to an ulcer. Several nodules then developed along the local lymphatic drainage. The *most reliable* method to identify the etiologic agent is:

  A. Culture of the organism in the laboratory
  B. Gram stain of smear prepared from the lesion
  C. India ink preparation
  D. Skin test for delayed hypersensitivity
  E. Stain the culture with potassium iodide

Answers

[44.1] **E.** *Aspergillus, Cryptococcus,* and *Histoplasma* infections routinely involve the respiratory system and form cellular components recognizable in the diagnostic laboratory. *Candida* species are usually endogenous flora that may be opportunistic under the right circumstances (immunocompromised patient, e.g.). Cutaneous and systemic infections are possible under these conditions. *S. schenckii* is typically introduced into the skin by trauma, often related to outdoor activities and/or plants. About three-fourths of the cases are lymphocutaneous, with multiple subcutaneous nodules and abscesses along the lymphatics.

[44.2] **A.** The most reliable method of diagnosing *S. schenckii* is by culture. Specimens are usually biopsy materials or exudate from granulose or ulcerative lesions and are usually streaked on a selective medium such as Sabouraud agar containing antibacterial antibiotics. Initial incubation is usually 25–30°C, followed by growth at 35°C and confirmation by conversion to the yeast form. Staining procedures are usually nonspecific unless fluorescent antibody.

MICROBIOLOGY PEARLS

 Sporothrix schenckii is a dimorphic fungus found in the soil of many areas of the world and associated with skin lesions following traumatic implantation most commonly from rose thorns.

 Cutaneous sporotrichosis is commonly treated with oral potassium iodide.

 Extracutaneous sporotrichosis, although rare, occurs in severely immunocompromised patients such as those with HIV.

REFERENCES

Fitzpatrick TB, Johnson RA, Polano MK, Suurmond D, Wolff K. Color atlas and synopsis of clinical dermatology, 2nd ed. New York: McGraw-Hill, 1992.

Gorbach SL, Bartlett JG, Blacklow NR. Infectious diseases, 2nd ed. W.B. Saunders, 1998.

Harmon EM, Szwed T. Aspergillosis. eMedicine, 2002. Available online at: http://www.emedicine.com/med/topic174.html

Mandell GL, Bennett JE, Dolin R, eds. Principles and practice of infectious diseases, 5th ed. Philadelphia: Churchill Livingstone, 2000.

Murray PR, Rosenthal KS, Kobayashi GS, Pfaller MA. Medical microbiology, 4th ed. St. Louis: Mosby, 2002.

Rex JH, Okhuysen PC. Sporothrix schenckii. In: Mandell GL, Bennett JE, Dolin R, eds. Principles and practice of infectious diseases, 5th ed. Philadelphia: Churchill Livingstone, 2000:22695–2702.

Shafazand S, Doyle R, Ruoss S, Weinacker A, Raffin T. Inhalational anthrax: epidemiology, diagnosis and management. Chest 1999;116(5):1369–76.

Todar K. University of Wisconsin-Madison Dept. of Bacteriology, 2002; http:www.bact.wisc.edu/bact330/lymelecture

An 8-year-old boy, a child of immigrants from El Salvador who moved to the southwestern United States three months ago, presents to the emergency room with abdominal pain and vomiting. He was ill for a day, but his symptoms have worsened in the past few hours, and his parents became panicked when they saw a worm in his vomitus. He has no significant medical history and has taken no medications. On examination, he appears very ill and in obvious pain. His temperature is 37.7°C (99.9°F), his pulse is 110 beats per minute, and his blood pressure is normal. His mucous membranes are dry, but his head and neck exam is otherwise normal. He is tachycardic, and his lungs are clear. His abdomen has high-pitched, tinkling bowel sounds on auscultation and is diffusely tender to palpation. There is, however, no rebound tenderness. An abdominal x-ray shows air-fluid levels consistent with a small bowel obstruction. His parents saved and brought in the worm that he vomited. It is 5 inches long and reddish-yellow in color.

◆ **What organism is most likely responsible for the patient's illness?**

◆ **How did the patient become infected?**

ANWERS TO CASE 45: *Ascaris*

Summary: An 8-year-old boy with a small bowel obstruction and who vomited a worm.

◆ **Most likely organism responsible for the patient's illness:** The nematode, *Ascaris lumbricoides.*

◆ **How did the patient become infected:** By ingesting eggs of the parasite that have matured to contain a larval form.

CLINICAL CORRELATION

Infections with *Ascaris* are frequently asymptomatic or may be accompanied by numerous symptoms. The pathology that underlies symptoms is conditioned by the number of worms harbored and the sequential location of larvae in the lungs and adult worms in the intestine.

Larvae released when ingested eggs hatch make a so-called "heart-lung circuit" in which they are carried via the blood to various tissues (Figure 45-1). Migrating larvae elicit eosinophilia and granulomatous lesions. During the larval migration stage, symptoms are associated mainly with larvae present in the liver and lungs. Larvae that reach the lungs may cause pneumonitis. Patients may cough up exudates that are blood-tinged and contain polymorphonuclear leukocytes, mainly eosinophils. Fever may accompany pneumonitis, which disappears when the larvae move to the small intestine. *Ascaris* is highly allergenic, stimulating inordinately high IgE levels. Therefore, pneumonitis may be especially severe in individuals who are sensitized by a prior infection and encounter a challenge or secondary infection. Increased severity is caused by immune-mediated inflammation.

Gastrointestinal (GI) symptoms depend on the number and location of adult worms. Light infection may cause GI upset, colic, and loss of appetite and impair digestion or absorption of nutrients. In heavy infections, the adult worms may ball up in the small intestine, resulting in physical obstruction, a rare but serious occurrence. From their location in the small intestine, adult worms infrequently migrate down and out of the anus or up and through the mouth or nose. Adult worms may cause symptoms by migrating to obstruct the bile ducts or penetrate the gallbladder or liver. Adult worms may be seen in the stool or vomitus.

Approach to Suspected *Ascaris* Infection

Definitions

Nematode: A helminth characterized by a cylindrical body and separate sexes, in contrast to cestodes and trematodes that are flatworms and generally hermaphroditic.

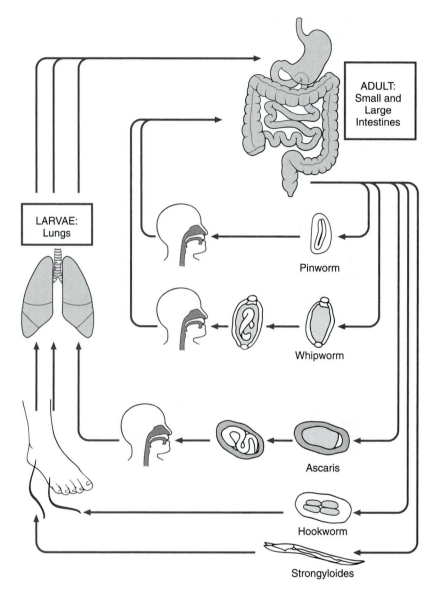

Figure 45-1. Life Cycle of Parasitic Nematodes, including *Ascaris lumbricoides.*

With permission from Barron S, ed. Medical microbiology, 4th ed. Galveston: University of Texas Medical Branch, 1996.

"Giant intestinal roundworm": common name for *Ascaris lumbricoides.*
Egg (ova), larva, and adult: sequential developmental stages in life cycle of helminths.
Larva: preadult or juvenile stage of helminths; nematodes have four larval stages in their life cycle prior to reaching the adult stage. Each stage is preceded by a molt.

Objectives

1. Learn the life cycle of *A. lumbricoides* and the epidemiology and clinical course of infection.
2. Be able to describe three basic aspects of infection: transmission, diagnosis, and treatment/prevention.

Discussion

Characteristics of *Ascaris*

***Ascaris* is one of several nematodes that infect the GI tract and, like all of these, develops through egg, larva, and adult stages.** *Ascaris lumbricoides* is very similar in size and life cycle to *Ascaris suum,* which is found in pigs. If a human ingests eggs of *A. suum,* the larvae will migrate to the lungs and die, but in the process can cause a serious form of "ascaris pneumonia." Adult worms of this species do not develop in the human intestine. Parasitologists debate the point that there is only one species of *Ascaris* that infects both pigs and humans. Other ascarids that infect humans are *Toxocara canis* and *Toxocara cati,* which are parasites of dogs and cats, respectively. Although humans can become infected by ingesting eggs of these species, neither worm develops to maturity. After hatching in the intestine, *Toxocara* larvae migrate chronically in visceral tissue, giving rise to the condition termed "visceral larvae migrans."

Infection Transmission

Typical of nematodes, *A. lumbricoides* has separate sexes and a life cycle that involves **egg, larva, and adult stages.** Growth involves **four larval stages.** Transition from one stage to another and to the adult stage is preceded by a molt or shedding of the cuticle or "skin." A person **becomes infected by ingesting eggs** that are usually acquired through hand-to-mouth transmission from the soil or via contaminated food or water. Eggs **hatch in the duodenum,** releasing larvae that **penetrate the small intestine to enter the blood stream.** Larvae are **carried hematogenously** to various organs. On reaching the **lungs, they penetrate into the alveoli.** Larvae reside in the lung for approximately three weeks, growing and advancing to a subsequent larval stage. They then **migrate up the bronchi and trachea, where they are then swallowed** and returned to the small intestine. In the **intestine, larvae develop to the adult**

stage and reach reproductive maturity in about 2 months. Adults can survive for up to 2 years and grow to 15–35 cm in length. A single female worm lays about 200,000 eggs daily that are passed in the feces. Eggs can survive for years in the soil, tolerating a wide range of temperatures and other environmental variables. Under optimal conditions, eggs reach an infective, larvated stage in 2–3 weeks. Development is arrested at this stage until the egg is ingested.

Ascariasis is a chronic disease of the small intestine and can be transmitted as long as adult worms are in the intestine and feces containing ascaris eggs are allowed to contaminate the environment. Ascariasis is more prevalent in tropical climates but is found in temperate regions of the world. It is most common where sanitation is poor and where human feces are used as fertilizer in agricultural practices. Infections occur in all ages but are more common in children. In endemic areas, most of the population has some worm burden. With the **exception of pinworm infection, ascariasis is the most common helminthic infection of humans.**

Diagnosis

A presumptive diagnosis may be based on clinical symptoms. However, symptoms are not pathognomonic. The **pneumonitis** phase of infection cannot be diagnosed as *Ascaris*-induced because it precedes the intestinal phase by several weeks. Intestinal symptoms are normally absent or mild and, in most cases, go undetected.

A definitive diagnosis is based on **identifying egg or adult stages.** As in this case (Case 45), the first clue of infection may be adult worms that are vomited or passed in a stool. Intestinal obstruction, especially in children, often prompts medical attention. Because of its uniquely large size, an adult *A. lumbricoides* is unmistakable. The adult females are reddish yellow in color and can measure up to 12–15 inches long (males are generally shorter) and one-fourth of an inch in diameter. Although a definitive diagnosis can be made by identifying adult worms, ascariasis is more commonly diagnosed by identifying eggs in the stool. Both fertile and infertile eggs are passed in the stool. Because female worms pass thousands of eggs daily, diagnosis can be made by direct examination of a stool sample without the need for techniques to concentrate eggs. The eggs are ovoid, measure 45 by 75 μm and have a thick transparent inner shell covered by an albuminous coat that is wrinkled and usually stained light brown by bile pigments. Unfertilized eggs are commonly seen in a stool. These are more elongated, measuring 40 by 90 μm. The inside of the unfertilized egg is amorphous instead of containing a well defined single cell of the fertilized egg.

Treatment and Prevention

Adult worms are the target of several drugs available to treat ascariasis. The drug of choice is **mebendazole,** a benzimidazole derivative that has a high therapeutic index. The effectiveness of treatment can be assessed by the disappearance of eggs in stool samples and alleviation of symptoms. In cases of intestinal obstruction, the first action should be directed at ridding the patient of worms through the use of chemotherapeutic agents, such as mebendazole. If the worms can be dislodged the patient may void them in the stool. If the bolus of worms cannot be dislodged, surgery may be an option. If surgery is chosen, it is imperative that the worms be killed or paralyzed with a drug such as piperazine prior to physically removing them from the intestine. The reason for this procedure is that a live, active worm releases an aerosol of eggs through its uterine pore. Eggs are invisible to the naked eye. However, if eggs fall on exposed viscera they elicit granulomatous lesions and adhesions that can lead to severe complications. Preventive measures relate to instructing the patient on how the infection was acquired and on the proper disposal of feces to avoid soil contamination and reinfection.

Comprehension Questions

[45.1] A definitive diagnosis of ascariasis can be made by observing which of the following?

A. An eosinophilia in a differential white blood cell count.
B. Motile larvae in a stool sample.
C. Larvae in x-ray of lungs.
D. An adult worm passed during a bowel movement.

[45.2] Ascariasis is most effectively treated with which of the following drugs?

A. Mebendazole
B. Metronidazole
C. Niclosamide
D. Praziquantel

[45.3] A person presents to his physician complaining of chronic GI symptoms. A diagnosis of *Ascaris lumbricoides* was made. Human nematodes infect individuals via different routes. This patient was most likely infected by which of the following?

A. Larvae penetrating unprotected skin
B. Ingesting larvated eggs
C. Eating uncooked pork
D. Internal autoinfection

Answers

[45.1]   **D.** Identification of adult worms passed by an individual can ensure a definitive diagnosis. Although an eosinophilia accompanies ascariasis, this condition can be caused by other infections and by various allergic conditions. Motile larvae in a stool are indicative of infection with *Strongyloides stercoralis.* Nematode larvae cannot be seen in an x-ray.

[45.2]   **A.** Mebendazole is a broad spectrum antihelminthic that is the drug of choice for treating *Ascaris* and several other intestinal nematodes. Metronidazole is used primarily to treat infections with protozoa, such as *Giardia lamblia* and *Trichomonas vaginalis.* Niclosamide is the drug of choice in treating most adult cestode or tapeworm infections. Praziquantel is used to treat infections with blood flukes or schistosomes and can also be used to treat adult tapeworms.

[45.3]   **B.** *Ascaris* is acquired by ingesting infective eggs, as are the whipworm, *Trichuris trichiura,* and the pinworm, *Enterobius vermicularis.* Filariform larvae penetrating unprotected skin is the route by which a person becomes infected by other intestinal nematodes, hookworms and *Strongyloides;* eating uncooked pork could lead to trichinosis; and internal autoinfection is caused only by *Strongyloides.*

Synopsis of Ascariasis

MICROBIAL PEARLS	Infective stage of etiologic agent	Location of Pathogenic stage	Laboratory diagnosis based on identification of:	Drugs used in treatment
	Egg of: *Ascaris lumbricoides*	Lungs (larvae, transient) Small intestine (adult, chronic)	Egg (stool exam) or Adult (vomitus; passed in stool)	Mebendazole

MICROBIOLOGY PEARLS

❖ The fertilized eggs are unsegmented when laid by the female worm.
❖ Mebendazole, one of several available benzimidazole compounds used to treat nematodes, is the drug of choice in treating *Ascaris* infection.

REFERENCES

Centers for Disease Control. DPDx. Laboratory identification of parasites of public concern. Ascariasis. Centers for Disease Control and Prevention, 2004. Available online at: http://www.dpd.cdc.gov/dpdx/HTML/Ascariasis.htm

Graphic Images of Parasites. Ascaris lumbricoides and ascaris suum (intestinal round worms of humans and pigs). Author, 2004. Available online at: http://www.biosci.ohio-state.edu/~parasite/ascaris.html

Medical Letter on Drugs and Therapeutics. Drugs for parasitic infections. New Rochelle, NY: Author, 2002. Available online at: http://www.medletter.com/freedocs/parasitic.pdf

A 32-year-old man with known HIV is brought to the hospital with diarrhea. He has had between 15 and 25 watery stools a day for the past 2 weeks. He has had a low grade fever and felt very fatigued, but denies vomiting. He has not passed any blood in his stool. He says that he has lost 8 lb in this time frame. He is on a "triple therapy cocktail" of AZT, 3TC, and a protease inhibitor for his HIV. His last CD4 cell count was 150 cells/mm^3. On examination, his temperature is 37.2° C (98.9°F), pulse is 110 beats per minute, blood pressure is 95/75 mmHg, and respiratory rate is 24 breaths per minute. In general, he appears cachectic. His eyes are dry and sunken. His mucous membranes are moist. His cardio-vascular exam is notable for tachycardia, and he has orthoscopic changes on sitting up from lying down. His abdomen has hyperactive bowel sounds, but is soft and only mildly tender. His stool is heme negative. A modified acid-fast stained stool sample reveals multiple red and pink, round oocysts.

◆ **What is the most likely cause of diarrhea?**

◆ **How is this infection most commonly acquired?**

ANSWERS TO CASE 46: *Cryptosporidium parvum*

Summary: A 32-year-old man with HIV and diarrhea. A modified acid-fast stained stool sample reveals multiple red and pink, round oocysts.

◆ **Most likely etiologic agent:** *Cryptosporidium parvum*

◆ **How is this infection most commonly acquired:** Ingestion of oocysts in contaminated water or food or fecal-oral transmission from infected animals or person to person.

CLINICAL CORRELATION

Cryptosporidium parvum belongs to a group of protozoans known as coccidians. The infective oocyst is about 3–8 μm in diameter. The parasite, on emerging from the oocyst, attaches to the surface of intestinal epithelium where it multiplies both asexually and sexually. The parasite causes changes in mucosa that include crypt hyperplasia and villous atrophy. Associated with its presence in the intestine, and after an incubation period of about 2–12 days, is an acute illness characterized by nausea, abdominal cramps, weight loss, anorexia, malaise, low-grade fever, and diarrhea. The frequency of diarrheal episodes and voluminous fluid loss is often debilitating. During infection there, may be periods in which symptoms are absent. In immunocompetent individuals, the disease will resolve on its own, usually within 7 to 14 days. In immunocompromised hosts, the disease is generally more severe and chronic, sometimes lasting for life. Five to ten percent of patients with AIDS acquire infection with *Cryptosporidium*. Persistence of infection in HIV-infected individuals is closely associated with CD4 lymphocyte counts of less than 180 cells/mm^3. Protracted diarrhea may lead to dehydration, wasting, and death. Severe intestinal distress, usually in immunodeficient individuals, is sometimes associated with pulmonary and tracheal cryptosporidiosis that is associated with coughing and low-grade fever. The strains that infect the intestine and lungs are, to date, indistinguishable.

Approach to Suspected *Cryptosporidium* Infection

Definitions

Coccidian: The specific taxonomic group of protozoans to which C. parvum belongs.

Oocyst: The stage in the life cycle of C. parvum that transmits the disease and is also sought in making a definitive diagnosis. Each oocyst contains four sporozoites.

Sporozoite: The stage released from the oocyst following ingestion and which initiates infection.

Zoonosis: A disease that is transmitted from lower vertebrate hosts to humans.

Acid-fast stain: A type of stain that renders oocysts highly visible in a fecal sample. It is used to support the microscopic diagnosis of the parasite.

Objectives

1. Learn the life cycle of *Cryptosporidium parvum* and the epidemiology and clinical course of cryptosporidiosis, and compare this disease with those caused by related organisms, such as *Cyclospora* and *Isospora.*
2. Be able to describe the three basic aspect of infection: transmission, diagnosis, and treatment/prevention.

Discussion

Characteristics of *Cryptosporidium* that Impact Transmission

Misdiagnosis with cyclosporiasis may be made, in part because clinical symptoms are similar. **Protracted, watery diarrhea is the hallmark of infection.** *Cyclospora cayetanensis,* which infects humans, has a worldwide distribution. Another related organism that causes diarrhea in humans is *Isospora belli.*

Cryptosporidium **species are ubiquitous, worldwide enteric pathogens of humans** and multiple other animal species. Of the many species of the genus, *C. parvum* is responsible for most clinical disease in humans and other mammals. The life cycle of *C. parvum* occurs within a single host and, like other coccidian, involves sexual and asexual reproduction.

The **small intestine is the usual host habitat for *Cryptosporidium,*** where it lives in a unique intraepithelial niche. The life cycle is initiated with the ingestion of oocysts that contain four sporozoites. When oocysts are ingested, they undergo excystation as the outer wall is removed by digestive processes. Sporozoites that are released attach to the host's intestinal epithelial cells and become surrounded by a host-derived membrane, making them intracellular but extracytoplasmic. Sporozoites undergo multiple fission to form meronts that contain multiple merozoites. The merozoites are released to infect other cells. Following another round of asexual division and on release of the second and subsequent generations of merozoites, they penetrate new cells to form gametes. Most gametes undergo enlargement into macrogametes (female). Some become microgametocytes that undergo fission multiple times to form sperm-like microgametes (male). Microgametes leave the microgametocyte and fertilize a macrogamete to form a zygote. The zygote then becomes covered by a wall, forming an oocyst that is highly resistant to chemical and physical changes in the internal and external environment. Sporozoites develop within the oocyst that are sloughed, along with intestinal epithelial cells, and voided in the feces. Because oocysts are passed in the feces in a sporulated stage (i.e., contain sporozoites), they are immediately infective and can retain infectivity for long periods because of their protective wall. In having oocysts that are immediately infective, *Cryptosporidium* is different from *Cyclospora,* which has oocysts that require 1–2 weeks to develop to an infective stage.

Presumably ingestion of one oocyst can initiate an infection that can be contracted by eating contaminated food or drinking contaminated water.

Touching the stool of infected individuals or animals or anything contaminated with feces and then not washing your hands before touching your mouth can also initiate infection.

Infection can be transmitted by ingestion of oocysts passed in feces of infected humans or animals. Thus, infection can be transmitted from one person to another or from animals to humans, from eating and drinking food or water contaminated with fecal material or from transfer of oocysts from contaminated material to the mouth or from person–to person.

Diagnosis

A **definitive diagnosis is based on identifying oocysts in a fecal sample.** A technique, such as sugar flotation, is used to concentrate the oocysts and acid-fast staining is used to identify them. A **fluorescent antibody technique** is also available to stain the isolated oocysts, augmenting visualization. **Oocysts contain four sporozoites.** It is important to make a differential diagnosis with *Cyclospora* oocysts, which are similar in size but are not sporulated when passed. *Cryptosporidium* oocysts contain four sporozoites and are about 8 μm in diameter. When sporulated, the oocysts of *Cyclospora* are the same size, but contain two sporocysts, each with two sporozoites. *Isospora* oocysts can also be found in the stool; however, they can be differentiated by their larger size, 15 by 30 μm ovoid. Like *Cyclospora,* oocysts of *Isospora* are excreted in an unsporulated stage, and, after becoming sporulated, contain two sporocysts, each with two sporozoites. **Pulmonary infections of *Cryptosporidium* are diagnosed by biopsy and staining** (Table 46-1).

Table 46-1
DIFFERENTATION OF HUMAN COCCIDAN OOCYSTS

SPECIES	NUMBER OF SPOROCYSTS	NUMBER OF SPOROZOITES	SPORULATED IN STOOL	SIZE OF OOCYST μM
Cryptosporidium parvum	0	4	Yes	4–8
Cyclospora cayetanensis	2	4	No	4–8
Isospora belli	2	4	No	12 x 30

Treatment and Prevention

No specific chemotherapeutic agent is available to effectively treat cryptosporidiosis. As noted, infection is self-limiting in immunocompetent hosts and chronic in immunosuppressed individuals. HIV infection makes a person vulnerable to infection with *Cryptosporidium*. Because of massive fluid loss due to diarrhea, infected individuals may require rehydration therapy.

Because there are **no effective agents to treat infection,** the best measure to control infection is avoidance of situations that are conducive to transmission. Thus, knowledge about sources of infection and how infection is transmitted is the key to prevention.

Most surface water, such as streams, lakes, and rivers contain some *Cryptosporidium* oocysts. Many public supplies of treated and filtered water derived from these sources are contaminated with low levels of oocysts. Although any individual may acquire infection, children in daycare centers and individuals with AIDS or HIV infection represent populations that are especially vulnerable to infection.

Cryptosporidiosis can be prevented by thoroughly **washing hands before eating** and after any contact with animals or soil or after changing diapers. In people with weakened immune systems, cryptosporidiosis can be life-threatening. These individuals must take extra precautions to drink only water that has been purified; wash with purified water; cook all food; do not swim in lakes, rivers, streams, or public pools; avoid sexual practices that might involve contact with stool; and avoid touching farm animals.

Comprehension Questions

[46.1] A 33-year-old woman has chronic diarrhea. A fecal sample is obtained. Microscopic identification of which of the following stages of the organism would provide the strongest evidence for cryptosporidiosis?

  A. Cyst
  B. Oocyst
  C. Egg
  D. Sporozoites
  E. Merozoites

[46.2] A 24-year-old male scientist is diagnosed with chronic cryptosporidiosis. He asks about the epidemiology of this disorder. Which of the following accurately describes the disease or the etiologic agent?

  A. Is self-limiting in immunocompromised patients
  B. Reproduces sexually and asexually in different hosts
  C. Can be acquired through sporozoites transmitted by an insect vector
  D. Is transmitted through drinking water contaminated with animal feces
  E. Is the only human parasite that produces oocysts

[46.3] Chronic, debilitating cryptosporidiosis is most likely to affect which of the following individuals?

A. Dairy farmers
B. Individuals with AIDS
C. Infants placed in daycare centers
D. Zoo animal handlers
E. Hikers who drink from streams and lakes

Answers

[46.1] **B.** Oocyst is the correct answer. Egg and cyst stages are not part of the life cycle of *Cryptosporidium*. Eggs are produced by helminths, and cyst stages are produced by other intestinal protozoans, such as *Entamoeba* and *Giardia*. Merozoites occur within infected epithelial cells but are not the target of diagnostic tests or procedures. Sporozoites are part of the life cycle and occur inside the oocyst but are not the object of the microscopic examination.

[46.2] **D.** Infection can be acquired from oocysts transferred from farm animals. In immunocompromised individuals, such as those with AIDS or cancer patients being treated with immunosuppressive agents, infection is not self-limiting but rather chronic and sometimes life-threatening. The life cycle of *Cryptosporidium* involves both asexual and sexual reproduction, but both forms occur in a single host. Sporozoites are stages in the life cycle that are released from ingested oocysts. There is no insect that serves as a biological or mechanical vector in the life cycle. Oocysts are also produced by other species of coccidians that infect humans *Isospora, Cyclospora, Toxoplasma,* and *Plasmodium. Toxoplasma* oocysts only occur in feline hosts; Plasmodium species cause malaria in which only the mosquito definitive host harbors oocysts; Isospora and Cyclospora are intestinal coccidian parasites that produce oocysts that are passed in the feces and must be considered in making a differential diagnosis.

[46.3] **B.** All individuals (A–E) are susceptible to infection. However, persons that are at high risk of severe, protracted infection are those with AIDS, or those who have cancer or organ transplants who are treated with drugs that weaken the immune system, or individuals who are genetically immunodeficient.

Synopsis of Cryptosporidiosis

MICROBIAL PEARLS	Infective stage of etiologic agent	Location of Pathogenic stage	Laboratory diagnosis based on identification of:	Drugs used in treatment
	Oocyst of: *Cryptosporidium parvum*	Small and large intestine	Oocyst (stool exam)	None satisfactory

MICROBIOLOGY PEARLS

❖ Often there is misdiagnosis between cryptosporidiosis and cyclosporiasis.

❖ Cryptosporidiosis does not respond to specific therapy, whereas cyclosporiasis responds well to a combination of trimethoprim and sulfamethoxazole.

REFERENCES

Centers for Disease Control. DPDx. Laboratory identification of parasites of public concern. Cryptosporidiosis. Author, 2004. Available online at: http://www.dpd.cdc.gov/dpdx/HTML/Cryptosporidiosis.htm

Graphic Images of Parasites. *Cryptosporidium parvum* (cryptosporidiosis). Author, 2004. Available online at: http://www.biosci.ohio-state.edu/~parasite/cryptosporidium.html

Medical Letter on Drugs and Therapeutics. Drugs for parasitic infections. New Rochelle, NY: The Medical Letter, 2002. Available online at: http://www.medletter.com/freedocs/parasitic.pdf

A 4-year-old girl is brought to the office by her mother because of anal itching. The mother has noticed her daughter scratching and rubbing her anal area frequently for the past few days. Her anal area has been getting red and raw from all the scratching. Mother has used some petrolatum and hydrocortisone cream, but it hasn't helped much. The child has not had any obvious skin rashes and is not scratching any other part of her body. She has not had diarrhea. She takes no medications and has no significant medical history. She attends daycare 4 days a week. On examination, she is a well-appearing child. Her vital signs and general examination are normal. Examination of her perianal area reveals some erythema and excoriation from scratching. You perform a microscopic examination of a sample collected by touching the perianal region with a piece of clear cellophane tape.

◆ **What diagnostic finding are you likely to see on this microscopic examination?**

◆ **What is the organism responsible for this infection?**

ANSWERS TO CASE 47: Pinworms

Summary: A 4-year-old girl has perianal pruritus. The diagnosis is made by microscopic examination of a sample collected by touching the perianal region with a piece of clear cellophane tape.

◆ **Diagnostic finding likely to see on this microscopic examination:** Thin-walled, ovoid eggs that are flattened on one side and contain a nematode larva.

◆ **Organism responsible for this infection:** *Enterobius vermicularis*

CLINICAL CORRELATION

Enterobius vermicularis, commonly called the pinworm, is the most common cause of helminthic infections in the United States and is endemic around the world. Humans are the only known host with *E. vermicularis,* but other vertebrates can be infected with different species of this nematode. Adult worms, approximately 1 cm in length, white and thread-like in appearance, inhabit the large intestine. Gravid females migrate to the perianal and perineal regions at night to lay eggs that are immediately infective. Infection is more common in children than adults and is often asymptomatic. However, a variety of symptoms are ascribed to pinworms. Atypically, worms are sometimes found in an inflamed appendix and there are rare reports of worms reaching the genital tract and producing vaginitis. By far the most common signs of infection occur in children and include restless sleep and tiredness during the day. However, more common symptoms consist of anal or perianal itching because of the adult worms crawling on the skin. The eggs can also cause local itching, which may be more intense in secondary infections as a result of allergic reactions to their coating. Frequent scratching results in transfer to the hands and areas under the fingernails. Eggs are frequently transferred to clothing, bedding, toys, and dust, where they can survive for several weeks. Through hand-to-mouth transmission, the eggs are ingested and hatch in the duodenum. Larvae released from eggs reach adult stage in about a month. Infections are acute, generally lasting 4–8 weeks. Considering the relatively short duration of a single infection, chronic enterobiasis is caused by reinfection.

Approach to the Suspected *Enterobius* Infection

Definitions

Pinworm: Common name for *Enterobius vermicularis.*

Cervical alae: An extension of a lateral cuticular protuberance or lateral line on the body surface of the pinworm that extends to the head region and appears microscopically as a "flared" region or collar. Cervical alae help in the identification of adult worms.

Nocturnal migration: Refers to the tendency of pinworms to migrate at night from the colon, out the anus, to the perianal and perineal regions to deposit eggs.

Larvated egg: Refers to eggs that contain a larval stage and are deposited by pinworms on the skin.

Objectives

1. Learn the life cycle of *E. vermicularis* and the epidemiology and clinical course of infection.
2. Be able to describe three basic aspects of infection: transmission, diagnosis, and treatment/prevention.

Discussion

Characteristics of *Enterobiasis* that Impact Transmission

A patient acquires infection by **ingesting the pinworm eggs containing infective larvae.** Ingested eggs hatch in the small intestine releasing larvae that migrate to the cecal area and mature into adult male and female worms that are free or insecurely attached to the mucosa. The period between ingestion of eggs to maturation takes about 3–4 weeks. Following copulation, the female pinworms produce eggs. Rather than release eggs in the colon, the **female worms migrate out the anus onto the surrounding skin and release eggs. Worm migration usually occurs at night.** Each female will lay 10,000–20,000 microscopic, larvated eggs. Pinworm eggs are infective within a few hours after being deposited on the skin. They can survive up to 2 weeks on clothing, bedding, or other objects. Individuals can become infected after accidentally swallowing infective pinworm eggs from contaminated surfaces or fingers. The duration of a single infection is 4–8 weeks.

Diagnosis

Although *Enterobius* is an intestinal parasite, eggs are rarely found during lab examinations of stools. If a person is suspected of having pinworms, the so-called **"scotch tape test"** should be used to identify the parasite. Transparent adhesive tape, sometime attached to the end of tongue depressor or "pinworm paddle," is pressed in the anal region. This procedure involves the help of a patient or parents of suspected children. The tape is then transferred to a glass slide, sticky side down. The slide should then be examined microscopically by an expert for eggs. Pinworm eggs are about 20×50 μm characteristically flattened on one side and usually contain an active larva. Because bathing or having a bowel movement may remove eggs, the scotch tape impression should be made on awakening in the morning. In children, samples taken from under the fingernails may also contain eggs because scratching of the anal area is common.

A definitive diagnosis may also be made on **recovery and identification of adult worms** seen directly in bedclothes or around the anal area. The **female** pinworm has a **sharply pointed tail and anterior alae** that form a **collar-like structure** around the mouth. The female worm is about 1 cm long with a diameter about .5 mm. In female worms that are gravid, the uterus filled with eggs is a common feature.

Treatment and Prevention

A highly effective drug in the treatment of enterobiasis is **mebendazole,** given as a single dose, with a repeat dose administered 2 weeks later. This is a broad spectrum antinematode agent that has a high therapeutic index. Close family contacts should be treated as well. If reinfection occurs, the source of the infection should be identified. Therefore, playmates, schoolmates, close contacts outside the house, and household members should be considered. Each infected person should receive the two-dose treatment and, if necessary, more than two doses. In short, the importance of determining infection in the entire family or contacts should be explained in terms of the life cycle of the worm and personal, and group hygiene should be stressed.

Comprehension Questions

[47.1] In which of the following life cycle stages is enterobiasis transmitted?

    A. Larva
    B. Egg
    C. Adult
    D. Cyst
    E. Oocyst

[47.2] Which of the following is the drug of choice in treating enterobiasis?

    A. Mebendazole
    B. Metronidazole
    C. Piperazine
    D. Praziquantel
    E. Chloroquine

[47.3] A parent of a child suffering from disturbed sleep and restlessness calls the family physician and states that her child is once again infected with pinworms and asks if she can administer the same medicine that was used to cure an earlier infection. After the physician is convinced that the pinworm infection is the problem, she advises on giving the same treatment and provides direction on how to clean up the environment to prevent further reinfection. The physician should have been convinced by the fact that the parent:

A. Knew that reinfection was a possibility
B. Had collected worms from bed linen and accurately described them
C. Described symptoms of enterobiasis
D. Had the child's stool examined by her veterinarian who identified tell-tale eggs
E. Noted that the family's pet cat continued to sleep on the child's bed.

Answers

[47.1]   **B.** The egg stage is the stage transmitted from person to person. A larval form (A) is found inside the egg but does not escape to initiate infection until the egg is ingested. Adult forms (C) live in the intestine but are not the stage directly responsible for transmission of the infection. Cyst (D) and oocyst (D) stages are not a part of the life cycle of *E. vermicularis.*

[47.2]   **A.** Mebendazole is the most appropriate of several available benzimidazole compounds to treat enterobiasis. This drug of choice is a highly effective, broad-spectrum antihelminthic. Metronidazole (B) is used to treat various protozoan infections, but is not efficacious in treating pinworms. Piperazine (C) is an anthelminthic that was used prior to the discovery of mebendazole to treat enterobiasis and is less effective, and its dose regimens are more complicated. Praziquantel (D) is effective in treating tapeworm and fluke (flatworms) infections but is not useful against pinworms or other nematodes. Chloroquine is a potent antimalarial drug but of no use against helminths.

[47.3]   **B.** Finding and identifying adult pinworms is one way to make a definitive diagnosis. Reinfection (A) is a definite possibility but not convincing evidence that the child is actually infected. Symptoms described (C) are associated with enterobiasis but are only presumptive, not definitive, evidence of infection. A stool exam (D) is not an appropriate or effective method to diagnose enterobiasis. Cats (E) are in no way associated with transmission of infection.

Synopsis of Enterobiasis

MICROBIAL PEARLS	Infective stage of etiologic agent	Location of pathogenic stage	Laboratory diagnosis based on identification of:	Drugs used in treatment
	Egg of : *Enterobius vermicularis*	Large intestine	Egg or Adult (anal swab)	Mebendazole

MICROBIOLOGY PEARLS

❖ The egg (larvated) is the infective stage.
❖ The life cycle is direct, meaning that the adults develop from larvae without leaving the gastrointestinal tract. Adult worms are the primary cause of pathology.
❖ Mebendazole, a broad spectrum antihelminthic, is the drug of choice.

REFERENCES

Centers for Disease Control. DPDx. Laboratory identification of parasites of public concern. Enterobiasis. Author, 2004. Available online at: http://www.dpd.cdc.gov/dpdx/HTML/Enterobiasis.htm

Graphic Images of Parasites. Pinworms (Enterobius vermicularis, Oxyuris species). Author, 2004. Available online at: http://www.biosci.ohio-state.edu/~parasite/enterobius.html

Medical Letter on Drugs and Therapeutics. Drugs for parasitic infections. New Rochelle, NY: Author, 2002. Available online at: http://www.medletter.com/freedocs/parasitic.pdf

A 50-year-old woman presents to your office with the complaints of fever, chills, nausea, and vomiting for the past 5 days. She is especially concerned because she just returned from a 3-week long church mission trip to central Africa during which she did not take the recommended malaria prophylaxis. She was careful about using insect repellent and wearing long-sleeved clothing, but she did not take the recommended weekly dose of mefloquine because it made her nauseous. Starting a few days after her return, she has had episodes of shaking chills followed by fever spikes as high as 39.7°C (103.5°F) and then profuse sweating. After these episodes she would feel so exhausted that she would sleep for hours. These severe episodes have been occurring every other day. In between these episodes, she has had low-grade fever, myalgias, nausea, vomiting, and diarrhea. On examination, she appears very fatigued and pale. Her temperature is 37.7°C (99.9°F), pulse 100 beats per minute, blood pressure 110/80 mmHg, and respiratory rate 18 breaths per minute. Other than signs of dehydration, her examination is unremarkable. A complete blood count shows her to be anemic. She has elevated blood urea nitrogen, creatinine, and lactate dehydrogenase levels. A thin-blood smear is sent to the laboratory, which shows erythrocytes with ring forms at the periphery of the cell and multiple erythrocytes with three or four ring forms present.

◆ **What is the most likely etiology of her infection?**

◆ **What findings on the thin blood smear are specific for this organism?**

ANSWERS TO CASE 48: *Plasmodium* species

Summary: A 50-year-old woman has fever and body aches. A thin-blood smear shows erythrocytes with ring forms at the periphery of the cell and multiple erythrocytes with three or four ring forms.

◆ **Most likely etiology of her infection:** *Plasmodium falciparum.*

◆ **Findings on the thin blood smear are specific for this organism:** Multiple ring forms in a single erythrocyte and ring forms located at the periphery of the erythrocytes.

CLINICAL CORRELATION

Malaria is caused by one of the four species of plasmodia and involve a mosquito-human-mosquito life cycle. Plasmodia are coccidian parasites of erythrocytes. Their life cycle involves asexual reproduction in humans and sexual reproduction in the mosquito. Human infection is initiated by the bite of an infected mosquito, which introduces sporozoites into the blood stream. The sporozoites travel to the liver where they mature and reproduce asexually by schizogony. *Plasmodium ovale* and *P. vivax* may also establish a dormant— hypnozoite—stage in the liver; *P. falciparum* and *P. malariae* are incapable of this. On completion of the hepatic growth and reproductive stage, merozoites are released from hepatocytes and infect erythrocytes, initiating the erythrocytic cycle. Asexual reproduction continues, resulting in rupture of erythrocytes and release of more infectious merozoites. The classic symptoms of malaria relate to the paroxysm of shaking chills, fever, and sweating and correspond with the cyclical lysis of erythrocytes and release of merozoites, although the actual cause of these symptoms is unknown. *Plasmodium vivax, P. ovale,* and *P. falciparum* species of malaria tend to produce paroxysms in 48 hour cycles (tertian malaria), whereas *P. malariae* causes paroxysms in 72 hour cycles (quartan malaria).

A series of paroxysms of decreasing intensity constitutes a primary malarial attack. After the primary attack, parasites tend to disappear from the blood. In infections with *P. falciparum* or *P. malariae* this would constitute a cure. In *P. vivax* and *P. ovale* infections, relapses may occur as a result of hypnozoites persisting in the liver.

Complicating pathologic changes such as anemia, hepatomegaly, and splenomegaly may occur. In the case of falciparum malaria, capillaries are blocked by infected erythrocytes that typically tend to become "sticky" and sequestered in capillary beds. Erythrocyte destruction leads to anemia. Capillary blockage leads to ischemia, anoxia, and subsequent organ damage. This is the basis for cerebral symptoms and kidney damage that leads to black water fever, a condition in which hemoglobin and erythrocytes appear in the urine and is associated with a poor prognosis. Falciparum malaria is the most virulent and lethal form of malaria, sometimes called malignant tertian malaria.

Approach to the Suspected Malaria Infection

Definitions

Relapse malaria: Infection derived from hypnozoites (hypnos = sleeping; zoites = animals) or residual liver stages that persist after a primary infection with *P. vivax* and *P. ovale.*

Appliqué form: Parasite on the periphery of erythrocytes, as in *P. falciparum* infection.

Ring stage: Stage in the life cycle of *Plasmodium* in an erythrocyte consisting of a thin ring of protoplasm with a nucleus at one side.

Schizogony: Asexual division or "splitting" carried out by all *Plasmodium* species.

Blackwater fever: A dangerous complication of malaria, especially falciparum, characterized by passage of red to black urine and associated with high mortality.

Objectives

1. Learn the life cycle of *Plasmodium* species and the epidemiology and clinical course of infection.
2. Be able to describe the three basic aspects of infection: transmission, diagnosis, and treatment/prevention.

Discussion

Characteristics of *Plasmodium* that Impact Transmission

Plasmodium is a genus in the phylum Apicomplexa, which contains other human parasites such as *Toxoplasma, Cryptosporidium, Cyclospora,* and *Isospora.* All of these organisms belong to a phylogenetic class in which all species are parasitic.

Malaria infections are endemic in **tropical developing countries.** Although endogenous malaria has occurred in the United States, most cases are imported by travelers. There are numerous species of *Plasmodium,* but only four species cause human malaria— *P. falciparum, P. vivax, P. malariae,* **and** *P. ovale.* All species are transmitted by an infected **anopheline mosquito.** *Plasmodium* **sporozoites** are the infective forms injected into the blood stream when the mosquito takes a blood meal. The sporozoites circulate in the blood stream and then invade **hepatocytes** to initiate a **preerythrocytic** cycle. In the liver parenchymal cells the parasite multiplies asexually by a process called schizogony or splitting. Asexual reproduction gives rise to multiple individual stages or merozoites. These **merozoites** become blood-borne and invade erythrocytes to initiate the **erythrocytic cycle.** In the case of *P. vivax* and *P. ovale,* the liver phase can be sustained for years by sporozoite-derived dormant stages known as **hypnozoites.** It is the prevalence of the hypnozoites that leads to relapses of malarial symptoms, possibly occurring several years after the first acute disease has been cured.

When merozoites parasitize erythrocytes, their development takes two routes. Some merozoites develop into micro (male) and macro (female) gametocytes. When a female anopheline mosquito bites an infected person and ingests the gametocytes, **fertilization of the macrogametocyte by the microgametocyte takes place in the mosquito** with the subsequent and sequential formation of diploid zygotes, oocysts, and, eventually, sporozoites. **Sporozoites travel to enter the salivary glands of the mosquito** where they are capable of initiating a new infection when the mosquito takes a blood meal. Through the second route in the erythrocytic cycle, the parasite develops successively through ring, trophozoite and schizont stages. As a result of schizogony, the erythrocyte breaks open and releases many new merozoites. These parasites then infect more erythrocytes, repeat the development cycle, ultimately causing the destruction of massive numbers of erythrocytes. The characteristic **chill, fever, and sweating paroxysm** occurs when the **parasites are released from the erythrocytes.** Because the release of parasites becomes synchronized and periodic, the paroxysms are also periodic, occurring at 48 or 72 hours depending on the species. The destruction of erythrocytes and release of cell and parasite debris contribute to pathological changes.

Diagnosis

Diagnosis is made by finding the **characteristic organisms on thick and thin blood smears.** Differential diagnosis rests on knowing the specific morphological characteristics of each species, which are revealed in a thin blood

Table 48-1
APPEARANCE OF MALARIA PARASITES
IN STAINED BLOOD SMEARS

CHARACTERISTIC	*PLASMODIUM* SPECIES
Crescent or sausage shapes present	*P. falciparum*
Trophozoites older than ring stages	*P. vivax, P. malariae, P. ovale*
Schizonts with more than 12 nuclei	*P. vivax*
Enlarged erythrocytes	*P. vivax*
Band forms	*P. malaria*
Ring stages only	*P. falciparum*
Fimbriated oval cell	*P. ovale*

smear. *Plasmodium vivax* and *P. ovale* appear as **ring shapes,** and in other advanced stages of development in enlarged erythrocytes that contain numerous **granules, known as Schüffner dots.** *Plasmodium malariae* has characteristic "band or bar" pattern and do not enlarge the host erythrocytes. *Plasmodium falciparum* can be identified by the presence of multiple ring forms within a single erythrocyte, in contrast to other plasmodia that will have only one ring form per erythrocyte. *Plasmodium falciparum* ring forms also tend to occur at the periphery of the erythrocyte; these "appliqué" forms are distinctive for this species. Mixed infections with more than one species of *Plasmodium* may occur.

Treatment and Prevention

From the perspective of patient management, drugs to treat malaria fall into three categories: **prophylactic, schizonticidal, and antirelapse.** Prophylactics are designed to prevent infection by attacking the sporozoite stages or preventing the development of clinical symptoms by preventing schizogony in the erythrocytic cycle. **Schizonticidal** compounds may be used in prophylactic measures and to effect a clinical cure in an acute infection. Antirelapse drugs are directed against hypnozoite stages, as in vivax infection. A radical cure in *P. vivax* and *P. ovale* infections requires the use of drugs that eradicate both the erythrocytic and exoerythrocytic schizonts in the liver.

 Chloroquine is a schizonticidal compound and drug of choice in treating clinical cases of malaria. Mefloquine, referred to in the case presentation, is used in prophylaxis and also to treat chloroquine resistant strains of *Plasmodium.* Drug resistance of certain strains of *Plasmodium* is a practical problem. In this case, back-up drugs are **quinine** or chemically related **mefloquine,** or a combination of **sulfadoxine** (a sulfonamide) and **pyrimethamine** (pyrimidine derivative). Antirelapse or tissue schizonticidal drugs are aimed at hypnozoites (liver schizonts). The drug of choice in this category is **primaquine.**

Comprehension Questions

[48.1] Microscopic examination of a thin blood smear from a patient suspected of having malaria reveals numerous normal size erythrocytes without stippling but with ring stages, many with multiple ring stages and appliqué forms. Several erythrocytes show developing trophozoites that are spread across the erythrocytes in a band fashion. Which of the following is the most likely cause of infection?

  A. *Plasmodium vivax*
  B. *Plasmodium malariae*
  C. *Plasmodium ovale*
  D. *Plasmodium falciparum*
  E. A mixed infection with two plasmodium species

[48.2] A patient in California was diagnosed with malaria acquired through a blood transfusion. A discussion of this case by physicians included the following statements. Which statement is correct?

A. The infected blood contained sporozoites.
B. The patient should be treated with chloroquine and primaquine.
C. The patient should be treated to eradicate the stages responsible for symptoms.
D. The blood donor had chloroquine-resistant malaria.
E. The patient would not be infective to mosquitoes.

[48.3] Cerebral malaria most commonly attends infection with which of the following?

A. Any two species of *Plasmodium*
B. *Plasmodium malariae*
C. *Plasmodium falciparum*
D. *Plasmodium ovale*
E. *Plasmodium vivax*

Answers

[48.1] **E.** Multiple ring stages and appliqué forms are indicative of *P. falciparum;* several erythrocytes show developing trophozoites that are spread across the erythrocytes in a band fashion that is indicative of *P. malariae* infection. Normal size erythrocytes without stippling (Schüffner dots) would exclude *P. vivax* and *P. ovale.*

[48.2] **C.** The primary goal should be to treat the patient to eliminate the erythrocytic cycle that is the cause of symptoms. This would constitute a radical cure because the liver phase only occurs if infection is initiated by sporozoites. Thus, treating with primaquine (B) is not necessary because the patient will not harbor hypnozoites. Likewise, (A) is not correct because sporozoites are only acquired from mosquitoes. Transfusion malaria is caused by schizonts and merozoites present in the transferred blood. There is no way to know that the malaria is chloroquine resistant until after treatment with chloroquine (D) and the patient, although not likely to occur, could transmit the infection to mosquitoes (E) because gametocytes would be present in the blood and susceptible *Anopheles* species occur in the United States.

[48.3] **C.** Cerebral malaria involves the clinical manifestations of *Plasmodium falciparum* malaria that induce changes in mental status and coma and is accompanied by fever. Without treatment, cerebral malaria is fatal in 24–72 hours and the mortality ratio is between 25–50 percent. The common histopathological finding is the sequestration of parasitized and nonparasitized red blood cells in cerebral capillaries and venules.

Synopsis of Malaria

MICROBIAL PEARLS	Infective stage of etiologic agent	Location of pathogenic stage	Laboratory diagnosis based on identification of:	Drugs used in treatment
	Sporozoite (injected by mosquito) of: *P. vivax* *P. malariae* *P. falciparum* *P. ovale*	Liver (primary schizogony) Erythrocytes (Schizogonic cycle)	 Blood smears (Stages in erythrocytes)	*Prophylaxis* Mefloquine *Acute* Chloroquine *Chloroquine Resistant* Quinine or Pyrimethamine +Sulfadoxine *Antirelapse* Primaquine

MICROBIOLOGY PEARLS

❖ In a laboratory diagnosis, in which blood smears are treated with Giemsa or Wright stain plasmodia can be identified when the nucleus and cytoplasm are seen.
❖ Chemotherapy is directed at erythrocytic stages to provide a clinical cure and hypnozoites in the liver to effect a radical cure.

REFERENCES

Centers for Disease Control. DPDx. Laboratory identification of parasites of public concern. Malaria. Author, 2004. Available online at: http://www.dpd.cdc.gov/dpdx/HTML/Malaria.htm

Graphic Images of Parasites. *Plasmodium* spp. (malaria). Author, 2004. Available online at: http://www.biosci.ohio-state.edu/~parasite/plasmodium.html

Medical Letter on Drugs and Therapeutics. Drugs for parasitic infections. New Rochelle, NY: Author, 2002. Available online at: http://www.medletter.com/freedocs/parasitic.pdf

A 40-year-old man presents for a routine examination. He is generally feeling well but complains of some mild dysuria and increasing urinary frequency. He has never had a urinary tract infection (UTI) and thought that the increasing urinary frequency was a normal part of aging. He has not seen any blood in his urine but says that the urine does appear darker than it used to look. He has no other complaints and his review of systems is otherwise entirely negative. He has no significant medical or family history. He smokes a pack of cigarettes a day and denies alcohol use. He is an immigrant from Egypt who has lived in the United States for 3 years. His vital signs and physical examination, including genital and prostate exams, are normal. A urinalysis shows many red blood cells, a few white blood cells, and oval-shaped parasite eggs with terminal spines.

◆ **What organism is the likely cause of his hematuria?**

◆ **How does this organism gain entry into humans?**

ANSWERS TO CASE 49: Schistosomiasis

Summary: A 40-year-old Egyptian man has hematuria. A urinalysis shows many red blood cells, a few white blood cells, and oval-shaped eggs with terminal spines.

◆ **Organism likely cause of his hematuria:** *Schistosoma haematobium.*

◆ **Method organism gains entry into humans:** Penetration through intact skin by the cercarial stage of the organism.

CLINICAL CORRELATION

Schistosomiasis is a human disease syndrome caused by infection with one of several **parasitic trematodes or flukes** of the genus *Schistosoma.* These parasites are known commonly as **blood flukes** because the adult worms live in blood vessels of the definitive host. The human disease syndrome is characterized by dermatitis that is caused by entry of the infective stage and by acute and chronic systemic symptoms caused by host responses to eggs deposited by adult worms. *Schistosoma hematobium, S. mansoni,* and *S. japonicum* are the major species that infect over 200 million humans in Asia, Africa, the Middle East, and South America. *Schistosoma japonicum* is considered a zoonotic infection. In addition to these three major species, others, such as *S. mekongi* and *S. intercalatum,* also with potential zoonotic properties, rarely infect humans. Schistosomes with avian or nonhuman mammalian hosts can cause severe dermatitis or swimmers itch in humans.

The disease syndrome parallels the development of the parasite in the definitive host. **Swimmers itch,** an allergic dermatitis, is caused shortly after humans make skin contact with microscopic, infective larval forms called **cercariae** that live in an aquatic environment. Following exposure to human schistosomes, the dermatitis is mild and may go unnoticed. However, when exposed to cercariae of schistosomes that normally infect birds, swimmers itch can present as an itchy maculopapular rash. Cercariae penetrate the intact skin, enter the circulation and **migrate to the liver** where they mature into adult male and female worms. The adult worms migrate via the blood stream to their final locations. *Schistosoma mansoni* and *S. japonicum* descend to the mesenteric veins and *S. haematobium* to the **vesical plexus.** Gravid female worms may release 300–3,000 eggs per day over a 5–10 year life span. Eggs of *S. haematobium* can work their way through the wall of the urinary bladder into the lumen and are eliminated in urine, while eggs of *S. mansoni* and *S. japonicum* work their way through the walls of the small intestine and colon and are voided in feces. **Acute schistosomiasis or Katayama's syndrome** develops one to two months after initial infection and includes **fever, chills, abdominal pain, lymphadenopathy,** and **hepatomegaly and splenomegaly.**

The etiology of acute schistosomiasis is not known. However, the association of its manifestations with heavy infection suggests that it is a form of serum sickness as a result of circulating antigen-antibody complexes. Chronic schistosomiasis results from the inflammatory response to eggs, with granulomas, fibrosis, and scar tissue occurring at the site where eggs are deposited in tissues. Chronic schistosomiasis results from the inflammatory response to the presence of eggs, with granulomas, fibrosis, and scarring around the eggs. Eggs in the bowel wall may result in symptoms of abdominal pain, diarrhea, and blood in the stool. Schistosomiasis of the bladder can cause **hematuria,** dysuria, frequent urination, and a reduction in bladder capacity. With **intestinal schistosomiasis,** the liver is frequently involved as a result of eggs being carried by the portal circulation and becoming trapped. Pathology involves **inflammation and fibrosis,** leading to **cirrhosis** with resulting **portal hypertension, splenomegaly, ascites, and abdominal and esophageal varices.** Ectopic lesions may rarely be associated with eggs reaching the brain and lungs.

Approach to the Suspected Schistome Infection

Definitions

Cercaria: Infective, aquatic larval form of schistosomes; characterized by a forked tail.

Miracidium: Ciliated larval form of schistosomes (and other flukes) that escapes from the egg and infects a snail intermediate host.

Intermediate host: The host in the life cycle of a helminth that harbors the larval stage(s) of the parasite.

Bilharziasis: A synonym for schistosomiasis.

Swimmer's itch: Dermatitis in humans caused by cercariae penetrating the skin, commonly involving cercariae of schistosomes that parasitize birds or mammals but which cannot complete their life cycle in humans.

Dioecious fluke: A fluke that has separate sexes, as opposed to hermaphroditic flukes.

Objectives

1. Learn the life cycle of blood flukes and the epidemiology and clinical course of infection.
2. Be able to describe three basic aspects of infection: transmission, diagnosis, and treatment/prevention.

Discussion

Characteristics of Schistosomes that Impact Transmission

The life cycle of all human schistosomes is similar, except in fine details. **Eggs voided in feces or urine hatch in fresh water,** releasing **ciliated miracidia** that penetrate a **snail intermediate host.** The species of snail varies with the species of schistosome. Miracidia undergo morphological development through other larval stages, eventually reproducing asexually. The product is hundreds of **cercariae** with forked tails that emerge from the snail and swim freely. On contacting humans that enter their environment, the **cercariae penetrate the intact skin, losing their tails in the process,** and enter the circulation and are **disseminated to all parts of the body.**

The cercariae, now termed **schistosomula,** are carried via the **portal vein** into the **intrahepatic portal system** where they mature in about 3–4 weeks. After maturing, the worms migrate against the blood current and move into branches of veins that drain the **urinary bladder** (*S. hematobium*) or the **lower ileum and cecum** (*S. japonicum*) or the **colon** (*S. mansoni*). Female worms lay several hundred eggs per day. The eggs of each species have characteristic morphology. All eggs leaving the host contain a fully developed miracidium.

Diagnosis

Infections can be definitively diagnosed by **finding characteristic eggs in the urine or feces.** Eggs of *S. hematobium* are in the shape of an **elongated oval with a terminal spine;** *S. mansoni* eggs are also oval shaped with a distinct lateral spine; and *S. japonicum* eggs are round to oval with a short lateral spine or knob that often is unseen. In suspected cases where stools are negative, eggs of *S. mansoni* may be seen in microscopic examination of a rectal biopsy.

Treatment and Prevention

Praziquantel is the drug of choice in the treatment of human schistosomiasis and is effective against all human species. Because the drug has been reported to be effective as a prophylactic, **larval stages and adult forms are presumed to be susceptible.** The treatment of cercarial dermatitis is symptomatic. Prevention is based on avoiding skin exposure to water in endemic areas.

Comprehension Questions

[49.1] Which of the following is a host in the life cycle of all trematodes that infect humans?

    A. Flea

    B. Mosquito

    C. Mollusk

    D. Flour weevil

    E. Sand fly

[49.2] An oil field worker who has lived in Brazil for 10 years has mild gastrointestinal symptoms. Brazil is the only country ever visited by the patient outside of the United States. The patient is diagnosed by his physician of having schistosomiasis mansoni because:

A. Round eggs with a prominent terminal spine were observed in a rectal biopsy.
B. Blood was detected in the stool.
C. Nonoperculated eggs with a miracidium inside were observed in stool samples.
D. Eggs were found in a urine sample.
E. Symptoms were relieved by treatment with praziquantel.

[49.3] A 12-year-old boy reports feeling tingling and itching of his legs 30 minutes after swimming in a lake. Over the next day, small papules develop followed by blisters of the legs. Dermatitis due to schistosome infection is diagnosed. What larval stage most likely caused the infection?

A. Filariform larva
B. Cysticercus
C. Cercaria
D. Miracidium
E. Sparganum

Answers

[49.1]   **C.** Snails are mollusks. All flukes have snails as intermediate hosts. Fleas, mosquitoes, flour weevils, and sand flies serve as intermediate or definitive hosts to various helminth and protozoan parasites, but not to flukes.

[49.2]   **C.** Eggs with a miracidium inside is indicative of a fluke infection; nonoperculated eggs are characteristic of schistosomes and differentiate them from all other human flukes, which have eggs with opercula. Also, *S. mansoni* is the only human schistosome endemic to Brazil and to the western hemisphere. A round egg with a terminal spine (A) is characteristic of *S. hematobium* but would not be expected in a rectal biopsy; furthermore, *S. hematobium* is not endemic to the western hemisphere. Blood in the stool (B) may be a finding in *S. mansoni* infection but would not be a definitive diagnosis. Finding eggs in a urine sample (D) is consistent with *S. hematobium* but not *S. mansoni* infection; again, *S. hematobium* is not endemic to the western hemisphere. Vague gastrointestinal symptoms are not pathognomonic of schistosome infections. Praziquantel (E) is used to effectively treat all intestinal tapeworms of humans, as well as schistosomes. Symptoms could have been caused by adult tapeworms.

Synopsis of Schistosomiasis

MICROBIAL PEARLS	Infective stage of etiologic agent	Location of pathogenic stage	Laboratory diagnosis based on identification of:	Drugs used in treatment
	Cercariae: *Schistosoma mansoni*	Adults: Mostly inferior mesenteric veins	Eggs (stool exam, rectal biopsy)	*Praziquantel*
	Schistosoma japonicum	Mostly superior mesenteric veins	Eggs (stool exam, rectal biopsy)	
	Schistosoma hematobium	Vesicular veins	Eggs (urine)	
	Swimmer's Itch— Cercarial dermatitis (*Various species of non human schistosomes*)	Skin	Clinical diagnosis	None specific

[49.3]   **C.** Forked-tail cercariae are infective for humans. A filariform larva
          is the infective stage for hookworm and strongyloides, both nematode
          parasites. A cysticercus larva (B) is the infective stage of *Taenia* species
          of tapeworms. A miracidium (D) is the stage of flukes that infects
          snails, not humans. A sparganum larva (E) is involved in the life cycle
          of pseudophyllidean tapeworms, such as the broad fish tapeworm.

MICROBIOLOGY PEARLS

❖ Swimmers itch is often transmitted by bird schistosomes.
❖ Pathology in clinical cases is caused by egg stages.
❖ Praziquantel is effective for all species and is also used to treat intestinal tapeworms.

REFERENCES

Centers for Disease Control. DPDx. Laboratory identification of parasites of public concern. Schistosomiasis. Author, 2004. Available online at: http://www.dpd.cdc.gov/dpdx/HTML/Schistosomiasis.htm

Graphic Images of Parasites. Graphic images of parasites. *Schistosoma* species (schistosomes or blood flukes; schistosomiasis). Author, 2004. Available online at: http://www.biosci.ohio-state.edu/~parasite/schistosoma.html

Medical Letter on Drugs and Therapeutics. Drugs for parasitic infections. New Rochelle, NY: Author, 2002. Available online at: http://www.medletter.com/freedocs/parasitic.pdf

CASE 50

A 19-year-old woman presents to the office for the evaluation of an itchy vaginal discharge that she has had for about a week. She has had no fever, abdominal pain, or dysuria. She became involved with a new sexual partner about 3 weeks ago. She takes birth control pills but does not regularly use condoms during intercourse. Her partner is asymptomatic. On examination, her vital signs are normal, and a general physical examination is unremarkable. On pelvic examination, her external genitalia are normal. After inserting a speculum you see a bubbly, thin, yellow vaginal discharge. Her cervix is erythematous but without discharge. She has no cervical motion or uterine or adnexal tenderness. A wet mount of the vaginal discharge examined microscopically reveals numerous motile, flagellated, pear-shaped organisms along with numerous white blood cells.

◆ **What is the most likely infectious cause of her vaginal discharge?**

◆ **What is the most likely source of her infection?**

ANSWERS TO CASE 50: *Trichomonas*

Summary: A 19-year-old woman with vaginal discharge, which on microscopy reveals numerous motile, flagellated, pear-shaped organisms along with numerous white blood cells.

◆ **Most likely infectious cause of her vaginal discharge:** *Trichomonas vaginalis.*

◆ **Most likely source of her infection:** Sexual contact with infected but asymptomatic partner.

CLINICAL CORRELATION

Trichomonas vaginalis is a **motile, pear-shaped protozoan with four flagella** and an **undulating membrane.** It multiplies by **binary fission** and exists only in its trophozoite form; no cyst form has been identified. It is a common cause of both symptomatic and asymptomatic infections. Many infected women are asymptomatic or have only a small amount of thin vaginal discharge. Others develop symptomatic disease with vaginal **inflammation, itching, and copious vaginal discharge.** The discharge may be white, yellow, or green, and bubbles are often seen. Cervical inflammation with punctate hemorrhages may produce a **"strawberry cervix."** The vast majority of infections in men are asymptomatic, although urethritis, prostatitis, and epididymitis can occur. The parasite is almost always passed by **sexual contact,** although fomite transmission has been documented. The diagnosis is most often made by the microscopic evaluation of a sample of vaginal discharge in a saline wet mount. Flagellated, motile trichomonads will be visible in most symptomatic infections. The diagnosis can also be made by the identification of organisms on Pap smears, by culture of the vaginal discharge, or by the use of specific monoclonal antibody stains or nucleic acid probes. This infection is usually treated with oral **metronidazole,** and both partners should be treated to prevent reinfection. Because of its route of transmission, the identification of infection with *Trichomonas* should prompt the consideration of evaluation for other sexually transmitted diseases.

Approach to the Suspected *Trichomonas* Infection

Definitions

Trophozoite: Feeding stage of protozoans.

Axostyle: A hyaline rod-like structure that runs through the length of *T. vaginalis* and exits at the posterior end.

Fomite: A substance other than food that may harbor and transmit infectious agents.

Objectives

1. Learn the life cycle of *Trichomonas vaginalis* and the epidemiology and clinical course of infection.
2. Be able to answer the three basic aspects of infection: transmission, diagnosis, and treatment/prevention.

Discussion

Characteristics of *Trichomonas* that Impact Transmission

The life cycle of trichomonads in general is the simplest of protozoan life cycle because the organism exists only as a trophozoite that divides by binary fission. Transmission is presumed to be by **direct transfer of trophozoites** because a cyst stage does not exist.

Sexual intercourse is considered the usual means of transmitting this infection that is common worldwide. The organism is transmitted cyclically from a woman to a man and back to the same or another woman. Infected men, who play a key role in transmission, are usually asymptomatic. *Trichomonas vaginalis* trophozoites in vaginal discharge are known to live for 30 minutes or more on toilet seats, supporting the possibility that some infections could be acquired through **fomites** such as towels and toilet seats. However, this means of transmission is not well supported by evidence.

Diagnosis

If infection with *T. vaginalis* is suspected, a first step is to diagnose infection by **microscopically examining a wet mount preparation** of vaginal discharge from the patient. The live parasite appears as a **pear-shaped trophozoite with active flagella** that give it motility. Sometime the undulating membrane provides a waving movement. Propagation and concentration of the organism in culture is a possibility if wet mounts are negative. However, examination of wet mounts is usually sufficient to find and identify the organism.

Treatment and Prevention

Metronidazole is effective in treating *T. vaginalis*. Treatment of both sexual partners is recommended to prevent reinfection. Using condoms correctly and consistently will lower the risk of individuals contracting trichomoniasis and other sexually transmitted diseases.

Comprehension Questions

[50.1] Trichomoniasis is transmitted through this stage:

    A. Cyst
    B. Oocyst
    C. Egg
    D. Sporozoite
    E. Trophozoite

[50.2] The drug of choice in treating vaginal trichomoniasis is:

    A. Metronidazole
    B. Mebendazole
    C. Mefloquine
    D. Niclosamide
    E. Niridazole

[50.3] Laboratory diagnosis of vaginal trichomoniasis is most commonly made by:

    A. Identifying cyst stages in an iodine stained preparation of vaginal secretion.
    B. Finding trophozoites in a saline wet mount of vaginal discharge.
    C. Using an acid-fast stain to highlight the parasite.
    D. Staining a thin blood smear with common blood stains.
    E. Testing for specific antibodies against *T. vaginalis* in the patient's serum.

Answers

[50.1] **E.** *Trichomonas vaginalis* exists only as a trophozoite; no cyst stage has been identified. A cyst (A), oocyst (B) and sporozoite (D) are stages involved in transmitting other protozoan infections, and an egg (C) is the means of transmission in a number of helminth infections.

[50.2] **A.** Metronidazole is the drug of choice. Mebendazole (B) is a broad-spectrum antinematode agent. Mefloquine (C) is used as a prophylactic drug to prevent malaria and also used to treat chloroquine-resistant clinical malaria. Niclosamide is a broad-spectrum agent effective in the treatment of adult tapeworm infections. Niridazole (E) is a drug used to treat schistosomiasis if praziquantel is not available.

[50.3] **B.** Trophozoites are usually visible in saline mounts of vaginal scrapings. Cysts (A) are not present in the *T. vaginalis* life cycle, and iodine is used primarily to observe cysts of intestinal protozoa. Acid-fast stains (D) are used to search for oocysts of coccidian intestinal parasites, such as *Cryptosporidium* and *Cyclospora.* Thin blood smears are used to diagnose malaria. Serological diagnoses (E) are helpful in the diagnosis of several "deep tissue" parasites but are not used in diagnosing *T. vaginalis.*

Synopsis of Vaginal Trichomoniasis

MICROBIAL PEARLS	Infective stage of etiologic agent	Location of pathogenic stage	Laboratory diagnosis based on identification of:	Drugs used in treatment
	Trophozoite *Trichomonas vaginalis*	Genito-urinary tract	Trophozoite (vaginal discharge)	Metronidazole

MICROBIOLOGY PEARLS

 Trichomonas vaginalis is an important sexually transmitted parasite throughout the world.

 Only trophozoite stages occur and frequently are difficult to find in a wet mount.

 Males and females are hosts, although males are generally asymptomatic.

 Metronidazole is the drug of choice for treating trichomoniasis.

REFERENCES

Centers for Disease Control. DPDx. Laboratory identification of parasites of public concern. Trichomoniasis. Author, 2004. Available online at: http://www.dpd.cdc.gov/dpdx/HTML/Trichomoniasis.htm

Graphic Images of Parasites. *Trichomonas vaginalis* (trichomoniasis, "trich" or "trick"). 2004. Available online at: http://www.biosci.ohio-state.edu/~parasite/trichomonas.html

Medical Letter on Drugs and Therapeutics. Drugs for parasitic infections. New Rochelle, NY: Author, 2002. Available online at: http://www.medletter.com/freedocs/parasitic.pdf

Listing of Cases

Listing by Case Number

LISTING OF CASES (BY CASE NUMBER)

CASE #	SYSTEM	CASE DESCRIPTION	DISEASE/CLINICAL CONDITION	PAGE #
19		*Salmonella/Shigella*	Diarrhea	141
20		*Streptococcus agalactiae*	Neonatal meningitis; neonatal pneumonia; neonatal sepsis	149
		Streptococcus pneumoniae	Meningitis; otitis media; pneumonia; sinusitis	
		Streptococcus pyogenes	Glomerulonephritis; Pharyngitis; rheumatic feber; scarlet fever; toxic shock syndrome	
		Streptococcus viridans group	Dental caries; endocarditis	
21		*Staphylococcus aureus*	Cystitis; cutaneous infections; endocarditis; gastroenteritis; meningitis; osteomyelitis; pneumonia; septic arthritis; sepsis	155
		Staphylococcus epidermidis	Endocarditis; skin contaminant	
22		*Treponema pallidum*	Syphillis	163
23		*Vibrio cholera*	Diarrhea	171
24	Viruses	Adenovirus/Rhinovirus	Conjunctivitis; upper respiratory infection (URI)	177
25		Cytomegalovirus	Congenital infection; mononucleosis; Pneumonia; retinitis	183
26		Epstein Barr virus	Mononucleosis	189
27		Hepatitis A,B,C,D,E	Hepatitis	195
28		Herpes simplex virus-1,2	Cutaneous infections	205
29		Human Immunodeficiency Virus	Viral induced immunocompromise	211
30		Human papillovirus	Cervical dysplasia and cancer; genital warts	219
31		Molluscum contagiosum	Cutaneous lesions	225
32		Mumps	Lymphadentisis	231
33		Parvovirus	Congenital infection; viral syndrome	237
34		Polio virus	Meningitus; paralytic poliomyelitis	243
35		Rotavirus	Diarrhea	249
36		Respiratory synctial virus	Bronchiolitis	255
37		Smallpox virus	Cutaneous infection	261
38		Varicella zoster virus	Chickenpox; shingles	267

CASE #	SYSTEM	CASE DESCRIPTION	DISEASE/CLINICAL CONDITION	PAGE #
39	Fungi	Aspergillus fumigatus	Hypersensitivity pneumonitis	273
40		Blastomycosis dermatitides Coccidioides immitis Histoplasmosis capsulatum	Hypersensitivity pneumonitis	279
41		Candida albicans	Diaper rash; thrush; vaginitis	285
42		Cryptococcus neoformans	Meningoencephalitis	293
43		Pneumocystis carinii	Pneumonia	299
44		Sporothrix schenkii	Sporotrichosis	305
45	Parasites	Ascaris lumbricoides	Gastrointestinal invasion	311
46		Cryptosporidium	Diarrhea	321
47		Enterobius vermicularis	Pinworms	329
48		Plasmodium falciparum Plasmodium malariae Plasmodium ovale Plasmodium vivax	Malaria	337
49		Schistosoma haematobium Schistosoma japonicum Schistosoma mansoni	Bladder venous invasion Intestinal venous invasion Intestinal venous invasion	345
50		Trichomonas vaginalis	Vaginitis	353

❖ INDEX

Note: Page numbers followed by f indicate figures; those followed by t indicate tables.